Avian (Poultry) Production

2nd Revised and Enlarged Edition

nipa books for everyone
PAPERBACKS

NIPA® GENX ELECTRONIC RESOURCES & SOLUTIONS P. LTD.
New Delhi-110 034

Avian (Poultry) Production

2nd Revised and Enlarged Edition

Editors

D Sapcota, MVSc, PhD. Post. Doc. (USA) FUWAI, FIPSA
Professor
Department of Poultry Science
College of Veterinary Science
Assam Agricultural University
Khanapara, Guwahati, Assam

D Narahari, MVSc, PhD., FFAO (USA), FNAVS
Retired Professor
Department of Poultry Science
Madras Veterinary College
Tamil Nadu Veterinary and Animal Science University
Chennai, Tamil Nadu

J D Mahanta, MVSc, PhD.
Professor
Department of Poultry Science
College of Veterinary Science
Assam Agricultural University
Khanapara, Guwahati, Assam

nipa books for everyone
PAPERBACKS

NIPA® GENX ELECTRONIC RESOURCES & SOLUTIONS P. LTD.
New Delhi-110 034

books for everyone
PAPERBACKS

NIPA® GENX ELECTRONIC RESOURCES & SOLUTIONS P. LTD.

101,103, Vikas Surya Plaza, CU Block
L.S.C. Market, Pitam Pura, New Delhi-110 034
Ph : +91 11 27341616, 27341717, 27341718
E-mail: newindiapublishingagency@gmail.com
www: www.nipabooks.com

For customer assistance, please contact
Phone: + 91-11-27 34 17 17
Fax: + 91-11- 27 34 16 16
E-Mail: feedbacks@nipabooks.com

ISBN: 978-93-86546-07-4

Composed and Designed by NIPA®.

Contents

ASSAM AGRICULTURAL UNIVERSITY

DR. K M BUJARBARUAH, ARS, PhD, FNAAS, DSc (Hc) Jorhat-785013
VICE-CHANCELLOR

FOREWORD

I am pleased to write foreword for the book, "Avian (Poultry) Production 2nd Edition". The book deals with the subject Poultry/Avian Science containing updated information as per revised VCI curriculum for under-graduate teaching in Veterinary Colleges. Altogether 30 authors from different Agricultural/ Veterinary Universities of India have contributed on different topics.

The massive expansion taking place in Indian poultry industry under commercial sector has been well reflected in the chapter: *Indian Poultry Industry*. However, emphasis has also been given on unorganized poultry sector which is a backbone of rural people for nutritional security, women empowerment and solution to unemployment problem; the book has well covered this area under the topic: *Backyard poultry under scavenging system*. Of late, it has been observed that consumers are becoming more health-conscious emphasizing on organic products; the book has covered this subject under: *Organic and Hill farming*. Yet another topic: *Designer egg and meat production* is well suited to the present-day need of food quality savy consumers. While poultry has taken slow stride from backyard to industry there appeared necessity to conserve indigenous germplasm; a chapter on this topic, "*Conservation of indigenous germplasm*" a quite appropriate. While dealing with conventional poultry species – chicken, an emphasis has been made in this book to other avian species like duck, quail, geese, turkey, guinea fowl, pigeon, emu etc.

The topics of the book are well planned, explained using simple language with coloured photographs, sketches, illustrations and tables, wherever necessary. For the benefit of students the book also contains certain guidance/tips for

Phone: (91)-376-2340013(O), 2340350 (R), Fax: +91-376-2340001
Email: kmbujarbaruah@rediffmail.com, vc@aau.ac.in

improving memory, increasing performance, excelling in examinations or relieving stresses. After each chapter a Question bank is given with answer key so as to benefit students for self-evaluation and preparation of examination. All the three editors are well experienced with long years of teaching stint. I am sure; this book will be well accepted by the student community not only for their academic pursuance but also for the preparation of competitive examinations both in public and private sectors. I appreciate the editors for their effort to write this book.

Place: Khanapara **K.M. Bujarbaruah**

Phone: (91)-376-2340013(O), 2340350 (R), Fax: +91-376-2340001
Email: kmbujarbaruah@rediffmail.com, vc@aau.ac.in

Preface to the Second Edition

It is a delightful occasion that our book, **Avian (Poultry) Production: A Text Book,** is on the brink of second edition. The readers of this book are spread all over India. Not only this, the leading academia of Agriculture and Forestry University (Rampur, Chitwan), Nepal have also appreciated the book and shown keen interest on the introduction of similar courses in their University. The book has been authored by 30 well experienced academia to match the syllabi *in vogue* prescribed by the Veterinary Council of India. In addition, we believe that it has also been useful to postgraduate students of Poultry Science and candidates appearing for JRF, SRF, ARS and NET examinations. Further, this book has also been prepared for the students of the Courses: Poultry Production & Business Management (PPBM), B. Tech, B.Sc Poultry Science and Poultry Science diploma.

The title is quite comprehensive and includes updated information on topics dealt with. The unique feather of this book is that at the end of each chapter there is a Question Bank with Answer key so as to help the students for self-testing and prepare for the examinations. This book also contains best quality photographs, figures and illustrations to reflect the course contents and explain the subject. We do hope that the book will be appropriate use for the students in particular and teachers, scientists and farmers in general.

Dated: Guwahati, the May 27/2017.

D Sapcota
D Narahari
J D Mahanta

Terminologies

Addled egg: A fertile egg containing a dead embryo, which has died during the early period of incubation.

Air sacs: Expandable membranes communicating with the lungs and the hollow bones. Help in respiration of birds and also gives lightness to birds.

Avian: Relating to birds.

Bantam: Dwarf variety of domestic fowl.

Blood ring: Observed in some hatching eggs, when the embryo has died during first few days of incubation.

Blood spot: A small blood clot attached to the membranes surrounding the yolk, or to the chalaza, or noticed in the albumen as a result of haemorrhage during ovulation. It can be detected by candling.

Bloom: A layer of protective coating on the external surface of egg; also called cuticle.

Breed: It is a group of birds that have usually the same general body shape; they are true to the type, carriage and characteristics of the name of the breed they carry. Eg. Leghorn, Rhode Island Red, Australorp, Aseel etc.

Brood: A group of chicks hatched out from the same batch of eggs.

Broodiness: Desire in a hen to sit on eggs, characteristic of desi hens.

Broiler or Fryer: Broilers are the young birds of either sex, upto 5 to 6 weeks of age and weighing 1.5 to 2.5 Kg body weight with soft pliable skin, tender meat and well developed breast bone cartilage.

BCC: Broiler Co-ordination Committee.

Candling: Visual examination to test eggs for freshness by holding them between the eye and a source of light.

Cannibalism: Vice that may occur in chickens of all ages. It includes feather picking, toe picking, vent picking, egg eating etc.

Capon: Castrated male chicken. Chickens are usually caponized between 3 and 4 weeks of age.

CARI: Central Avian Research Institute.
Chick: Young one of chicken, quail or pheasant from day old to 8 weeks of age.
Chicken: It is a term used to designate domestic fowl- *Gallus*.
Clutch: Term expressing the sequence of egg laying or number of eggs laid on consecutive days.
Cock or Roaster: These are adult male chicken above 1 year of age.
Cockerel: These are male chicken above 08 weeks but below I year of age.
Cygnet: Young one of swan.
Dead-in-shell: Embryo that has died at any stage of incubation.
Down: Initial hairy covering of baby chicks, duckling etc. Also the fluffy part of the feather below the web.
Drake: Adult male duck.
Droppings: The faecal excretion of birds.
Dubbing: The process of trimming or removing the comb of breeder males to improve their virility and vigour. Preferably done at day-old age.
Duck: Adult female duck.
Duckling: Young one of duck.
Forced moult: Deliberate moulting of birds, by drastic changes in food and environment. Done after the first laying cycle is completed to help increase egg production in the second cycle.
Fowl: It has three meanings- 1. Live poultry, 2. A mature chick, 3. Any large bird OR Any bird, but more commonly referred to larger ones.
FSSAI: Food Safety and Standards Authority of India.
Gander: Mature male goose.
Giblets: The edible viscera of the bird, comprising its gizzard, heart and liver.
Goose: Mature female goose.
Gosling: Young one of goose.
Grower: Chicks of either sex between 9 to 18 weeks of age.
Hen: These are female chicken above 1 year of age.
Inbred line: A bird resulting from four or more generation of inbreeding.
Keel bone: Breastbone of birds; the sternum.
Keets: Young one of guinea fowl.
Layers: These are chickens which lay eggs. Generally chickens lay eggs at the age of 5.0 to 5.5 months (20-22 weeks).
Management: It is the art and science of combining ideas, facilities, processes, material and labour to produce or market a worthwhile product or service.
Morbidity: Sick rate
Mortality: Death rate
NAFED: National Agricultural Co-operative Marketing Federation of India.
NECC: National Egg Co-ordination Committee.
Oviposition: Act of laying of egg.

Poult: Young one of turkey.

Poultry: The term 'Poultry' indicates all domesticated species of birds reared for economic purpose. It includes chicken, duck, turkey, Japanese quails, guinea fowl, geese, pigeon, ostrich, emu etc.

Poultry management: It is the art and science of organization and operation of farms so as to obtain maximum amount of continuous net income.

Pullet: These are female chicken above 08 weeks but below I year of age.

Roaster: These are the young chicken (usually 3 to 5 months of age) of either sex that is tender meated with soft, pliable, smooth textured skin and breast bone cartilage that may be somewhat less flexible than that of a broiler.

Squab: Young one of pigeon.

Starter: Chicks of either sex between 0 to 8 weeks of age.

Strain: Strains are closely related inbred flocks with definite economic characters. A strain is the name given by a breeder who has done breeding on the birds and introduced certain economic characters in the birds. A breed or a variety may have several strains and may be phenotypically alike but often differ on their production performance depending on breeding history. Eg. Babcock, Hyline, BV-300, BV-380, Bovans, Hisex, Cobb, Hubbard, Ross, Hybro erc.

Straightrun: Means chickens irrespective of male and female.

Table bird: Means 'meat birds' which are specially bred for this purpose. Eg. Broilers, turkeys, capon etc.

Tom: Adult male turkey.

Vaccine: A product which contains living disease producing organisms which have been weakened or attenuated so as to lose much of their virulence and power and injected into the body of a healthy bird to produce a mild attack of the disease and induce production of anti-bodies.

Variety: A variety is a sub-division of a breed distinguished either by plumage colour, plumage pattern or comb type. Eg. White Leghorn, Single Comb White Leghorn, Barred Plymouth Rock, Black Minorca etc.

List of Contributors

A. Jalaludeen
Former Professor and Special Officer
Faculty of Poultry Science of KVASU
Pookode, Kerala
Email id: jalalabdulrazak@gmail.com; pfso@kvasu.ac.in.

Amitav Bhattacharyya
Assistant Professor
Department of Poultry Science
Dairy Farm Campus, DUVASU
Mathura - 281 001, UP
Email id: amitav16@rediffmail.com

Ashok Kumar
Director
Students' Welfare, BAU
Sabour, Bhagalpur, Bihar
Email id: drashoklpm@gmail.com

Asma Khan
Associate Professor and Head
Division of Livestock Production
Management. SKUAST, Jammu, J&K
Email id: asmakhan_70@yahoo.co.in

B. Mohan
Professor and Head
Poultry Disease Diagnosis and Surveillance Laboratory
Veterinary College and Research Institute Campus
Tamil Nadu Veterinary and Animal Sciences University, Namakkal – 627 002
Email id: mohan.balusamy@gmail.com

D. Narahari
Former Professor and Head
Poultry Science Department, 31/15, 3rd Floor
First Main Road East, Shenoy Nagar
Chennai – 600 030, Tamil Nadu
Email id: narahari.devareddy@gmail.com, dnarahari@scientist.com

D. Sapcota
Professor
Department of Poultry Science
CVSc, AAU, Khanapara – 781 022, Assam
Email id: debensapcota@yahoo.com

H.N. Narasimha Murthy
Dean
Hassan Veterinary, College of KVAFSU
(B) 1320, First Floor, 24th Main, 9th Block
Jayanagar, Bangalore – 560 069, Karnataka
Email id: hnnm2007@gmail.com

I.U. Sheikh
Associate Professor
Division of LPM, F.V.Sc & A.H.
SKUAST-K, Shuhama
Srinagar – 190 006, J&K.
Email id: iusheikh@rediffmail.com; sheikhiu@ gmail.com

J.D. Mahanta
Professor
Department of Poultry Science
CVSc, AAU, Khanapara – 781 022
Assam
Email id: mahantajd@gmail.com

Jyoti Palod
Professor, College of Veterinary and Animal Sciences
G.B. Pant University of Agriculture and Technology,
Pantnagar– 263 145, Uttarakhand
Email id: palod_jyoti17@rediffmail.com

M. V. Dhumal
Professor, Department of Poultry Science
MAFSU, Parbhani – 431 402
Maharastra
Email id: dhumalmv@gmail.com

M. Tufail Banday
Professor and Head
Division Livestock Production Management
Faculty of Veterinary Sciences & Animal Husbandry, Srinagar. Shuhama, J&K.
Email id: drtufailbanday@yahoo.co.in, mtbanday@gmail.com

Mihir Sarma
Jr. Scientist
Livestock Research Station, Mondira
AAU, Kamrup Dist. Assam
Email id: mihirsarma21@gmail.com

Mukund M Kadam
Assistant Professor
Department of Poultry Science
Nagpur Veterinary College
MAFSU, Nagpur, Maharastra
Email id: mukundkadam@gmail.com

N. Panda
Associate Professor
College of Veterinary Science and Animal Husbandry, OUAT
Bhubaneswar-751003
Email id: npandaouat@gmail.com

P.K. Shukla
Professor and Head
Dean PG Studies and Scientific and Technical Advisor to the Vice Chancellor
DUVASU, Mathura-281001, UP
Email id: hukla_pankaj2004@rediffmail.com, pksmathura@yahoo.co.in

Prashant Shinde
Technology Application Manager at Cargill Feed & Nutrition
Maharastra
Email id: prashant_shinde@cargill.com

R. Prabakaran
Former Vice-Chancellor
TNVASU, Chennai, Tamilnadu
Email id: rpkaran@mail.com, karanmgk@gmail.com

Rahul M. Warhadpande
I/C Assistant Commissioner of Animal Husbandry
Taluka Veterinary Mini-Polyclinic
Deori and Livestock Development Officer
TMVPC, Deori Dist. Gondia, Maharashtra
Email id: dr.rahulwarhadpande@gmail.com

Ranjana Goswami
Assistant Professor
College of Veterinary Sciences and Animal Husbandry
C.A.U. Selesih, Aizawl, Mizoram
Email id: sksthakur2007@ rediffmail.com

S.C. Edwin
Professor and Head
Department of Poultry Science
Veterinary College and Research Institute
Namakkal – 627 002, Tamilnadu
Email id: drscedwin@yahoo.com, drscedwin@rediffmail.com

S.J. Manwar
Associate Professor and Head
Department of Poultry Science
Post Graduate Institute of Veterinary and Animal Sciences, Akola, MAFSU
Maharastra.
Email id: satishmanwar@rediffmail.com, vetsatish@yahoo.com

S.C. Mishra
Former Dean Extension Education and Prof. & Head
Department of Poultry Science, College of Veterinary Science and Animal Husbandry
OUAT, Bhubaneswar-751003
Email id: scmishraouat @gmail.com

S. George Paradis
Associate Professor
PJN. College of Agriculture and Research Institute
Karaikal, Puducherry
Email id: georgeparadis2000@yahoo.com

S.T. Viroji Rao
Principal Scientist and Head
AICRP on Poultry Breeding, S.V.V.U.
Hyderabad – 500 030, Telengana
Email id: virojiraosindhe@yahoo.co.in

Sarbjit Singh Nagra
Director, Instructions
Central Agricultural University
Imphal, Manipur
Email id: snagra52@rediffmail.com

Sujit Nayak
Assistant Commissioner
Department of Animal Husbandry Dairying & Fisheries
Ministry of Agriculture, Government of India
39-C, Krishi Bhawan, New Delhi – 110 001
Email id: sujit.nayak@nic.in

T. Srilatha
Assistant Professor
Department of Poultry Science
College of Veterinary Science
Korutla, S.V.V.U., Telengana.
Email id: srilatha.mangalam@gmail.com

V. Ravinder Reddy
Professor and Head
Department of Poultry Science
College of Veterinary Science
Rajendranagar, S.V.V.U.
Hyderabad – 500 030, Telengana
Email id: vangoorravinder@yahoo.co.in

Stimulating Memory Tips

Brain gym – Simple Exercises for a Better Mind and Body

- Brain Gym is a programme of physical activities that enhances the development of neural pathways in the brain through movements.
- It comprises of easy body movements, designed to coax the two hemispheres of the brain to work in synchronisation.
- It could help your brain function better, making you sharper, smarter – and far more confident.
- It can do everything from speeding up your reading to boosting self-esteem and creativity. It improves communication skills, helping you make better decision maker.
- It is observed that very simple body movements could help to improve brain function. The Brain Gym can help everyone, even those who think they have perfectly normal brain function will help perform even better.
- For details one can search Google.

Drink Water to Drive-Out Stress

- More of the brain is comprised of water (about 85%). Drinking water during class can help '*grease the wheel*'.
- Brain function depends on having abundant access to water.
- Water gives the brain the electrical energy for all brain functions, including thought and memory processes.
- Drinking water is very important before any stressful situation tests as we tend to perspire under stress, and dehydration can affect our concentration negatively.

Relieve Stresses, Improve Performance

1. Sit relaxed.
2. Close your eyes.
3. With the fingertips of each hand gently touch the point above each eye halfway between the hairline and eyebrow.
4. Take slow and deep breaths.
5. Your memory blocks will be released, stresses will be relieved, thinking will be cleared, speaking abilities will be improved!

Memory Improvement Tips

- **Give attention**: Concentrate on the information you are trying to learn. Grow interest. This is especially true if you are trying to learn a new skill or subject. Give it your undivided attention.
- **Play games**: Use your brain just like every other muscle of your body; the more you exercise it the better it will function.
- **Be active:** If your attention is diverted take a moment and get up and move around the room. Try some deep knee bends or body stretching.
- **Eat brain foods**: Our *brain* accounts for only 2 percent of your body weight but *consumes* roughly 20 percent of our *calorie intake.* As it operates at its peak it needs to have the proper nutrients. Eating food rich in omega -3 fatty acid will help as will increasing the amount of antitoxins that you consume.
- **Use as many senses as possible**: When trying to remember information the more senses you can incorporate the better. For example, if you read louder so that you hear as well as see the information.
- **Drink water**: When your body gets dehydrated you actually lessen your ability to focus. Stay away from coffee and sugar filled drinks. Water is the best way to hydrate your body.
- **Use acronyms, initialism** or **pseudo-blend**: You can use acronyms, initialism or pseudo-blend to remember words or facts. The first letter of other words or phrases come together to create ***acronyms***. e.g., *SARS* = severe acute respiratory syndrome. **initialism** is an abbreviation pronounced wholly or partly using the names of its constituent letters, e.g., CD =compact disc, pronounced *cee dee*. **Pseudo-blend** is an abbreviation who's extra or omitted letters mean that it cannot stand as a true acronym or initialism, e.g., *UNIFEM – United Nations Development Fund for Women.*

- **Re-read and Review**: Underline or highlight the information into point form and read and re-read over a number of days. This will help to create long term memories.
- **Take more oxygen**: If you are working for long periods of time the brain cells may become fatigue. Take a break and practice few deep breathing. This will help you to relax get more oxygen to your brain.
- **Room System**: To use the technique, imagine a room that you know, such as your sitting room, bedroom or classroom. Within the room are objects. Associate images represent0ing the information you want to remember with the objects in the room. To recall information, simply take a tour around the room in your mind, visualizing the known objects and their associated images. The idea is to associate the new items with stable old memories.

1

Indian Poultry Industry

D. Narahari

The modern commercial poultry production in India is barely 50 years old, although backyard poultry keeping dates back to pre-historic period. In between 1955 to 1965, some Christian Missionaries had imported White Leghorn, Rhode Island Red and White Rock breeds, to upgrade the local chicken, having very high disease resistance power; but highly broody. Later, hybrid broiler (Arbor Acres) and layer (Babcock) strains were brought to India in early seventies, to start modern poultry industry. Among the two, the layer industry took wings early and registered a spectacular growth rate between 1970 and 1985. The broiler industry came to existence five years later and showed 25 -100% annual growth rate initially and 10-20% growth rate subsequently; between 1975 – 2005. The growth indicators of poultry development in India are presented in Table 1.

In addition to the modern hybrid layers and broilers, India is having a huge (300 -500 millions) population of indigenous chicken in the backyard or free range; which provides pin money to the housewives. The Japanese quail farming is also growing at a rapid rate, as an alternative to chicken, by small farmers and entrepreneurs. Native ducks and a few Khaki Campbell X native crosses are reared in the north eastern states and in Kerala, mostly in the free range.

The poultry industry is owned by farmers and several private companies; with good technical support from agricultural and veterinary universities and financial support from nationalized banks. The present poultry industry in India is a US$ 16 billion industry; providing direct employment to about two million people and many more, indirectly. The layer and broiler sectors are recording an annual growth rate of five and nine percent, respectively. Now India ranks 3rd and 5th in the world in egg and broiler production, respectively. Most (>80%) of the modern poultry industry is concentrated in the southern states of Andhra Pradesh, Karnataka, Maharashtra and Tamilnadu; besides Punjab in the north.

India is self sufficient in poultry production as well as in all farm inputs; except pure lines, grandparent stock and amino acids. Now India is exporting incubators, cages, feed mills, all other farm equipment, medicines, vaccines, feed supplements, day old chicks, hatching eggs, table eggs, egg powder, dressed chicken, soybean meal, corn and other feedstuffs, mostly to Afro-Asian and few European countries. The contribution of poultry sector to total value of outputs from livestock sector in India has gone up from 2.2 % in 1951 to about 28.5 % in 2013. The poultry industry is contributing about 2% to the national G.D.P.

Table1: Growth of poultry industry in India

Year	Production by hybrid chicken			Per capita availability	
	Eggs (Billions)	Broilers (Millions)	Broiler Meat (X1,000T)	Chicken Eggs (No.)	Poultry Meat (g)
1961	2.88	<1	81	7	188
1971	5.34	4	121	10	220
1980	12.50	30	179	18	266
1985	16.13	75	274	22	365
1990	23.30	190	412	28	498
1991	23.66	215	440	28	521
1992	22.74	210	427	26	493
1993	24.80	235	454	28	517
1994	26.29	275	507	29	566
1995	28.13	330	578	31	633
1996	30.30	400	659	32	707
2000	35.50	800	980	36.6	1020
2003	39.50	1250	1600	40.3	1360
2004	41.90	1400	1900	41.4	1660
2005	43.30	1600	2200	42.5	1900
2006	44.70	1800	2500	43.8	2200
2007	46.20	1900	2680	44.7	2500
2008	52.23	2040	2854	47.9	2650
2009	56,09	2203	3109	49.2	2810
2010	59,56	2348	3344	51.0	2940
2011	63,12	2465	3428	52.4	3080
2012	65.32	2588	3513	53.6	3170

Egg Production

The commercial egg production in India was started in early seventies, with introduction of Babcock chicken. Later, other hybrids like Bovans, Hisex, Hyline, Keystone and Lohmann were introduced into the Indian market. All hybrids are laying white shell eggs only. On the contrary, the native chicken as well as the cross breeds developed by the Agriculture / Veterinary Universities, produce brown shell eggs; which constitute nearly 16% of the total eggs produced in India.

India has developed its own technology in poultry housing suitable for tropics, cages, other farm equipment, incubators, feed mills, farm /feed automation equipment at low cost; which are not only efficient, but also durable. This has not only reduced the cost of production of eggs, but also improved the production standards. The egg production technical standards in India are presented in Table 2.

Besides chicken eggs, duck eggs contribute about 5% and Japanese quail eggs about 2.5% of the total eggs produced in India. The duck eggs are mostly produced in the free range system; whereas the quail eggs are produced in organized farms, mostly in cages. Nearly 12% of the farm eggs produced in India is exported to Afro-Asian countries and Europe; either as shell eggs or egg powder.

Table 2: Egg production standards in India 2013

Details	Standards	Remarks
Table egg production-farm eggs	55.2 billion	3rd rank
Free range / backyard egg production	10.1 billion	17%
Duck egg production- mostly free range	2.6 billion	5.0%
Japanese quail egg production	1.3 billion	2.5%
Total table egg production	69.2 billion	—
Export of shell eggs	3.3 billion	Afro-Asian countries
Export of egg powder	35,200 tonnes	From 2.82 billion eggs,100% export
Per capita chicken egg consumption	53.6 eggs	One of the lowest in the world
Per capita other eggs consumption	4.2 eggs	—
Average commercial layer farm size	30,000 layers	—
Flock depreciation (0-20 wks)	5%	Low mortality rate
Flock depreciation-(21-80wks)	7%	—do—
Age at culling	80-85 wks	Some flocks are force moulted & kept >100 wks.
Hen-day egg production	86%	Some flocks produce >80% @ >75 wks.

(Contd.)

Details	Standards	Remarks
Peak egg production	95%	Very good production
Hen-housed egg production up to 80 wks.	355 eggs	—
Feed /hen /day	108 g	Mostly own feed
Feed / egg	127 g	—
Annual growth rate	5%	—
Cost of production /100 eggs	US$ 5.12	One of the lowest
Market price for 100 eggs	US$ 5.55	—do—

Most of the layers are reared in 3-tier Californian cages erected on elevated platforms in open sided houses of 20,000 to 50,000 layers capacity, with automatic feed trolleys. Eggs are manually collected, due to cheaper labour. The rate of egg production by hens is mostly above the standards recommended by the breeder companies, due to better management, feed quality and health care. *E.coli* infection, mycotoxins, coryza and wing rot are some of the health problems faced by layer farmers; but they overcome these problems within two weeks; with least loss. Prompt veterinary services are available in all poultry pockets, within few hours of any disease outbreak. Farms with >100,000 birds are employing their own poultry veterinarians.

Broiler Production

Commercial broiler production in India was started around 1974, with the import of Arbor Acres and Cobb broiler grandparent stocks. Later, Hubbard, Hybro, Marshall and Ross hybrid G.P. stock were introduced. Besides hybrid broilers, few indigenously developed cross bred coloured broilers and local free range birds are having about 18% market share. These birds fetch premium price due to their strong game flavour, lean and tough meat; which is likened by locals. In addition to these meats, the culled hens, egg-type cockerels, broiler breeders and egg-type breeders are also utilized as low value meat. The per capita poultry meat consumption in India is one of the lowest in the world (2.35kg), due to more vegetarian population.

Unlike the layer industry, the broiler industry is a highly integrated operation. The integrator is the owner of the bird, who owns the breeding stock, hatchery, feed mill, processing plant and the marketing network. The farmer will rear six batches of broilers per year on "all-in-all-out basis" for contract in his / her farm, for a commission. Despite of integration, the poultry processing industry is still in its infancy; due to preference of hot fresh chicken by the consumers, instead of chilled or frozen chicken. This trend is slowly changing .Hence a big boom in the poultry processing sector is to be expected in the next decade. The broiler integrators' business volume ranges between 100,000 to 7,000,000 broilers per week. Some of them have their own pharmaceutical unit, poultry house fabrication section, incubator and other equipment manufacturing section. The broiler production standards in India are presented in Table 3.

Table 3: Broiler production and standards in India-2013

Details	Standards	Remarks
Total broiler chicken production	2.59 billion	4th in the world
Broiler meat production	3.51 mill. tons	— do —
Culled hen, breeders & cockerel meat production	0.20 mill. tons	Sold at reduced cost
Back yard and free range chicken meat production	0.28 Mill. tons	Sold at premium price
Poultry, other than chicken meat production	0.14 m.t.	—
Total poultry meat production	4.13 m.t.	—
Poultry meat exports	0.05 m.t.	Negligible
Per capita poultry meat consumption (all poultry)	3.17 kg	One of the lowest in the world
Annual growth rate	8%	Fair growth rate
Housing and Rearing system	Deep litter	Open sided house
Average farm size & batch system	10,000 birds	All- in-all out under integration & batch system in own farms
Growing period	38days	—
Average body weight	2kg	—
Mortality	5%	—
Feed conversion ratio (FCR)	1.7	—
Source of feed & chicks	—	Own or integrators
Marketing	Own	Live or dressed chicken
Cost of production / 2 kg live broiler	US$ 1.00	Low for integrators
Cost / kg dressed chicken in the retail market	US$ 2.22	Varies with the supply & demand

Breeder Farms and Hatcheries

India is having three pure line breeding farms and >10 grandparent stock farms; all under private sector. Many Agricultural and Veterinary Universities are having their own pure line breeding farms, to supply dual purpose chicken to small farms. There are more than 500 parent stock farms and > 1,000 hatcheries, to supply necessary commercial broilers and egg –type pullets to the farmers.

Unlike in other countries, most of the layer and broiler breeding stocks are reared in cages in open sided houses and artificial insemination is done twice a week. This will ensure high rate of fertility particularly in the old flock as well as in summer, especially in broiler breeders; resulting in more number of chicks per dam. Slat–cum deep litter system has become obsolete, due to high cost and low fertility. Few small breeding stock owners are having their breeders on deep litter, with plans to shift them to cage houses soon. Cage rearing of breeders is having several advantages like:

- Better fertility rate, resulting in more chicks per dam
- Lesser feed/bird/egg/chick
- Lesser mortality
- Lesser capital cost and cost of production

Rubber or plastic mats are provided on the bottom of the cages, to prevent hair cracks to the eggs; which will affect the hatchability. India is exporting large number of hatching eggs and day-old chicks to Afro-Asian countries. The performance of breeders in India is presented in Table 4.

Table 4: Breeders' performance and standards in India-2013

Details	Broiler breeder	Layer breeder
Housing & rearing system	Elevated cages in open sided houses	Elevated cages in open sided houses
Average flock size	10,000 hens + cocks + growers	20,000 hens + cocks + growers
Age at culling	65 weeks	75 weeks
Flock depreciation- 0-20 wks.	9%	4%
—do—— = >20 wks.	12%	6%
Source of feed	Own	Own
Source of parent stock	Own or from G.P.farms	Own or from G.P. farms
Hatching eggs /hen	180	300
Day old salable chicks /hen	150 unsexed chicks	125 pullet chicks
Fertility	90%	95%
Hatchability of total eggs set	85%	88%
Feed/hatching egg (includes sires' share)	470g	150g
Feed/chick	543g / unsexed chick	340g/ pullet chick
Cost of production/100 hatching eggs	US$ 20.00	US$ 10.00
Cost of production/100 chicks	US$ 25.00	US$ 23.00

Non-Chicken Poultry Farming in India

Besides chicken, Japanese quails and emus are reared in India on a commercial scale, following modern scientific methods. Other species of poultry like ducks, geese, turkeys and pigeons are still reared by traditional methods in a small scale to supply the local market.

Japanese Quail Farming

Japanese quails are reared for meat and eggs; both in cage and deep litter systems of rearing. Most of the Japanese quail farms are having their own hatchery and breeding stock. Such farms will have a total stock of 10,000 and above. They obtain an average hatchability of 80%. Large farms are preparing their own feed and others are purchasing quail feed crumbles from feed manufacturers. Three types of feeds are given to J. quails; namely starter feed from 0-2 weeks of age, grower feed from 3-5 weeks of age and layer / breeder feed from 6 weeks of age. They are ready for market at 4 weeks of age, with a body weight of 150– 180g. They start laying eggs from 6 weeks of age and the hatching eggs are collected from 8 weeks of age. The egg weight is around 10g and sold at Rs150/ 100 eggs for table purpose and Rs250 /100 hatching eggs.

The mortality rate during 0-4 weeks of age is around 6 % in cages and 8% in deep litter system. The major causes of mortality during growing period are chilling, drowning, stampeding, huddling and starvation; which can be controlled by using right brooding temperature, right size feeders and waterers, combined with proper management. Egg peritonitis and egg bound are the major cause of mortality in laying quails and cannibalism in adult males. Under integrated quail operation, with own breeding stock, hatchery, feed mill, farm and direct marketing, the Japanese quail farming is highly economical in India.

Emu Farming

Prior to 1990, emus were reared in India in zoological parks only. The commercial emu farming was first stared in Andhra Pradesh in 1992. By the end of 2007, there were about 10,000 commercial emu farms in India, out of which nearly 50% are in Andhra Pradesh alone. The number of emus in each farm ranges from four to 10,000 birds; with an average of 60 birds per farm. Now few big corporate entrepreneurs are entering into emu farming business for valuable oil and skin production.

Management, feeding, breeding and hatching procedures for emu rearing are standardized for Indian conditions. The emu farms are able to achieve the technical standards reported in Table 5. Specialized emu incubators, with capacities ranging from 10 to 1000 eggs are fabricated locally, which are giving hatchability up to 80%. Due to high prices and demand for emu oil, the processing of emu has started as per HACCP standards. The skin, feathers and meat are also fetching remunerative prices. Based on such demand, many farms will expand and new farms will emerge in India, as alternative to chicken farming.

Previously chicken or quail feeds were given to emus; but at present specialized emu feeds are given, in order to achieve better growth rate and egg production. Both mash and pellets feeds are offered to the birds. Big farms are preparing their own feed; while small farms are buying feed from nearby big farms. Each adult bird is fed 750 – 1250 g of feed per day, depending on the season. Besides feed, fresh green grass or legumes are also fed to the birds. In addition to regular feeds, a special fattening feed is also given prior to slaughter, to obtain more emu oil; which fetch good price.

Of late emus are better managed to achieve lower rate of mortality. Leg weakness and injuries are mostly avoided. After initial outbreak of Newcastle Disease six years back, all farms are vaccinating their emus for ND several times, periodically. They are also deworming their birds, to avoid intestinal parasites. Coccidiostats are added in feed, to avoid coccidiosis. Common causes of mortality in emus are omphalitis, enteritis, coccidiosis, impaction, conjunctivitis, injuries and ND. Expert veterinary aid is available for all farms. Health insurance is done for all birds.

Table 5: Technical standards on emu farming in India

Sex ratio /mating type	Pairs, trios or flock mating
Laying season	August – February.
Daily feed intake /adult bird	800 – 1000g
Annual egg production	20 – 50 eggs- (average=30 eggs)
% Hatchability	60 – 80%
Incubation period	50 -60 days
Egg weight	400 –700g
Chick weight at hatch	330 – 550g
Mortality during first month	<5%
Age at slaughter	16 – 20 months
Floor space (breeding)	500 – 1000 sq.ft. / pair
Floor space (slaughtering)	50 – 100 sq.ft. / bird
Dressed meat yield obtained	40%
Oil obtained from one bird	5 – 6 liters

Duck Farming

Duck eggs are popular in north –eastern states, West Bengal and Kerala; where they are mostly reared in free range system. Some farms are rearing Khaki Campbell X indigenous cross bred ducks on bamboo slat / cages and deep litter floors for better egg production. Indigenous ducks are highly disease resistance and can survive by grazing in the rice fields, canals, ponds, marshy lands, irrigation tanks and rivers. Hence they are more popular than Khaki Campbell ducks. Meat –type ducks are not popular; hence the surplus males are utilized for meat. Fish and duck combined farms are also available in north-eastern states.

Duck farmers of Kerala are mostly nomadic type. They take ducks to marshy areas and paddy (rice) fields soon after harvest; for feeding the fallen paddy, insects, crabs, small fish, toads, weeds etc. There will be no supplemental feeding of these ducks, except during dry season, when are fed with whole paddy grains (rice with husk intact).

The indigenous ducks (Chara and Chemballi from Kerala) are maintained for 2 to 3 years. Each year, they lay 120 to 180 extra large eggs, bigger than Khaki Campbell eggs. The egg weight will be 65-80g, depending on the breed / variety. Since the ducks are mostly fed in the range with natural feeds, mycotoxin problems are not there. The major disease challenging the ducks are duck plague, for which all the ducks are vaccinated periodically, starting from two months of age. Duck eggs are sold at a premium price of 50-100% more than the cost of the chicken egg; but duck meat is only a byproduct of the egg industry.

Turkey Production

Turkey farming is not as much commercialized as that of quail and emu farming. The turkeys available in India are not hybrids. Beltsville small, bronze and their crosses are available; which will attain a body weight of 7 to 10 kg only, at 10 months of age. Turkeys are reared in deep litter houses, similar to broilers and fed with broiler or turkey feeds. Due to high cost of feed combined with poor feed efficiency, turkeys are often fed with vegetable, kitchen and slaughter house waste. Small flocks are maintained in the free range or pen-cum–run system; with free access to range.

Geese Farming

In India there is no commercial goose production for meat or eggs. Small flocks or even a pair of Chinese geese are maintained as pets, ornamental birds, de-weeders or watch dogs in orchards, gardens, parks and backyards. Goose eggs are hatched in chicken /duck egg incubators and sometimes even under a broody hen. During brooding period, the goslings will be fed with other poultry feeds for a month and then left in the open yard, where they eat grass, greens, vegetable and kitchen waste. Therefore, in places where lots of grass or vegetable waste is available, geese can be reared economically. Since there is no demand for goose meat or eggs in India, feeding geese with balanced feed is not economical. Goslings are sold as pets to other farmers or pet lovers, who have enough space in the back yard.

Guinea Fowls Farming

In some pockets of India, guinea fowls are reared and sold for breeding or meat purpose. They are flying type and good grazers in the ranch. The keets are brood and fed with chick mash for one month. Thereafter they are allowed in the free range to gather their feed like weeds, insects, fallen grains and other agro waste. Since their egg production is very low, scientific feeding is not economical. Hence they are reared in the free range, supplemented with a mixture of kitchen waste, vegetable and slaughter house waste, for economic egg and meat production.

Pigeon Production

Pigeons are reared in India for racing purpose as well as for squab production and as pets. The racing pigeons are very expensive, compared to pets or squabs; costing Rs 2687- 13436/ pair. Pigeon races and betting are going on in some places. The owner will train the pigeon for races and once they win any race, the owner will earn a good income and the bird's price will go up. They are reared in pairs and two pigeon holes are provided for each pair. The young ones are fed with pigeon milk by their parents until the market age of four weeks. Hence they don't need any special feeding. However, the breeding pairs are fed with a mixture of peas, soya seeds, pigeon pea, sunflower seeds, chick peas and other legumes, depending on the local availability. No separate pigeon feeds are available in the market. Shell grit or lime stone and drinking water are provided in separate hoppers during breeding season. The pigeons are not confined; but allowed to fly freely. They will come back to the owners' house during nights. Paralysis and other nervous disorders are common in pigeons. Hence racing pigeons are injected with vitamin B-complex, liver tonics during training period and racing season. Pigeon meat is popular in North Eastern Region, Sikkim as well as in West Bengal.

Poultry Feed Production

During the year 2012, India has produced about 21.5 million tons of poultry feed, to produce the specified number of eggs and meat mentioned in Tables 1 to 3, above. India is self sufficient not only in feedstuffs and animal feed production; but also in feed mill manufacturing. India has produced around 10 million tons of soy extractions and 50 million tons of coarse grains in 2012, of which 25 metric tons is corn. India is exporting corn, soy and other feedstuffs as well as mash and pellet feed mills of various capacities, to Afro-Asian countries. Only amino acids are imported.

Poultry feeds are mainly corn – soy based; but lots of sunflower meal (5 – 17%) and fish (5-12%) are also used, depending on the relative cost and availability. More than 90% of the poultry feed is prepared by poultry farmers and integrators for own use and the remaining by the feed manufacturers for sale. Due to own use the feed quality is excellent and giving highly satisfactory performance by the birds. Various types of chicken, quail and emu feeds are prepared. Very little quantities of other poultry feeds are prepared, in small pockets.

Summary

- The Indian poultry industry is just four and half decades old.
- Most of the poultry activities are in the southern states of Andhra Pradesh, Karnataka, Maharashtra and Tamilnadu and in the northern state of Punjab.
- Within this period, India has not only became self sufficient in poultry production, but also capable of exporting eggs, egg powder, meat, vaccines, medicines, cages, incubators and other poultry equipment.
- The poultry houses and cages are designed to suit the local conditions at low cost, but with excellent results and durability.
- Management, feeding, health care and marketing strategies are standardized for optimal performance of the birds at low cost.
- The overall performance of the birds, especially egg production, chick production and Japanese quail growth rate are above the standard recommended levels.
- Indigenous chicken in free range is contributing 16% of total eggs and meat; which fetch premium price.
- The per capita egg (53.6 eggs) and poultry meat consumption (3.17kg) in India is one of the lowest in the world, due to more vegetarian population.
- The production cost and market price of eggs in India is one of the lowest in the world.
- The poultry processing industry is not well developed, due to preference of live and hot chicken by Indians, instead of chilled / frozen chicken. This trend is changing now.
- Japanese quail farms are emerging as alternative to chicken for egg and meat production, due to lesser capital and growing demand for quail eggs and meat; which are considered as aphrodisiac and good for T.B. and H.I.V. patients.

- Emu farms with full integration are coming up for valuable oil and skin production

Question Bank

Q. 1. Fill in the blanks with appropriate word (s).

i) India ranks .... and ....in the world in egg and broiler production, respectively.

ii) The poultry industry is contributing about .... per cent to the national G.D.P.

iii) Duck eggs contribute about ....per cent of the total eggs produced in India.

iv) Japanese quails are reared for both............ and ....

v) The total table egg production in India is .... billion in 2012.

vi) In India, the per capita availability of poultry meat is .... kilogram.

vii) By the end of 2012, there were about............... commercial emu farms in India.

viii) Duck farmers of Kerala are mostly ....type.

ix) Emu farms with full integration are coming up for valuable .... and skin production.

x) Indigenous chicken in free range is contributing .... per cent of total eggs and meat.

Q. 2. Write True or False against the following statements.

i) The Indian poultry industry is just four and half decades old. (T)

ii) The production cost and market price of eggs in India is one of the highest in the world.(F)

iii) During the year 2012, India has produced about 21.5 million tons of poultry feed.(T)

iv) Young pigeons are called keets. (F)

v) Turkey farming is not as much commercialized as that of quail and emu farming. (T)

vi) Young ones of geese are called goslings. (T)

vii) The indigenous ducks (Chara and Chemballi) are maintained for one year only. (F)

viii) India is exporting hatching eggs and day-old chicks to Afro-Asian countries.(T)

ix) The commercial egg production in India was started in early sixties. (F)

x) Quail eggs weight is around 15-18 g (F).

Q. 3. Describe briefly about the development of poultry industry in India.

Q. 4. Write about the recent Table Egg Production Standards in India.

Answer Key

I (i) 3rd, 4th (ii) 2 (iii) 5 (iv) meat, egg (v) 65.32 bill. (vi) 3.17kg (vii) 10000 (viii) nomadic (ix) oil (x) 16

2

Classification and Common Breeds of Poultry

D. Sapcota

The modern breeds of chicken have known to be descended from the wild jungle fowl. India, Nepal, Bangladesh, Myanmar, Thailand, Sri Lanka and Malaysia are the homeland to these jungle fowls. There are four known species of jungle fowl viz. *Gallus gallus* (Red jungle fowl), *Gallus lafayetti* (Ceylon jungle fowl), *Gallus sonnerati* (Grey jungle fowl) and *Gallus varius* (Java jungle fowl). The domestic breeds of chicken/fowl have originated from *Gallus gallus*.

Classification of Fowl

Kingdom	-	Animalia (as opposed to plant kingdom)
Sub-kingdom	-	Metazoa (bodies consisting of specialized cells)
Phylum	-	Chordata (axial skeleton with notochord)
Sub-phylum	-	Vertebra (well developed brain and axial skeleton)
Class	-	Aves (feathered, warm blooded vertebra with 4-chambered heart)
Sub-class	-	Neornithes (without teeth)
Order	-	Galliformes (bird with short wings, legs and toes adapted for running and scratching)

Family - Phasianidae

Genus - Gallus (cock like bird)

Species - Domesticus (breeding under domestic condition). The domestic fowl is called *Gallus gallus domesticus*.

Birds of distinct type and colour patterns admitted to the standard are termed as *standard breed.* The British Poultry Standard listed more than 225 breeds and varieties of chicken, ducks and turkeys. They are further classified as follows:

1. **Class** - It is a group of breeds which have been developed in certain regions or geographical areas. e.g. American, English, Mediterranean, Asiatic etc.
2. **Breed** - It is a group of birds that have usually the same general body shape, they are true to the type, carriage and characteristics of the name of the breed they carry e.g. Leghorn, Rhode Island Red. etc.
3. **Variety** - Varieties represent a sub-division of a breed, distinguished either by plumage colour, feather patterns or comb type e.g. Single Comb White Leghorn, Rose Comb Leghorn, Brown Leghorn, Barred Plymouth Rock etc.
4. **Strain** - A strain refers to line, family or a group of birds within a variety bearing a name of a place or person connected and produced by a breeder through a specialized breeding programme, which reproduces uniform characteristics with marked regularity. e.g. HH – 260, Babcock-300, ILI-80, B-77, BV-300 etc.
5. **Lines** - These are sub classes of strains which are engaged for production of commercial hybrids.

Classification of chicken

1. Standard or official classification based on the place of origin.
2. Classification based on utility, economics or commercial value.

I. Classification based on the place of origin

1. Asiatic - i.e,. Brahma, Langshan, Cochin, Kadaknath, Aseel
2. American - i.e,. Plymouth Rock, Rhode Island Red, Wyandotte
3. Mediterranean - i.e,. Leghorn, Minorca, Ancona
4. English - i.e,. Orpington, Sussex, Cornish

5. Continental - i.e,. Houdans, Hamburg, Polish, Campines, Lackvelders
6. Oriental - i.e,. Malays, Yokohama, Sumatra, Cubalayas
7. French, South American (or) Latin American - i.e,. Araucana
8. African: i.e,. Negro, Jago
9. Miscellaneous - i.e,. Bantams

II. Classification based on utility

This classification is based on utility or commercial value; such as

1. Egg-type: i.e,. White Leghorn, Minorca, Ancona.
2. Meat-type: i.e,. Cornish, Plymouth Rock, Brahma.
3. Dual purpose: i.e,. Rhode Island Red, New Hampshire, Australorp,
4. Game type: i.e,. Aseel
5. Fancy variety or Exhibition type: i.e,. Silky, Frizzled, Bantam
6. Desi type: i.e,. Aseel, Kadaknath, Naked neck, Chittagong

Standard classes, breeds, and varieties of fowl

Classes and their characteristics	Common breeds and their characteristics	Varieties	Commercial importance
A. American class 1. Clean shanks 2. Yellow skin 3. Red earlobes 4. Medium size 5. Brown-shelled eggs	**1. Rhode Island Red (R.I.R.)** Origin : Rhode Island in New England (US) after crossing with the Red Malay Game, Leghorn and Asiatic native stock i) Long rectangular body ii) Back is flat and the breast is protuded well forward. iii) The plumage is rich dark or brownish red in colour iv) Shanks are yellow v) Standard weight : Cock – 3.8 kg Hen – 2.9 kg vi) Annual egg production : 225 to 260 eggs hen-housed per bird.	Single Comb (S.C.) Rose Comb (R.C.)	Dual purpose
+	**2. New Hampshire** Origin : American i) Broad, deep and rounded body. ii) The plumage is chestnut red iii) Shanks are yellow iv) Standard weight : Cock – 3.8 kg Hen – 3.1 kg v) Mostly used as female line in broiler breeding.	Single Comb	Meat purpose

(Contd.)

Classes and their characteristics	Common breeds and their characteristics	Varieties	Commercial importance
	1. Plymouth Rock Origin: America. i) Long body and have good depth of body ii) In general, the plumage is grayish white, each feather crossed by almost black bars iii) Shanks are yellow iv) Standard weight : Cock – 4.2 kg Hen - 3.3 Kg vi) White variety is extensively used as male line in broiler breeding.	Barred, White, Buff, Partridge plumage	Meat purpose
B. English class 1. Clean shank 2. White skin 3. Red earlobes 4. Meat purpose 5. Medium to large size 6. Single comb 7. Brown shelled eggs	**1. Australorp** Origin : Australia. i) Deep oval body ii) Black shanks, white skin and red earlobes. iii) Plumage is lustrous greenish black in all the sections. iv) The back is long and the body slopes gradually towards the tail. v) Standard weight : Cock – 3.8 kg Hen – 3.0 kg.	Black plumage.	Dual purpose
	2. Cornish Origin : England i) Heavily meated compact body with a good depth.	White, Dark, Buff plumage.	Meat purpose

(Contd.)

Classes and their characteristics	Common breeds and their characteristics	Varieties	Commercial importance
	ii) Body is well rounded all sides and carried higher in front than rear. iii) Pea comb is present iv) Yellow shank v) Standard weight : Cock – 4.6 kg Hen – 3.5 kg. vi) Used as male line in broiler breeding.		
	3. Sussex Origin – England i) Long rectangular body. ii) Standard weight : Cock – 4.0 kg Hen – 3.1 kg	Light red	Meat purpose
	4. Orpington Origin: England i) Body in deep and well rounded ii) Full breast and broad back iii) Standard weight: Cock – 4.5 kg Hen – 3.5 kg	White, Black and Buff	Meat purpose
C. Mediterranean class 1. Clean shank 2. Yellow or white skin 3. White earlobes	**1. Leghorn** Origin : Italy i) It is the world's No.1 egg producer ii) It has small, oval and compact body iii) It has relatively long neck, prominent breast and long shanks.	Out of 12 varieties of Leghorn 3 varieties are popular i.e. S.C. White	Egg purpose

(Contd.)

Classes and their characteristics	Common breeds and their characteristics	Varieties	Commercial importance
4. Small size 5. Egg purpose 6. White-shelled eggs.	iv) All varieties have yellow beaks, skin, shanks and toes. v) Plumage may be white, dark, brown or light brown. vi) The single comb of the male should be of medium size and should stand erect with 5 uniform deeply serrated points. The front point of female should stand erect; but remainder of the comb gradually slopes to one side. vii) Standard weight : Cock – 2.7 kg Hen – 1.8 kg viii) Annual hen-housed egg production per bird is 290-320 eggs.	S.C. Buff S.C. Light brown	
	2. Minorca Origin : Spanish i) Largest and heaviest of Mediterranean breeds of poultry. Long rectangular body, white skin. ii) Long strong bodies, large comb, large white earlobes (Red in Black Australorp) iii) Beak, shank and toes are black.	S.C. & R.C. Black S.C. & R.C. White	Egg purpose

(Contd.)

Classes and their characteristics	Common breeds and their characteristics	Varieties	Commercial importance
	iv) Standard weight : Cock – 4.1 kg Hen – 3.0 kg		
D. Asiatic class 1. Feathered shank 2. Yellow skin 3. Red earlobes 4. Massive size 5. Meat purpose 6. Brown shelled egg	**1. Brahma** Origin : America i) Circular shaped and massive in appearance. ii) Eggs are tinted brown iii) Matured weight : Cock - 5.3 kg Hen - 4.4 kg	Pea comb Light dark and buff	Meat purpose
	2. Cochin Origin : China i) It is a fancy bird ii) Colour of shank is yellow iii) Standard weight Cock - 5.2 kg Hen – 3.7 kg	Single comb Buff Black White	Meat purpose

Breeds of duck: Ducks are reared for eggs and meat. They belongs to –

1. Class- Aves
2. Order- Anseriformes
3. Family – Anatidae
4. Genus – Anas
5. Species – Platyrhynchos

Sl. No.	Name of breeds and their characteristics	Commercial importance
1.	**Khaki Campbell**	
	Origin : England (developed by Mrs. Campbell) from crosses among: Rouen, White Indian Runner and Mallard	Egg purpose
i)	Plumage colour is khaki	
ii)	The size of head of male is larger than that of female	
iii)	Bills and shanks are black in colour	
iv)	Light body weight	
v)	Egg production: 280 to 300 eggs per bird per year	
vi)	Standard weight – Duck : 2.0 to 2.2 kg Drake : 2.2 to 2.4 kg	
2.	**Indian Runner**	
	Origin : Indonesia	Egg purpose
i)	It is a second good layer, next to Khaki Campbell	
ii)	White, white-penciled and fawn are the three standard varieties	
iii)	Body is broader in front and slightly tapering at back	
iv)	The outstanding feature of this breed is its perpendicular carriage which gives a lean appearance with wedge-shaped bill	
i)	Egg production: 250 to 280 eggs per bird per year	
ii)	Standard weight – Duck – 1.5 - 2.1 kg Drake – 2.0 - 2.6 kg	
3.	**Pekin**	
	Origin : China	Meat purpose
i)	The white variety is most popular for meat purpose	
ii)	It has creamy white plumage, yellow flesh, long, broad and deep body with bills and legs deep orange	
iii)	The white Pekin attains 2.2 to 2.5 kg body weight in 7 weeks of age with a feed conversion of 1:2.6 - 3.0 kg	
iv)	Egg production: 160 eggs per bird per year	
v)	Standard weight : Duck – 3.3- 3.6 kg Drake – 3.8- 4.2 kg	
4.	**Aylesbury**	Meat purpose
	Origin : England	
i)	The plumage of both sexes is white	
ii)	The legs and feet are bright orange and bill is yellow.	
iii)	It is regarded as deluxe table bird because of its light bone and high percentage of creamy white flesh	
iv)	Standard weight : Duck – 4.0 – 4.2 kg Drake – 4.3- 4.6 kg	

Sl. No.	Name of breeds and their characteristics	Commercial importance
5.	**Rouen** Origin : France i) It is good for roasting ii) Eggs are light blue in colour iii) Standard weight Duck – 4.0 kg Drake – 4.5 kg	Meat purpose
6.	**Muscovy** Origin : South America i) There is still doubt whether it is duck or goose ii) It grazes like goose. Like goose, males have no such curled feathers in the tail iii) There are no feathers on the face and the skin is bright red in colour with caruncles around the eyes iv) Drake has a knob on head which gives the appearance of a crest. Voice is not characteristic of sex v) Incubation period of egg: 35 days vi) Muscovies when crossed with other breeds produce sterile ducks called 'Mule ducks' vii) Standard weight : Duck – 2.2 to 3.1 kg Drake – 4.5 to 6.4 kg	Meat purpose

Breeds of Quail

Japanese quail belongs to:

Family – Phasianidae

Genus – Coturnix

Species – *Coturnix japonica.*

Bobwhite quail comes under a different sub-family and species – *Colinus virginianus.*

Quail farming is popular in Indian, Japan, Hongkong, Korea, France, Italy, Germany and Britain. Japanese quails were introduced in India by CARI in 1974 from California.

These birds do well in laboratory cages and are used for experimental studies. Commercial farms are also gaining popularity. Females (150–180 g) are heavier than the males (120–130 g). They lay eggs at the age of 6 weeks and egg weight is around 10 g. Quails lay about 210 eggs per year. The colour of the feathers in the breast region of male is plain rust in colour while in the female it is speckled. They are very easy to raise and can be maintained in minimum space. The eggs are mosaic patterned. They produce a greater volume of eggs per unit of weight and in a shorter time. They reach maturity in 42 days. Meat is very delicious.

Breeds of turkey

1. Class – Aves
2. Order – Galliformes
3. Family – Meleagridae
4. Genus – Meleagris
5. Species – Gallopavo

Turkeys originated from Northern and Central America and were domesticated about 300 years ago by the Europeans colonized in North America. These are kept only for meat. In India turkeys are almost non-existent and constitute less than 1% of total poultry population. Turkeys are most popular in USA and are not classified into breeds like chicken and ducks.

The popular standard varieties are

i) Broad Breasted Bronze

It is the most popular and heaviest variety of turkey with a broad and prominent chest region and bronze coloured feathers. The males and females at maturity weigh 15-18 kg and 12-13 kg. respectively.

ii) Beltsville White

It is a medium sized turkey having white feathers. They produce more eggs compared to Broad Breasted Bronze and therefore included in breeding programmes. The toms generally weighs 10-12 kg. at maturity and hens 7-8 kg.

iii) White Holland

It is most commonly found in European countries. It is bred and developed in Holland after importing several varieties from North America. They are also used as crosses with the local basic turkey to improve their growth rate and reproductive ability. The toms weigh 10-12 kg. and the hens 6-8 kg. at maturity.

iv) Naragansette

This is a popular variety in Europe next to White Holland, mostly reared in Germany, Italy etc. Most of the hybrid turkeys available in Europe are crosses of White Holland or Naragansette.

Hybrid Turkey

Most of the present day hybrid turkeys are crosses of different strains of Broad Breasted Bronze or Beltsville white. All are meat-type. Examples: Nicholas turkey, British United Turkey

Breeds of Guinea Fowl

Guinea fowl (*Numida meleagris*) are native to West Africa. These were imported to Indian sub-continent about 600 years back and are being maintained in small holder backyard system of production. Of late, there has been an increasing demand for guinea fowl because of its pleasant manner, attractive plumage and value as a table bird with gamy - flavored meat. There is very little difference between male and female. Sexing based on physical appearance is not possible before 12 weeks of age. The guinea fowl has also been used in protecting the farm flock from intruders and predators because of its loud, harsh cry and its nervous disposition. There are three domesticated varieties: the Pearl, the White and the Lavender. Among these the Pearl is the most popular.

Table 6: Nomenclature of various species of poultry on the basis of age and sex

Sl. No.	Species	Adult		Young
		Male	Female	0-8 weeks
1.	Chicken	Cock	Hen	Chick
2.	Duck	Drake	Duck	Drakeling Duckling
3.	Goose	Gander	Goose	Gosling
4.	Turkey	Tom turkey	Turkey hen	Poult
5.	Quail	Quail cock	Quail hen	Quail chick
6.	Guinea fowl	Guinea fowl	Guinea fowl	Keet
7.	Pigeon	Pigeon	Pigeon	Squab

Question Bank

1 . Choose the Correct Answer

i) The domestic breeds of chicken/fowl have originated from *Gallus gallus/ Gallus lafayetti / Gallus sonnerati/ Gallus varius*. (*Gallus gallus*).

ii) Modern fowl falls under the family: Neornithes/ Galliformes/ Phasianidae. (Phasianidae).

iii) Rhode Island Red is a dual purpose/ meat-type/egg-type breed. (dual purpose).

iv) Leghorn breed produces brown/white/tinted eggs. (white).

v) The incubation period of Muscovy duck egg is 25/35/45 days. (35).

vi) A quail lays about 180/200/210 eggs per year. (210).

vii Quails reach maturity in 35/38/42 days. (42).

viii) Among the standard varieties, Broad Breasted Bronze/ Beltsville White/ White Holland turkey is the most popular and heaviest. (Broad Breasted Bronze).

ix) Among the three domesticated varieties of guineafowl, the Pearl/the White/the Lavender is the most popular. (The Pearl).

2 . True/False

i) Babcock-300 is a commercial hybrid strain of broiler chicken. (False).

ii) The skin colour of Rhode Island Red is yellow. (True).

iii) The earlobes of New Hampshire are red. (True).

iv) Australorp produces brown shelled eggs. (True).

v) Brahma breed has clean shank. (False).

vi) The Indian Runner is originated in India. (False).

vii) Pekin is a popular meat-type duck. (True).

viii) The Muscovy duck is originated in Moscow. (False).

ix) Females quails are heavier than the males (True).

x) The male turkey is called as Tom. (True).

xi) The young duck is called as duckling. (True).

3. Fill in the blanks

i) The modern breeds of chicken have known to be descended from the ....fowl. (wild jungle).

ii) .... and .... (countries) are the home lands of wild jungle fowls. (India, Nepal, Bangladesh, Myanmar, Thailand, Sri Lanka and Malaysia).

iii) There are four known species of jungle fowl viz................................ and............................ (*Gallus gallus, Gallus lafayetti ,Gallus sonnerati* and *Gallus varius).*

iv) The Cornish breed is originated in ....(England).

v) The Leghorn breed is originated in .... (Italy).

vi) .... (breed) is the world's No.1 egg producer. (Leghorn).

vii) The scientific name of duck is .... (*Anas platyrhynchos).*

viii) The Khaki Campbell is produced by crossing among three breeds:....................and .... (Rouen, White Indian Runner and Mallard).

ix) The scientific name of Japanese quail is .... (*Coturnix japonica).*

x) Quails lay eggs at the age of .... weeks and the egg weight is around ....g. (6, 10).

xi) Turkeys originated from .... and ....America. (Northern and Central).

xii) Guinea fowls are native to................................ (West Africa).

xiii) The scientific name of Guinea fowl is .... (*Numida meleagris)*

3

Indigenous Fowls of India

Islam Uddin Sheikh

The word indigenous, originates from the Latin work, *indigena*, implies that the individual and its ancestors originated from a specified country or continent. Presently, certain synonymous words used for indigenous chicken are: 'native', 'local' or 'village chicken'. The indigenous fowls are well adapted to the local climate, need less input and produce tasty egg and meat at the least possible cost through scavenging. The birds require no scientific feeding, health care, housing and management and thus make the indigenous birds suitable for backyard poultry farming. Indigenous birds are normally handled by women, can significantly contribute to farmers' livelihoods through increased food security and cash income. These breeds are self-propagating; contribute to poultry diversity and cultural heritage. Because of their local origin they are less prone to disease or predator attacks, and their cultural and sporting values secure additional income. The prices of egg and meat of local birds are 100-150 percent higher than that of commercial counterpart. Some of these fowls are described in brief, as below.

1. Ankleshwar

The breed is originated from the Ankleshwar region of district Bharuch (Gujarat). It is also found in Narmada district of Gujarat. These birds are traditionally reared by tribal communities in South Gujarat. The comb type is single. The bird attains sexual maturity at 181 days with annual egg production of 81 and average egg weight of 34.3 g. The standard body weight at 12 weeks for male is 885 g and female is 772 g.

2. Aseel

This breed (Fig.1) is famous for its fighting nature and is mostly found in coastal Andhra Pradesh (Seemandhra) and in the Dantewada district of Chhattisgarh. The standard weight of cock ranges from 3- 4 kg and of hen, 2-3 kg. It is a tall bird measuring 28 inches (70 cm) from back to toe. The age at sexual maturity is 196 days. The annual egg production is 92 numbers with average egg weight of 50 g at 40 weeks. The Aseel is reared under backyard system of management and is a vital source of meat and income for small scale poultry rearers.

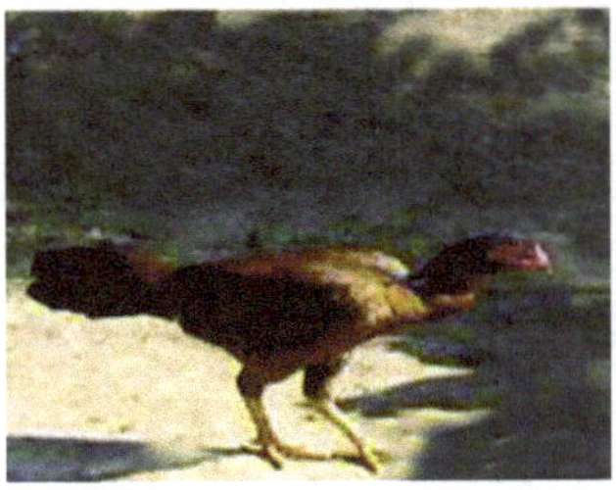

Fig. 1: Aseel

3. Busra

A small to medium sized bird found in Maharashtra and Gujarat. Plumage is mostly white, mixed with black feathers on the neck, back, tail and reddish brown feathers on shoulders and wings. Comb is red, single, small to medium in size, stands erect. Beak is yellow and wattles are red with a yellow shank. The standard weight varies from 0.85 - 1.25 kg for males and from 0.8 - 1.2 kg for females. The bird attains sexual maturity at 5-7 months with annual egg production of 40 - 55 numbers. The hatchability of eggs is 60 - 85%. The eggs are small, weighing about 28 - 38 g. The shell colour is primarily light brown. The birds are reared in a free range system for home consumption as well as for sale live or for eggs. The bird is preferred as a meat bird, since the egg laying capacity is poor.

4. Chittagong (Malay)

The breed is found in the North Eastern states of India bordering Bangladesh, also known as Malay as it was originally a native of Malayan peninsula. Adult male weighs 3.5 – 4.5 kg and female 3 – 4 kg. It is a large bird very strong and hardy with a quarrelsome temperament and possesses all the characteristics of good game bird. The head is long with single comb. The colour of the adult bird is white with splashes of gold colour markings on the wings. The wattles and earlobes are red in colour.

5. Denki

It is a large sized bird found in Andhra Pradesh bordering Odisha. The bird is attractive in appearance due to red glossy and lustrous plumage. Cocks have shining bluish black feathers on wings, breast, tail and thighs. The neck is darker compared to the rest of the body. Wattle is absent. Comb is red, pea type and compressed. The average weight of male is 3.12 kg and female is 2.22 kg. The birds start laying at 6-8 months with annual egg production of 25 – 35 numbers and average egg weight of 46.16 g. The Denki is basically used as a fighter bird.

6. Daothaigir

This breed (Fig.2) is found in Kokrajhar, Chirang, Udalguri and Baksa districts of Assam, reared particularly in Bodo tribe dominated areas. The males are mostly yellowish brown/ red in colour whereas; the females are barred with black and white stripes. Comb is red, single, erect and large in size. The average weight of cock is 1.79 kg and hen is 1.63 kg. The birds lay 60 – 70 numbers of eggs annually with average egg weight of 44.42 g.

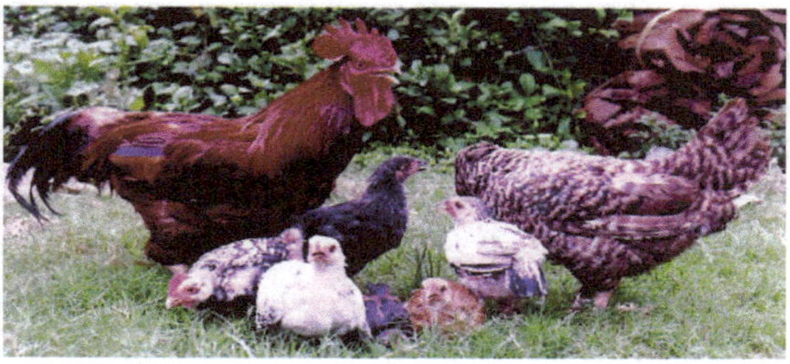

Fig. 2: Daothaigir breed

7. Dumasil

It is a dual purpose bird mostly found in Odisha. Birds are active, alert and fairly large, about 80 cm in length and 70 cm in height. Black and brown varieties are found mostly. The plumage colour of entire body including wings is black with a greenish sheen in black variety. The plumage colour is uniformly lustrous dark brown from head to tail in brown variety. Pea comb is common. Wattles are red in colour, moderately sized in males. The standard weight for cock is 3 - 3.6 kg and hen is 2 - 2.5 kg. The females attain sexual maturity at 6 months with average annual egg production varies from 100 - 150 numbers. Shell colour is light to medium brown. The hens are less broody compared to other indigenous domestic chickens.

8. Ghagus

The breed is reared mostly by the nomads of Karnataka and Andhra Pradesh. The plumage colour is mainly brown, followed by black. The colour pattern is usually patchy in males and spotted in females. Shining bluish black feathers are found on the breast, tail and thighs of cocks. The neck is covered with golden feathers. Wattle is absent. Comb is red and pea or single type. The bird attains age at sexual maturity at 5–7 months with annual egg production of 45 - 60 numbers. The body weight of cock is 2.16 kg and hen is 1.43 kg. The birds are maintained largely for eggs and/or game purposes.

9. Gujuri

It is a dual purpose bird, active and alert with a well-proportioned body found in Odisha. Plumage colour varies from dark brown to maroon, throughout the body. Buttercup comb is very common which is big in size and well developed in both sexes. Standard weight for male is 2.5 kg and for female is 1.5 kg. Their age at sexual maturity is 6 months with annual egg production 80 - 100 numbers. The shell colour is light to medium brown. They are also known locally as Thusuri, Kadamkhadia, Khairi, Kalua and Bansabania. Males are good fighters and hence used for cock fighting.

10. Harringhata Black

These are a small bodied-black bird with typical features of a layer, reared throughout West Bengal and are jet black in colour with red comb and wattles; while the shanks are white in colour. The average weight of cock is 1.5 kg and hen is 1.2 kg. The annual egg production is 130 numbers. The breed is very alert, highly mobile, and capable of escaping predator attack while scavenging. The breed's strong broodiness and mothering ability is used by farmers to hatch and brood eggs of other fowls including ducks. The breed is resistant to common diseases.

11. Kadaknath

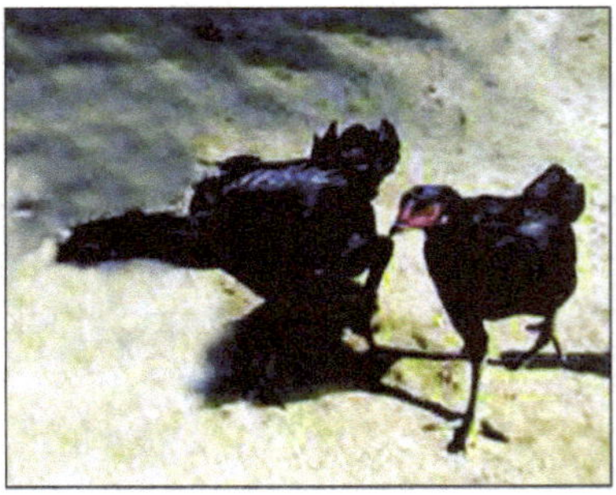

Fig. 3: Kadaknath

The breed (Fig.3) is mostly found in western Madhya Pradesh and adjoining districts of Rajasthan and Gujarat. The original name of the breed is Kalamasi, meaning a fowl with black flesh. The meat even though not very appealing to the eye but is very tasty. Adult plumage varies from silver and gold-spangled to bluish-black without any spangling. The skin, beak, shanks, toes and soles of feet are slate like in colour. Most of the internal organs of this breed show intense black colouration, which is also found in trachea, thoracic and abdominal air-sacs, gonads and at the base of the heart and mesentery. The blood is darker than normal. The black pigment is the result of melanin deposition. Average adult body weight of cock is 1.5 kg and hen is 1.0 kg. The annual egg production is 80 numbers with average egg weight of 46.8 g. The eggs are light brown in colour. Kadaknath chicken is said to contain many kinds of amino acids, hence a powerful source of protein and vitamins.

12. Kalahandi

It is a dual purpose bird, small to medium in size with proportioned body found in Odisha. Based on plumage colour three different varieties are seen such as Brown or Khairi, Black or Kabri and Barred or Chitri. Single comb with five serrations is very common. Wattles are fairly large and well-rounded and red in colour. The standard weight of cock is 2 - 3 kg and hen is 1.3 - 1.7 kg. The bird attains sexual maturity at 5 - 6 months and lays 100 - 150 white shelled eggs, annually.

13. Kalasthi

It is a meat type bird found in Andhra Pradesh. The common plumage colour is bluish black but brown birds are also noticed. The colour pattern is generally patchy in males and spotted in females. Cocks possess shining golden feathers on the neck and wings. Legs are proportionately longer. Wattle is absent. Comb is red, pea type and compressed. Adult body weight of cock is 2.48 kg and hen is 1.85 kg. Average age at first egg is 6 - 8 months. The annual egg production ranges from 30 - 40 numbers with average egg weight of 42.91 g.

14. Kashmir Faverolla

It is an indigenous chicken of Kashmir thrives at an altitude of 1,500 - 2,000 meters above mean sea level. They are small sized birds with small single comb and wattle. Feathered comb is the peculiarity of this breed. Average adult weight of cock is 1.72 kg and hen is 1.25 kg. This breed is most suitable for cold climate and mountainous terrains.

15. Miri

This bird is an inhabitant of Sibsagar, Dhemaji and Lakhimpur districts of Assam mostly reared by the Miri (*Mising*) tribes. Majority of the birds have white plumage followed by brown and black, however, some mixed coloured

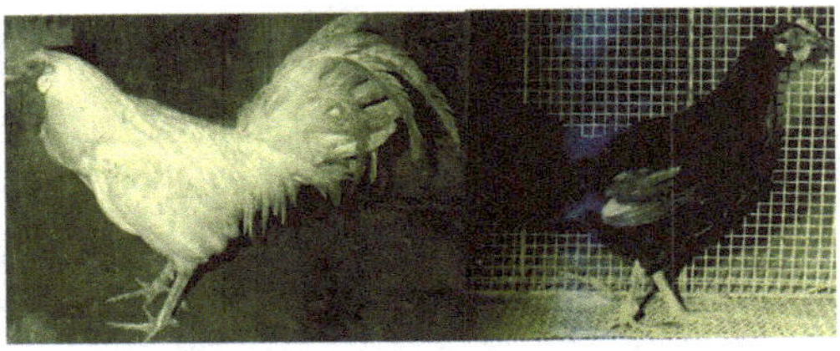
Fig. 4: Miri male and female

birds are also available. The shanks are white or yellow in colour, earlobes are mostly red. The birds have single comb with brown eyes. The standard body weight of cock ranges from 1.2 - 1.3 kg and of hen 0.9 - 1.0 kg. The ASM is 168 days, annual egg production is 60 - 70 numbers per bird with egg weight of 29-42 g.

16. Nicobari

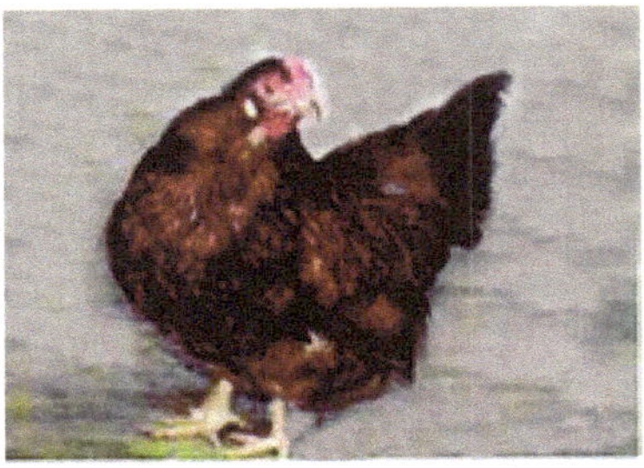
Fig. 5: Nicobari

This bird (Fig.5) is native to the Nicobar Islands and is locally known as "tekniet hyum", means short legged chicken. There are 3 strains: Brown, Black and White. It has a comparatively a smaller sized, short legged bird, somewhat round and compact body with a stout neck. Under free range systems, a hen can lay about 140 -150 eggs annually and attains sexual maturity in 177-200 days. The weight of female at maturity is 1024.7 g. The bird is well adapted to the tropical environment. It is the highest egg producer among all native breeds.

17. Punjab Brown

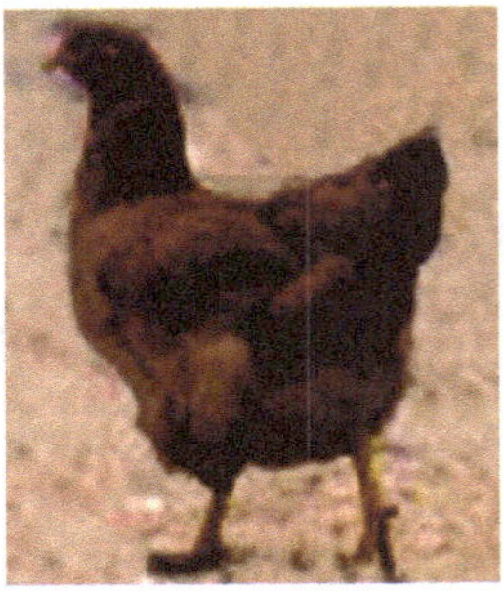
Fig. 6: Punjab Brown

This breed (Fig.6) is found in rural areas of Punjab and Haryana. It is a meat type bird having brown plumage with yellow beak and feet. Males in particular have black spots/stripes on their neck, wings and tail. The average weight varies from 3 - 4 kg in male and 2 - 2.5 kg in female. The age at sexual maturity is 5 - 6 months with annual egg production of 60 – 80 numbers. Egg shell colour is mostly light brown.

18. Phulbani

It is a dual purpose bird mostly found in certain districts of Odisha. Birds of both sexes are alert, active and vary from small to medium in size. Plumage colour is varied, predominant being black with various shades of brown and white. Based on comb type two varieties are recognized – rose comb and single comb. Combs are fairly large in males. Wattle is poorly developed. The standard weight for cock ranges from 1.2 - 1.5 kg and hen 1.0 - 1.2 kg. It reaches sexual maturity in 6-7 months with average annual egg production of 40 numbers. Egg shell colour is white. Females are broody, hence used for hatching and rearing of chicks.

19. Tellicherry

It is a small bird more or less round in shape found mainly in Kerala and Puducherry. Plumage color is black with a shining bluish tinge on hackle, back and tail feathers. Comb is red, single and large in size. They lay 60–80 numbers of tinted eggs annually with average weight of 40 g.

20. Vezaguda

The breed is widely distributed in tribal and rural areas of Odisha and adjoining areas of Andhra Pradesh. Adult cocks are fairly large with majestic gait and high stamina. Predominant plumage colours are black, brown and white. Comb, wattles, face and ear lobes are red in colour, head is light red and beak is yellow. Pea comb is common, fairly large in size and firmly set. The standard weight for cock is 2.5 - 3.5 kg and hen is 1.6 - 2.5 kg. The age at sexual maturity is 7 - 8 months with average annual egg production of 50 - 60 numbers. The shell colour is light brown. Males are mainly used for cock-fighting

Based on the feather pattern following indigenous varieties are available

1. Frizzle Fowl

This bird (Fig.7) is found in hot and humid coastal region and north eastern India. This dual purpose variety has varying plumage colour from red to black and white. The rachis of feather is curved due to presence of dominant frizzle gene (F) and thereby heat dissipation is increased. Single comb is predominant. The birds lay 70 - 80 brown eggs in a year having an average weight between 40 - 50 g. The age at sexual maturity is 25 - 28 weeks. Adult body weight in female varies from 1.25 - 1.40 kg while in male, from 2 - 2.5 kg. The birds are well adapted in tropical climate, especially for the arid zones.

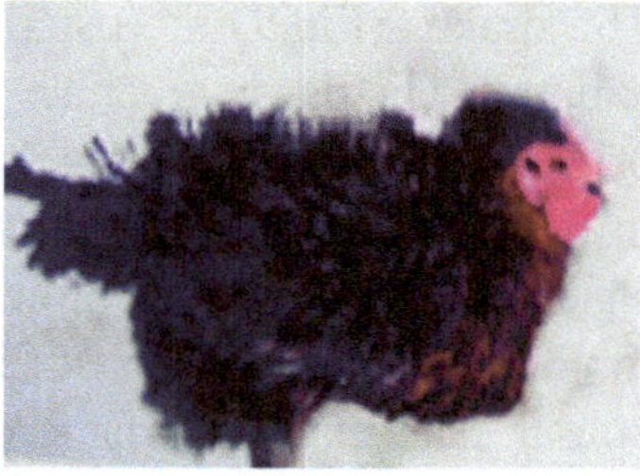

Fig. 7: Frizzle fowl

2. Naked Neck

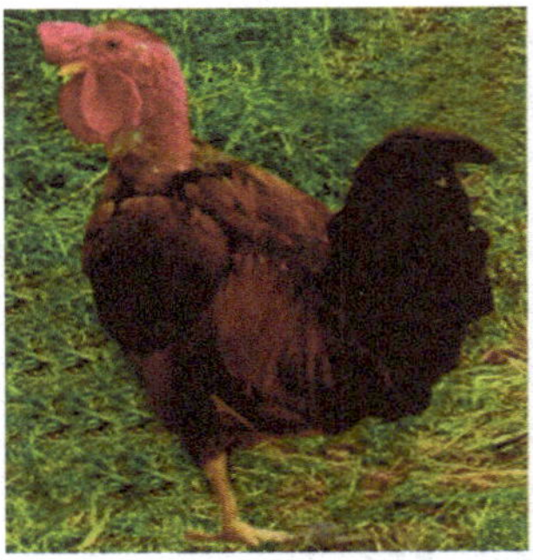

Fig. 8: Naked Neck

It is medium sized dual purpose bird (Fig.8) having rectangular shaped body with single or pea comb. Feather colour is variable with red and black tending to dominate. The birds are found in hot and humid coastal and northeastern regions of India. The neck of the bird is fully naked or only tufts of feathers are seen in front of the neck, above crop. The resulting bare skin become reddish, particularly in males as they approach sexual maturity. Hens lay 75 - 90 eggs in a year with average weight of 40 - 50 g. The age at sexual maturity is 6 - 6.5 months. The body weight of pullet varies from 1.4 - 1.6 kg whereas of cock, 2 - 3 kg at maturity. It lays the largest sized eggs among all the Indian native breeds of chicken.

Indigenous Duck Varieties of India

1. Nageswari

It is one of the important egg type native varieties of duck presently confined to a few pockets of Assam. Original homeland of this breed is Sylhet district of Assam (now in Bangladesh). It lays eggs with bluish tinge.

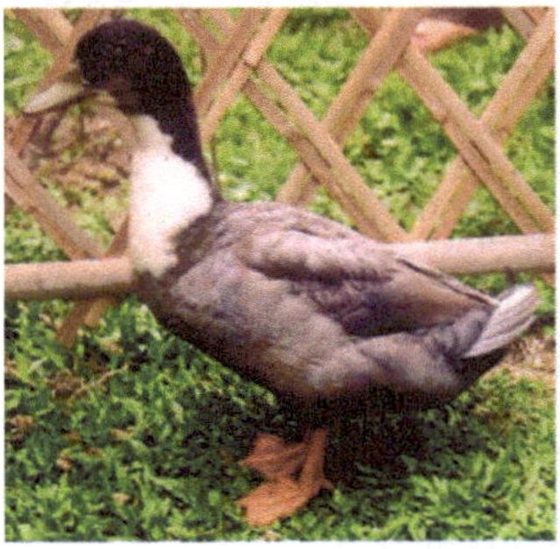

Fig. 9: Nageswari drake

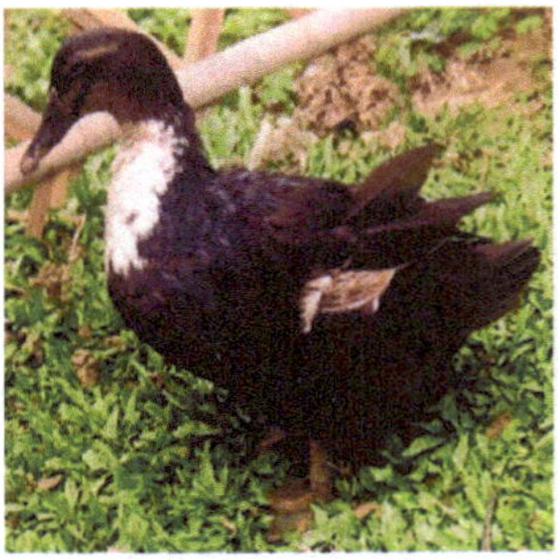

Fig. 10: Nageswari duck

The drakes (Fig.9) are usually erect in posture and gait. The bill is greenish yellow and feet are bright orange. The head is dull, brownish black in colour. The neck has white plumage with a shade of brownish black plumage tapering on the top of the neck. The breast feathers are white in colour. The major plumage colour of back and tail is grayish black. The ducks (Fig. 10) are normally squat in posture and gait. The general plumage colour of female is blackish brown in back, tail and wing, wherein blackish brown is predominant over brown and black. Adult body weight of drake is 1.42 kg and duck is 1.26 kg. The age at sexual maturity is 174-198 days. The annual egg production ranges from 100-120 numbers with average egg weight of 60g.

2. Chara

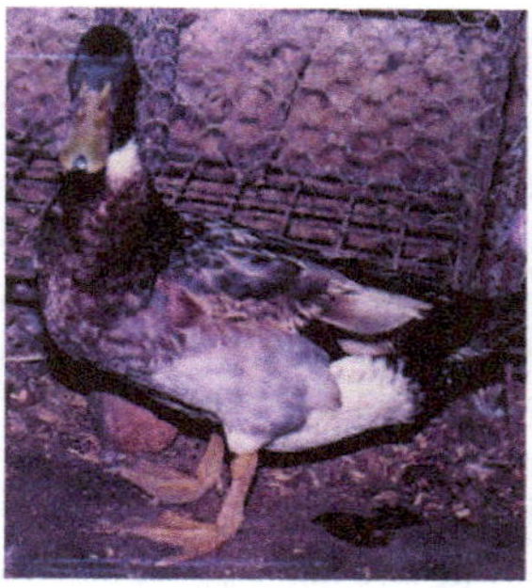

Fig. 11: Chara drake

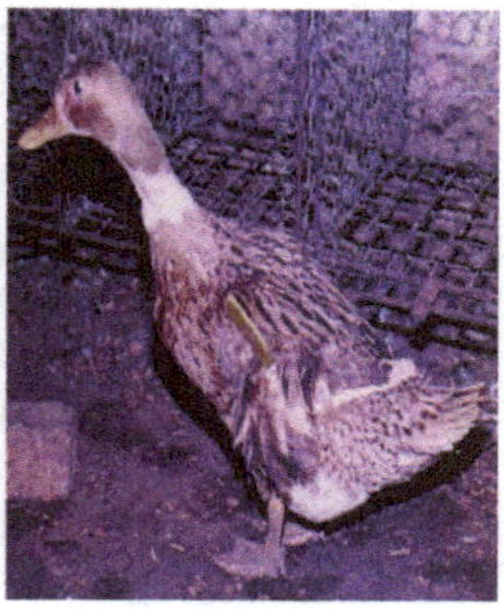

Fig. 12 : Chara duck

This variety of duck is indigenous to Kerala. This duck so named by the duck farmers based on their plumage colour. The drakes (Fig. 11) are usually squat in posture and gait. The head is lustrous greenish black in colour. The major plumage colour is brownish black. The females (Fig. 12) have an erect gait and squat in posture. The general plumage colour of female is blackish brown, wherein black was predominant over brown. Adult body weight of drake is 1.57 kg and duck is 1.49 kg. The age at sexual maturity is 147 days. The annual egg production is 150-180 numbers with average egg weight of 69 g.

3. Chemballi

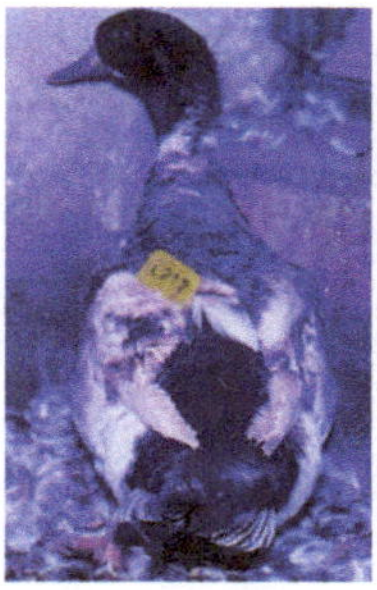

Fig. 13: Chemballi drake

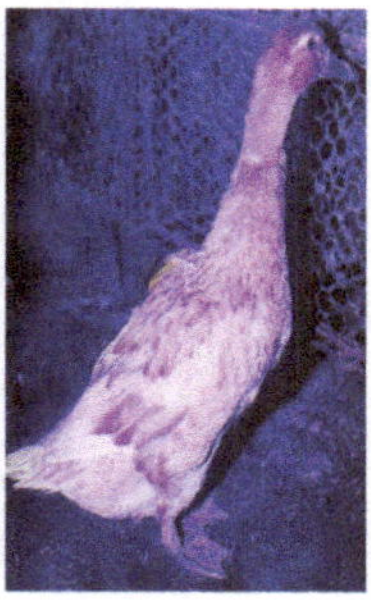

Fig. 14 : Chemballi duck

This variety of duck is indigenous to Kerala. The drakes (Fig. 13) are usually squat in posture and gait. The head is dull greenish in colour with brownish black plumage over the back region and sometimes light brown plumage is also observed. The females (Fig. 14) have erect gait and little squat in posture. The general plumage colour of female is brownish black and brownish grey in back, tail and wings, wherein brown is predominant over the black and grey. The adult body weight of drake is 1.56 kg and duck is 1.47 kg. The age at sexual maturity is 147 days. The duck lays 180-200 eggs annually with average egg weight of 68g.

Table 7: Indigenous chickens of India

Sl No.	Name of the breed	Native tract	State
1.	Ankleshwar	Bharuch and Narmada districts of Gujarat.	Gujarat
2.	Aseel	Most parts of Andhra Pradesh, especially the East Godavari, Visakhapatnam, Viziangaram districts and in the Dantewada district of and Chhattisgarh.	Andhra Pradesh Chhattisgarh.
3.	Busra	Nandurbar and Dhule districts of Maharashtra and Surat district of Gujarat.	Maharashtra and Gujarat.
4.	Chittagong (Malay)	North Eastern states of India bordering Bangladesh	North Eastern states.
5.	Denki	Vizianagram and Srikakulam districts of Andhra Pradesh and bordering Odisha	Andhra Pradesh and Odisha.
6.	Daothaigir	Kokrajhar, Chirang, Udalguri and Baksa districts in Assam.	Assam.
7.	Dumasil	Karaya and Jashipur blocks of Mayurbhanj district in Odisha.	Odisha
8.	Frizzle fowl	Hot and humid coastal region north eastern region of India.	Andaman and Nicobar Islands and North Eastern States
9.	Ghagus	Kolar district and adjoining locations of Karnataka and Andhra Pradesh.	Karnataka and Andhra Pradesh.
10.	Gujuri	Baripada and Khunta blocks of Mayurbhanj district in Odisha.	Odisha
11.	Haringhata Black	Reared throughout West Bengal	West Bengal
12.	Kadaknath	Jhabua and Dhar Districts of western Madhya Pradesh.	Madhya Pradesh.
13.	Kalahandi	Bhawanipatna, Khariar and Nawapara subdivisions of Kalahandi district of Odisha.	Odisha.
14.	Kalasthi	Chittoor district and adjoining regions of Nellore district in Andhra Pradesh.	Andhra Pradesh.
15.	Kashmir Faverolla	Kashmir.	Jammu and Kashmir
16.	Miri	Dhemaji, Lakhimpur and upper Assam regions.	Assam
17.	Naked Neck	Hot and humid coastal and northeastern region of India.	Andaman and Nicobar Islands and North Eastern states
18.	Nicobari	Nicobar Islands.	Nicobar Islands.
19.	Phulbani	Districts of Phulbani and Boudh in Odisha.	Odisha

(Contd.)

Sl No.	Name of the breed	Native tract	State
20.	Punjab Brown	Gurdaspur in Punjab and in Ambala and Yamunanagar in Haryana.	Punjab and Haryana
21.	Tellicherry	Calicut (primarily), Kannur and Malappuram districts of Kerala and adjoining Mahe region of Puducherry.	Kerala and Puducherry.
22.	Vezaguda	Malkangiri district and Jeypore subdivision of Koraput district of Odisha and adjoining areas of Andhra Pradesh.	Odisha and Andhra Pradesh.

Courtesy: http://sapplpp.org/indigenous-poultry-breeds-of-india

Table 8: Indigenous ducks of India

Sl No.	Name of the breed	Native tract	State
1	Nageswari	Barak valley of Assam bordering Meghalaya, Tripura, Mizoram and neighbouring country Bangladesh.	Assam
2	Chara	Distributed throughout the state of Kerala.	Kerala
3	Chemballi	Distributed throughout the state of Kerala.	Kerala
4	Pati	Distributed throughout the state of Assam.	Assam
5	Sanyasi	Distributed sporadically throughout the state of Tamil Nadu.	Tamil Nadu
6	Keeri	Distributed sporadically throughout the state of Tamil Nadu.	Tamil Nadu
7	Arani	Distributed throughout the state of Tamil Nadu.	Tamil Nadu

Question Bank

Q. 1. Fill in the blanks with suitable words.

i) The Aseel is famous for its ....nature.

ii) Wattle is absent in .... and .... breeds.

iii) The Chara duck is a native of the state............

iv) Butter cup comb is seen in .... breed.

v) The colour pattern in Kalasthi is .... in males & ....in females.

vi) Feathered comb is the specialty of ....

vii) The intense black colouration of internal organs of Kadaknath is due to ....

viii) Strong broodiness and mothering ability is seen in ....

Q. 2. State True/False.

i) The native tract of Nageswari Duck is Assam.

ii) Chemballi ducks are reared by nomadic tribes of Odisha

iii) The annual egg production of Chara duck is 80-90 numbers per duck.

iv) Punjab Brown is a meat type bird having brown plumage.

v) Daothaigir bird is reared by Missing tribes of Assam.

Q. 3. Choose the correct answers

i) Which of the following breed is found in Assam

a) Ankleswar c) Daothigir

b) Aseel d) Ghagus

ii) Hens of the following which breeds are less broody

a) Freezle fowl c) Dumasil

b) Chittagong d) Naked neck

iii) Golden feather on the neck is found in

a) Haringhata c) Miri

b) Ghagus d) Kadaknath

iv) The bird most suitable for cold climates and mountainous terrains is

a) Kashmir faverolla c) Kalahandi

b) Tellicherry d) Nicobari

v) The native tract of Miri bird is

a) Maharastra c) Assam

b) Gujarat d) Orissa

vi) The annual egg production of Nicobari hen is

a) 140-150 c) 90-100

b) 130-140 d) 120-130

Q.4 Write down the distinguishing features of the following

i) Aseel

ii) Nicobari

ii) Kadaknath

iv) Frizzle fowl

v) Nageswari duck

Answers

Q.No.1.

(i) fighting (ii) Ghagus & Kalasthi (iii) Kerala (iv) Gujuri (v) Patchy & Spotted (vi) Kashmir Faverolla (vii) Melanin (viii) Harringhata

Q. No.2.

i) True

ii) False

iii) False

iv) True

v) False

Q. No.3.

i) c

ii) c

iii) b

iv) a

v) c

vi) a

4

Reproduction in Fowl

S. George Paradis

Male Reproductive System

Male reproductive system (Fig. 15) consists of testes, epididymis, vas deferens and papillae.

Cocks have two ovoid creamy white testes, of which the left one is slightly larger than the right. Testes are located in the fore end of the kidneys in the abdominal cavity. Closely attached to the testes is short epididymis that continues as vas deferens which ends in the cloaca. The copulatory apparatus consists of two papillae and a rudimentary copulatory organ, the phallus which is located on the median ventral portion of one of the transverse folds of cloaca. Accessory reproductive organs like seminal vesicles, prostrate and Cowper's glands are absent in the cocks. The phallus is small and has associated lymph glands that produce a fluid which is added to the semen.

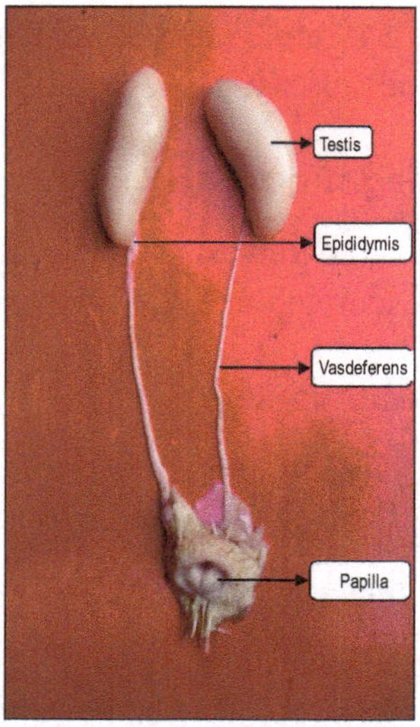

Fig 15: Male Reproductive System

The spermatozoa pass through the epididymis and are stored in the distal end of the vas deferens. The sperm after mating is stored in the folds in the oviduct of the hen to effect fertility up to six days. The spermatozoa of the cock have a long cylindrical head with a pointed acrosome, a short mid-piece and a long tail. Cocks produce about 0.5 -1 ml of whitish semen per ejaculate with a sperm concentration of 2- 4 billion.

Female Reproductive System

The female reproductive system (Fig. 16) consists of the ovary and oviduct. Only the left ovary and oviduct develop structurally and functionally in the fowl.

Ovary

The ovarian tissue appears as a cluster of ova or yolks at various stages of development. The ovum is enclosed in the vitelline membrane which is surrounded by a highly vascular coat of connective tissue called the follicle. The larger follicles are spherical, yellow coloured and loosely connected to the ovary by peritoneum. When the yolk matures, the follicle ruptures along stigma, the line that lacks blood vessels. Ovulation occurs but no corpus luteum is formed.

Oviduct

Oviduct is a long convoluted tubular structure between ovary and the cloaca. It is 65-80 cm long in the laying hen. It consists of five distinct portions viz., infundibulum, magnum, isthmus, uterus and the vagina that opens into the cloaca.

Infundibulum

It is a funnel shaped structure of 7 cm length that picks up the ovum from the body cavity. The egg stays here for 15 minutes and it is the site of fertilization.

Magnum

It is the longest (40 cm) portion of the oviduct, where the egg-white (albumen) is secreted and the egg stays here for 2-3 hours.

Isthmus

It is 9 cm long. It is the region of inner and outer shell membrane formation and the shape of the egg is determined here. The egg stays here for an hour.

Uterus: (Shell gland):

It is 8 cm long. Here water along with minerals is added to the albumen for plumping followed by calcareous shell formation and shell pigments addition. Egg stays here for about 20 hours.

Vagina

This is a muscular region of 7 cm length where the outer sealing protective layer called the cuticle is added to the egg. The egg is held here until it is laid.

Utero-vaginal Junction

This is a narrow portion between the uterus and the vagina with special tubular glands (sperm host glands) which are capable of storing and preserving the spermatozoa up to 3 weeks after mating.

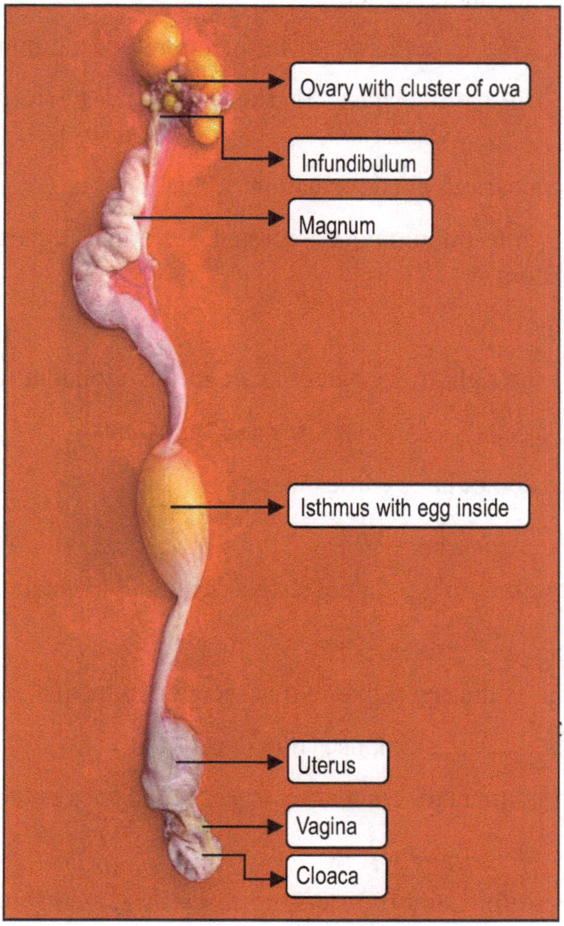

Fig 16: Female Reproductive System

Question Bank

Q.1. Fill in the blanks

i) Yolk is enclosed in a delicate sac called ....which maintains its spherical shape. (vitelline membrane)

ii) When the yolk matures the follicle ruptures along————the line that lacks blood vessel. (stigma)

iii) ....is the longest portion of the oviduct (Magnum)

iv) Uterus of the oviduct is otherwise called as .... (Shell gland.)

v) The sperm-host glands are present in the..................... (utero-vaginal junction)

vi) .... is the site of fertilization (infundibulum)

vii) The outermost part of the egg, the cuticle is produced in............(vagina)

viii) The calcarious shell formation occurs in ....(Uterus)

ix) Egg white (albumen) is secreted in .... part of the oviduct (magnum).

Q.2. True or false

i) Only the right ovary and oviduct are functional in fowl.

.... False (It is the left ovary).

ii) Birds do not have corpus luteum.

.... True.

iii) Infundibulum is a funnel shaped structure to catch the yolk.

.... True.

iv) White of the egg (albumen) is secreted in the uterus.

.... False (It is in magnum)

v) The rudimentary copulatory organ of the cock is the phallus.

.... True.

vi) Developing embryo gets its nourishment through the latebral apparatus of the yolk.

.... True.

vii) The sperm after mating is stored in folds of oviduct to effect fertility up to 6 days.

.... True.

viii) Sperm host glands are capable of preserving semen up to 3 weeks after mating.

.... True.

Q. 3. Draw a neat diagram of the female reproductive system of fowl and label its parts.

5

Formation and Structure of Egg

S.C. Edwin

A hen can produce eggs without mating by a cock. Such an egg is edible but infertile and will not hatch. If the hen is naturally or artificially inseminated with poultry semen, the spermatozoon unites with the ovum to form a fertile egg that will hatch after incubation. Unlike mammals, the embryo of birds grows independently within an enclosed hard structure called shell and thus, all nutrients required for embryonic development are contained in the egg. The yolk, albumen, shell membrane and shell protect the developing embryo apart from providing well balanced nutrients.

When viewing the internal structures of laying hen (Fig. 17), one can appreciate a cluster of developing yolks (ova) and a tubular structure called oviduct. The ovary of a laying hen contains a hierarchy of follicles in four categories viz. small white follicles, large white follicles, small yellow follicles and large yellow follicles.

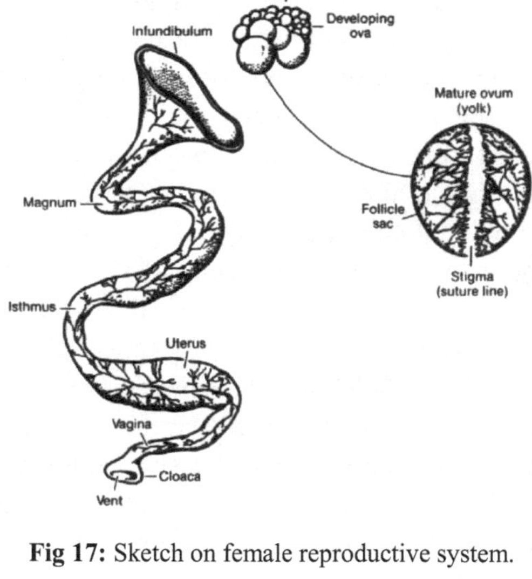

Fig 17: Sketch on female reproductive system.

The albumen, shell membrane and shell are assembled over yolk when it traverses through oviduct. It requires the coordinated functions of hypothalamus, pituitary gland, ovary, liver, bone and oviduct.

1) Formation of Yolk

The ovary and oviduct are small and underdeveloped in the immature chicken. The development of the ovarian follicles is stimulated by *follicle-stimulating hormone* (FSH) produced by the anterior pituitary gland. The ovarian sensitivity for FSH increases when chicken attains about 12 weeks of age that facilitates the deposition of yolk material in the ovarian follicles. Photostimulation also increases the concentration of FSH and thus birds subjected to photostimulation during growing period attain early sexual maturity. About 11 days before laying first egg, the FSH causes the ovarian follicles to increase in size. In turn, the active ovary begins to generate gonadal hormones, viz. estrogen, progesterone, and androgen (testosterone). Estrogen causes the oviduct to develop and increase the blood calcium, proteins, fats, vitamins and other substances necessary for egg formation. Estrogen also initiates the development of medullary bone, and also stimulates yolk protein and lipid formation by the liver. The yolk material is laid down to the germinal disc for about 10 days and the germinal disc continues to remain on the surface of the globular yolk mass. Deposits of yolk material increases as the ovulation time comes nearer. The yolk materials are utilized to sustain the life of the developing embryo from the germinal disc called *blastoderm.*

The characteristic yellow colour of the egg yolk is due to carotenoid pigments. It includes cryptoxanthin, alcohol soluble xanthophylls, vitamin A and carotenes. The pigment is transferred first to the bloodstream, then quickly to the yolk. More carotenoids are deposited when the hen is eating than during rest period (at night). This gives rise to deposits of dark and light layers of yolk material, depending on the dietary pigment available. Seven to eleven concentric rings are found in each yolk. Progesterone acts on the hormone-releasing factors in the hypothalamus to cause the release of *luteinizing hormone* (LH) from the anterior pituitary. The yolk is enclosed in the follicular membrane, which is attached to the ovary. This membrane is well supplied with blood vessels. The components of the yolk must be transferred from the blood across this membrane into the yolk itself. During ovulation, the mature ovum (yolk) ruptures through a visible streak, lacking blood vessels, called the stigma. If any blood vessel cross the stigma, a small drop of blood may be deposited, called *blood spot*. Any tissue sloughed from the follicular sac or the oviduct can be included in the developing egg as it passes through the oviduct. These bits of tissue darken with age and are known as *meat spots*. Many blood spots darken too, and are often incorrectly classified as meat spots.

The yolk is surrounded by the vitelline membrane. The next ovulation is regulated by *oviposition* (laying) of the first egg and occurs about 15 to 40 minutes after the first egg passes through the vent. The time necessary for an egg to traverse the oviduct varies with individuals. Most hens lay successive eggs with time intervals of 23 to 26 hours. If the time is greater than 24 hours, each successive egg will be laid later in the day, and the ovulation of the yolk for the next egg will also occur later in the day. Eggs laid in the afternoon have spent several more hours in the oviduct than those laid in the morning. Eventually eggs are laid so late that the rhythm is broken and an ovulation is skipped.

Normally, only one yolk is ovulated per day, but occasionally two may be released which is called as *double ovulation*. If the oviduct picks up both the yolks simultaneously, a *double yolk egg* will result. The *androgen* (testosterone) is responsible for the red waxy comb and wattles of the normal laying chicken and controls the secretion of albumen by the oviduct. This is the reason for the presence of red waxy comb in high egg laying hens. The ovulated egg yolk is engulfed by the infundibulum of the oviduct. About 15 minutes required to complete this process. Sometimes, the infundibulum does not pick up the yolk released from the ovary and thus the yolk is lost in the abdominal cavity and is eventually reabsorbed. Hens that do this routinely are called "*internal layers*" and appear to be in laying condition, although they never lay a completed egg. Occasionally, normal layers even fail to 'catch' an ovulated egg in the infundibulum.

2) Formation of Albumen

After the yolk is engulfed by the infundibulum, *fertilization* occurs. The continuous fertilized egg production for certain period in a hen after single insemination can be achieved by the presence of spermatozoa stored in *sperm storage tubules* located at *the junction of the uterus (shell gland) and the vagina* and in the *infundibulum*. Albumen (egg white) is formed around the yolk when the egg stays in the *magnum* portion of the oviduct for a period of *3 hours*. Magnum is the longest portion of the oviduct, about *33 cm* in length.

The albumen in an egg is composed of four layers. They are:

1. The chalazae and chalaziferous layer (inner thick albumen)
2. Inner thin albumen
3. Outer dense or thick albumen
4. Outer thin albumen

While all four are produced in the magnum, the outer thin white is not completed until water is added in the uterus. The albumen secreted in the magnum appears to be homogeneous, but the addition of water and turning and twisting of the egg later during egg formation seem to be responsible for the separation of the albumen into these four layers. The chalazae, the twisted cordlike structures extending out from the yolk, are formed as the egg is rotated in the lower portions of the oviduct. Twisted in opposite directions, the chalazae tends to keep the yolk centered in the egg after it is laid.

The dense nature of thick albumen is due to presence of more quantity of *mucin fibres*. The amount of thick albumen secreted in the magnum is large but the breakdown of mucin fibres and addition of water when the egg moves through the oviduct tend to reduce the amount of thick albumen later. Even after laying, there is a constant change in the internal contents of the egg. The thick albumen gradually loses its viscous composition and decreases its volume, while the thin albumen becomes watery and increases in quantity. The decrease in the amount of thick albumen is one of the best indicators of ageing (freshness) of the egg.

3) Formation of Shell Membranes

After leaving the magnum, the egg spends about 1.5 hours in the isthmus where the shell membranes are added. These membranes are made up of intermeshed protein fibrils coated with a glycoprotein matrix and are somewhat permeable to both water and air. Two membranes are formed, inner and outer shell membranes. These are rather loose-fitting membranes when first formed. Water and salts are added to the egg in the uterus to '*pump out*' the egg into its final shape. The membranes normally adhere to each other except at the large end of the egg, where they are separated to form the *air cell*. When the egg is laid, normally it has no air cell. Immediately after oviposition, the air cell is formed as a smaller one but progressively increases in size as the egg cools and as water later escapes from the contents by evaporation through the membranes and the shell.

4) Egg Shell Formation

The final stage is the formation of eggshell. Eggshell is formed in the uterus or shell gland for a period of 19 to 20 hours. 94% of the eggshell is made up of calcium carbonate ($CaCO_3$), which is deposited on an organic matrix consisting of protein and mucopolysaccharide. Eggshell calcification begins just before the egg enters the uterus from isthmus as small clusters of calcium appear on the outer shell membrane. Initially, shell is deposited over these sites to form the inner shell layer. Then hard chalky layer is added, which is composed of calcite crystals. Shell protects the embryo from mechanical damage and regulates gas exchange between the developing embryo and the external environment, especially prevents contamination by bacteria and other pathogens. It also provides calcium to the developing embryo. Chicken egg contains about 2 g of calcium and 8000 pores. The final layer of the shell is known as the cuticle, an organic material covering the surface of the egg. The cuticle seals the pores and is useful in reducing moisture losses and in preventing bacterial penetration through the eggshell.

Pigmentation of shells is the consequence of the deposition of pigments that are derived from the metabolism of haemoglobin. The capacity to produce and deposit the pigments is genetically controlled. The brown colouration of the eggshell is due to the deposition of porphyrin. The green or blue shell colour of Araucana breed of chicken is due to the production of biliverdin. The pigments are deposited during the later half of shell formation and at an increasing rate as oviposition (the act of laying egg) approaches. The fully formed egg is normally held in vagina for few minutes. Vagina has no role in egg formation and only serves to expel the egg once it leaves the uterus.

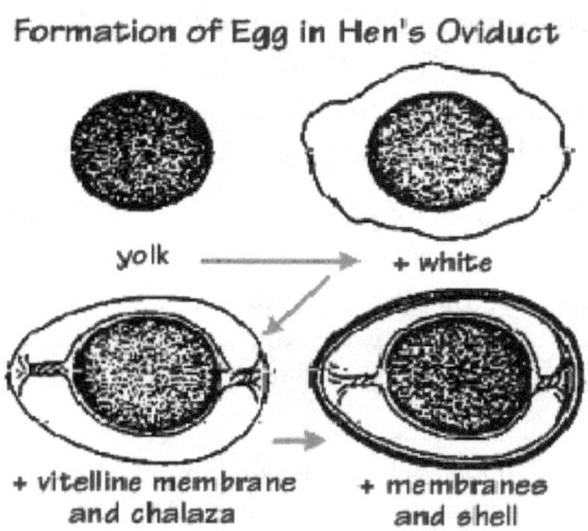

Shell Formation During Summer

The presence of adequate quantity of calcium ions (Ca^{2+}) and carbonate ions (CO_3^{2-}) in the shell gland fluid is required for shell formation. The major source of carbonate ions for shell formation is CO_2 from the blood. The enzyme, carbonic anhydrase is responsible for the formation of bicarbonate ions ($HCO3^-$) from CO_2 and H_2O in the shell gland mucosal cells. Any factor that affects acid-base balance of the blood may influence the process of shell formation.

During hot summer, the hen pants to dissipate body heat by way of water evaporation from the respiratory tract. Along with water evaporation, excessive quantity of CO_2 also exhaled and causes a reduction in CO_2 and HCO_3^- ions in the blood. The low HCO_3^- ions in the blood lowers its buffering capacity and may result in poor buffering of the H^+ ions produced during shell formation.

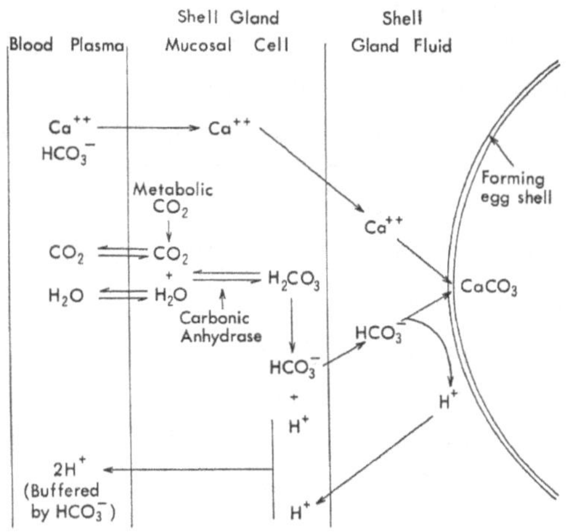

This may again interfere with CO_3^{2+} production and leads to less $CaCO_3$ deposition. This is the reason why hens lay eggs with thin shells in hot weather.

Laying of the Egg

Eggs are normally formed with small end first as they move down the oviduct. If the hen is not frightened, the egg will rotate horizontally just prior to *oviposition* and will be expelled large end first. However, if something disturbs the bird prior to rotation, the egg will be laid quickly and forced through the vent small end first.

The time of oviposition varies greatly among domestic fowl. Chickens lay most of the eggs in the morning; turkeys in the afternoon; ducks early in the morning and Japanese quail in the evening (4.00 to 7.00 p.m.).

S.No.	Part of the oviduct	Functions	Duration of developing egg stays	Length (cm)
1	Infundibulum	Picking and engulfing the yolk	15 minutes	9
2	Magnum	Secretion of thin and thick albumen	3 hours	33
3	Isthmus	Formation of shell membranes	1 hour & 15 minutes	10
4	Uterus	Formation of shell	18 to 21 hours (Average 20 hours)	10
5	Vagina	Oviposition	2 to 5 minutes	6
	Total	24 hours & 35 minutes		68

The egg has four main parts namely (1) Yolk, (2) Albumen, (3) Shell mem-branes and (4) Shell (Fig. 18).

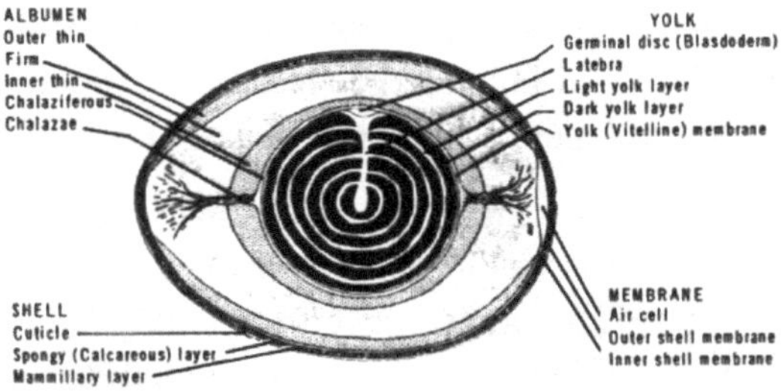

Fig. 18: Sketch on structure of an egg.

1) Yolk

The yolk is normally held centrally by the chalazae. The two chalazae are attached to the chalaziferous layer of albumen around the yolk and one to each pole of the egg and anchored in the outer thick albumen. The yolk is enclosed in a colourless membrane called *yolk membrane or vitalline membrane.* In the centre of the yolk, a small and nearly circular score of light coloured fluid, which does not completely harden on boiling is called *Latebra.* The yolk is about 31% of the total weight of an egg. Germinal disc is the reproductive cell present on the surface of the yolk. If fertilized the germ cell is then called as *blastoderm* and if not it is called as blastodisc.

2) Albumen

The lysozyme, present in the egg albumen can kill certain bacteria which invade it, thus helps to extend the shelf-life of the egg. Albumen or white of the egg surrounds the yolk. The albumen protects the blastoderm. It keeps blastoderm from coming in contact with the shell and lessens the force of jarring. Another function of the albumen is to prevent the entrance of bacteria to the yolk or germ cell. There are four layers of albumen amounting to approximately 58% of the total volume of the egg. The inner layer immediately around the yolk and extending on both sides of the yolk are called *chalaziferous layer* and *chalaze*, respectively (inner thick albumen). The thin layer immediately around the chalaziferous layer is called *inner thin albumen.* The middle portion of the albumen is called *outer thick albumen*, which holds the inner contents (thin albumen, chalaziferous layer and yolk) like an envelope and hence, otherwise called as *albumenous sac.* This layer is normally used for assessing the albumen quality when grading eggs. The outer low viscosity layer fills up the remaining space and is called *outer thin albumen*, which lies in-between the outer thick albumen and the shell membranes. The physical composition of different layers of albumen is;

The lysozyme, present in the egg albumen can kill certain bacteria which invade it, thus helps to extend the shelf-life of the egg.

1.	The chalazae and chalaziferous layer (Inner thick albumen)	02.7%
2.	Inner thin albumen	16.8%
3.	Outer dense or thick albumen	55.5%
4.	Outer thin albumen	25.0%

3) Shell Membranes

The outer shell membrane is about 3 times thicker than the inner one (0.050 *vs.*0.015 mm). The thickness of outer membrane is about 0.050 mm thick, whereas, the inner is 0.015 mm. The shell membranes allow transmission of gases to and from the egg contents. The size of the air cell increases as the age of the egg increases. The air present in the air cell provides first breathe to the fully developed embryo during pipping (the act of breaking open the eggshell by the fully developed embryo to hatch out).

5) Shell

Shell consists of approximately 10 to 12% of the chicken egg's weight. The eggshell consists of the following:

1. Mammillary layer
2. Spongy or Pallisade layer
3. The cuticle or bloom
4. The pore system

The internal shell layer is the mammillary layer that consists of knobs of calcium which are perpendicular to the surface of the shell. It is a dense layer, approximately one-third of the total shell. The next layer is spongy or pallisade layer, approximately two-third of the total shell thickness. It consists of calcium crystals set at right angles to the surface of the shell. It looks spongy appearance after the shell protein is removed by acid soaking. The cuticle or bloom is the extreme outer coating of an eggshell, consisting of mucous coating deposited on the surface of the shell. Chicken egg contains as many as 8000 pores, which may vary greatly in number and size. Shell pores facilitate exchange of gases between internal egg contents and the outside environment.

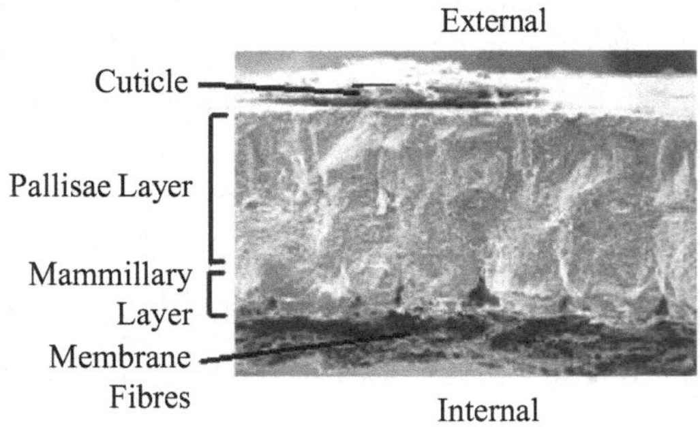

The shell colour is characteristic of breed that may be white, brown or green.

Brown colour is due to the presence of a pigment called *Oophorphyrin*.

Question Bank

1) Multiple choice questions – Choose the correct answer

i) Photostimulation during growing period leads to

a) Delays sexual maturity
b) Early sexual maturity
c) Abnormal egg production
d) Moulting

ii) The germinal disc in the fertile chicken egg lies

a) In the albumen
b) On the top of the yolk
c) On the bottom of the yolk
d) At the centre (middle) of the yolk

iii) The time taken for the formation of albumen (egg white) around the yolk in the oviduct is,

a) 1 hour
b) 2 hours
c) 3 hours
d) 4 hours

iv) Longest portion of chicken oviduct is

a) Infundibulum
b) Magnum
c) Uterus
d) Vagina

v) Major portion of eggshell is made up of,

a) CaOH
b) CaCl
c) $CaCO_3$
d) $CaHCO_3$

vi) The calcium content of average size chicken egg is,

a) 2.0 g
b) 4.0 g
c) 6.0 g
d) 8.0 g

vii) The green or blue shell colour of Araucana breed of chicken is due to the production of

a) Oocyan
b) Xanthin
c) Bilirubin
d) Biliverdin

viii) The enzyme responsible for eggshell formation is

a) Amylase
b) Carbonic anyhdrase

c) Lysozyme d) Cellulase

ix) Japanese quail lays most of the eggs during

a) 8.00 – 10.00 a.m. b) 12.00 – 2.00 p.m.

c) 4.00 – 7.00 p.m. d) 8.00 – 10.00 p.m.

x) Shell membrane is formed in

a) Infundibulum b) Isthmus

c) Magnum d) Vagina

Ans: i) b; ii) b; iii) c; iv) b; v) c; vi) a; vii) d; viii) b; ix) c; x) b

2) Fill in the blanks with suitable answer

i) The hormone responsible for the development of ovarian follicles in the growing birds is ....

ii) The characteristic yellow colour of the egg yolk is due to...........................

iii) .... is responsible for the red waxy comb and wattles of the normal laying chicken

iv) Albumen is secreted in the .... portion of the oviduct

v) The dense nature of thick albumen is due to presence of more quantity of .... fibres

vi) The brown colouration of the eggshell is due to the deposition of .... pigment

vii) The pigment, oophorphyrin is responsible for .... colour of the chicken egg.

Ans: i) Follicular stimulating hormone (FSH); ii) Carotenoid pigments; iii) Androgen (testosterone); iv) Magnum; v) Mucin; vi) Porphyrin vii) Shell.

3) Write "True" or "False" for the questions given below

i) A hen can produce eggs without mating by a cock ( )

ii) Gonadal hormones are FSH and LH ( )

iii) Estrogen stimulates yolk protein and lipid formation by the liver ( )

iv) The decrease in the amount of thick albumen is one of the best indicators of ageing (freshness) of the egg ( )

v) When the egg is laid, normally it has no air cell ( )

vi) Albumen provides calcium to the developing embryo ( )

Ans: i) True; ii) False; iii) True; iv) True; v) True; vi) False

4) Define or explain in a few lines

i) Stigma

ii) Blood spot

iii) Meat spot

iv) Oviposition

v) Double ovulation

vi) Chalazae

vii) Albumenous sac

viii) Pipping

5) Write short notes about "internal layers".

6) Why do hens lay eggs with thin shells during hot weather.

7) Mention the different portions of albumen in an egg.

8) Write about the physical composition of an eggshell.

9) Explain in details about the formation of a chicken egg.

10)Write in brief about the structure of chicken egg with a neat diagram.

6

Economic Traits in Poultry

A. Jalaluddin

In modern poultry farming, successful management relies on accurate and complete daily record keeping. Some of the traits may influence the profit of farm, thereby affecting the economics of the farm than the other traits, and hence they are called economic traits. Economic traits can be defined as those traits which are economically important and improvement in these traits would increase the profit of the farm. These traits are generally assumed to be controlled by the genes at larger number of loci. Some of the economic traits in egg and meat type chickens are as follows:

Egg Type Chicken

1. Egg Production

The egg production of a chicken is a result of many genes. With appropriate environmental conditions (nutrition, light, ambient temperature, water, free from diseases etc.), the many genes controlling all the processes associated with egg production can act to allow the chicken to fully express its genetic potential. Generally the egg production is considered as a composite trait largely influenced by five characteristics They are age at sexual maturity, intensity of production or rate of laying, broodiness, clutch size and pauses in laying and persistency of production. The egg production can be measured as follows:

a. Hen housed egg production per bird

$$= \frac{\text{Number of eggs laid}}{\text{Number of birds housed}}$$

b. Hen housed egg production per cent

$$\frac{\text{Number of eggs laid x 100}}{\text{Number of birds housed}}$$

c. Hen day egg production per cent

$$= \frac{\text{Number of eggs laid}}{\text{Number of hen days}} \text{ x 100}$$

d. Hen day egg production per bird

$$= \frac{\text{Number of eggs laid}}{\text{Average hen days}} \text{ x 100}$$

e. Average hen days

$$= \frac{\text{Total hen days}}{\text{Number of days}} \text{ x 100}$$

Egg production is a lowly heritable trait. To produce a hybrid cross having good egg number along with egg weight, one of the parent lines (usually female) is selected exclusively for egg number, while the other line is selected for both egg weight and egg production.

i) Age at Sexual Maturity (ASM)

This can be defined as the age in days when the bird laid its first egg and in chicken, the age at sexual maturity is around 150 days. Very early maturity is also not preferred as it results in the production of small sized eggs and a very late maturity is also not ideal either, as it ends up with less number of eggs. Early maturity increases the incidences like uterine prolapse and other complications. Sometimes the pullets are prevented by restricting light and feed to delay eggs at an early age so that production of small size eggs could be prevented. ASM is a moderately heritable trait ranging from 0.15 - 0.25.

ii) Intensity of laying (rate of lay)

This trait is an important contributing factor to the annual egg record. This is the ability of birds to lay at a high rate at any given point or a period of time. It has been found that hens at high intensity of lay, produce larger number of eggs per clutch and are usually better layers than birds which lay fewer eggs per clutch. The rate of laying is lowly heritable. The rate of laying can be measured in terms of hen-day and hen-housed egg production.

$$\text{Rate of lay (\%)} = \frac{\text{No. of eggs laid up to a that date or age}}{\text{No. of days that date}} \times 100$$

iii) Broodiness

When the birds are in brooding they are not laying. Hence, a minimum of broodiness is desired. The Mediterranean breeds like White Leghorn, Minorca, Ancona and a few others are on the whole non-broody, whereas the heavy breeds or Asiatic are very broody. English and American breeds derived from these contrasting groups are usually intermediate in broodiness. This trait is highly heritable and therefore can be eliminated by selection. Broodiness has high negative correlation with the egg production. Therefore, when a stock is selected for egg production, this character is eliminated from the flock. Modern commercial egg laying strains are devoid of this character However, broodiness and mothering ability are the two desirable characters in poultry for backyard rearing for self replication and survival

iv) Persistency

Persistency is a measure of the length of a laying year. The laying is ordinarily terminated at around 72 weeks of age and this is called laying cycle or biological cycle. After this the bird will enter into moulting, a physiological process by which the old feather are shed and renewed with new ones. During this process the bird will go out of production before entering into the next cycle of laying. In commercial layers, birds are culled after first biological cycle as they are uneconomical in the subsequent cycles. The good layer moults late and rapid, while the poor layer is early and a slow moulter. *Fecundity* is the another term, which may be defined as the number of eggs produced in an agreed period of time regardless of other characters such as egg size, hatchability etc. In practice, this period is considered as pullet year.

v) Clutch size and pause

The eggs are laid in a daily sequence and the number of eggs laid in a sequence without any break is called as *clutch size.* The bird will skip a day or two from production before entering in to the next clutch. In good producers, the clutch size is big with a short clutch interval. When this interval is considerably long, then, this is called as pause. Pause is not a desirable character in good layers. The bird may pause producing eggs in climatic extremities like winter and summer. Selection for high annual egg production ends up the elimination of this character from the population. The low producers and *desi* birds usually have frequent pauses, during which period they exhibit the maternal behaviour or broodiness.

2. Egg Size

This is measured in terms of egg weight. There appears to be a direct relationship between body size of birds and the size of the eggs laid. Eggs are smaller in the beginning of laying and there is gradual and steady increase in size for 6 to 7 months. Considerable variation in size of eggs has been observed between breeds, strains and lines. The egg weight varies from 40 to 60 grams and the heritability of the trait is approximately 50 per cent. Therefore genetic improvement for this trait can easily be brought in a population by individual selection. However, its strong negative correlation with egg number necessitates a careful approach in breeding programmes. In cross breeding programmes, the pressure for egg weight is usually given in the male line.

3. Egg Colour

The Mediterranean class of chicken lay white eggs and most of the other class of chicken lay brown eggs. The shell colour in Andalusian chicken is blue. The cross between chickens of brown and white eggs will produce tinted or light brown shell colour. To evolve a white egg layer, the common breed used is White Leghorn. Different elite strains of this breed can be crossed to produce a hybrid white egg layer. For brown eggs, breeds like RIR, Plymouth Rock and New Hampshire are used in different combinations.

4. Feed Efficiency

In commercial layers, the feed efficiency of per kilogram egg mass and of a dozen eggs is around 2.35 and 1.70 respectively. Measuring feed efficiency by recording individual feed intake is laborious and therefore selection for feed efficiency is also impractical. Both egg production and egg weight have a high positive correlation with feed efficiency; therefore, selection for these characters improves feed efficiency as a correlated response.

5. Body weight

The body weights at maturity (20 weeks) as well as of adult (40 weeks) are of significance in layer breeding. The optimum mature and adult body weights for medium egg type layer are 1.2 and 1.6 kg respectively. Selection for egg weight tends to increase the body weight as these traits are positively correlated. Restricted selection index can be used to check any untoward change in body weight.

6. Egg quality Traits

Egg quality characters like shell thickness, albumen index, Haugh unit and blood and meat spots are lowly heritable traits. Nevertheless they are not included in the selection programmes also. Shell thickness is the only quality trait which is having economic importance and this trait is negatively correlated with the size of the egg.

7. Viability

One of the most serious problems confronting in layer production is the mortality among laying pullets. Both genetic defects and infectious diseases are causes of death. Gross genetic defects are not a matter of concern as they are usually eliminated. However, efforts are required for breeding and selection of stains resistance to infectious diseases. Strains as well as crosses differ considerably in their susceptibility to different diseases. Mortality rates of 5 and 3 % are allowable at chick and grower stages. At layer stage mortality rate of one per cent per month is permissible. The mortality per cent can be measured as

$$\text{Mortality per cent} = \frac{\text{Number of chicks died}}{\text{Number of chicks hatched}} \times 100$$

8. Fertility and Hatchability

It is difficult to distinguish between low fertility and high incidence of embryonic death. Therefore, fertility and hatchability of fertile eggs are usually considered together as hatchability of eggs set. The heritability of fertility and hatchability is very low. The fertility and hatchability traits can be measured as given below:

a. $$\text{Fertility (\%)} = \frac{\text{Number of fertile eggs}}{\text{Number of eggs set}} \times 100$$

b. Hatchability per cent (TES) $= \dfrac{\text{Number of chicks hatched}}{\text{Number of eggs set}} \times 100$

c. Hatchability per cent (FES) $= \dfrac{\text{Number of chicks hatched}}{\text{Number of fertile eggs set}} \times 100$

9. Sex-linked dwarfism

Dwarfism, which causes an animal to be subnormal in size, is well known in chickens. Both egg producers and broiler producers are interested in sex-linked dwarfism. Hens that carry the sex-linked dwarf genes are about one third smaller than normal body size, but their egg size is about 8% smaller. The objectives in these 'mini' layers are to lower body maintenance requirements and thereby increase the efficiency of feed utilization.

Meat Type Chicken

In broilers, the trait of utmost importance is body weight at marketing age or juvenile body weight. The other traits of importance in selection programmes are body conformation and hatching egg production in the parent line. In broiler breeding, the female line should be one which produces high number of chicks. Therefore apart from juvenile body weight, the female parent line is also selected for hatching egg production. The other traits like colour of skin, plumage colour and rate of feathering in the hybrid can be decided by using appropriate breeds/ strains in the breeding programme. Compared to layer, broiler breeding is relatively easier because selection can be done as early as 6 weeks of age based on the body weight.

1. Body Weight

It is one of the most important characters of broiler production, and it is highly heritable at marketing age. Therefore, it is relatively easy to make progress genetically by individual selection. It is easy to measure and it is also known to be positively correlated with body conformation, feed efficiency and dressing loss. Hence if the growth rate is improved other carcass quality characters will also improve. However, it should be borne in mind that body weight is negatively correlated with egg production. Separate lines of males and females are developed with considerable high pressure of selection on body weight and egg production.

2. Feed Efficiency

In modern commercial broilers, a feed efficiency of 1.6-1.8 is achievable at sixth week of age. Measurement of feed efficiency on individual basis in breeding stock is very difficult and laborious therefore its inclusion in the selection programmes is also not possible. However, selection for growth rate automatically improves feed efficiency since both the traits are highly positively correlated.

$$\text{Feed efficiency} = \frac{\text{Amount of feed consumed in a period}}{\text{Total gain in body weight in the period}}$$

3. Meat Yield

Meat yield can be expressed as carcass yield or dressing percentage, yield of specific carcass parts and yield of specific tissues such as lean, fat, skin and bone. Meat quality can be assessed by several methods: by carcass conformation or grade, sensory evaluation or flavor, juiciness and tenderness of the cooked carcass or carcass part and by chemical composition of the carcass to determine the amounts or proportions of protein, fat, moisture and ash. Carcass yield or dressing percentage is expressed as weight of the carcass as a percentage of the weight of the live chicken.

$$\text{Dressing percentage} = \frac{\text{Dressed weight}}{\text{Pre-slaughter live weight}} \times 100$$

4. Viability

In commercial broilers under standard management, mortality rates of 3 and 2 per cent are allowable, respectively at starter and finisher stages. Mortality in broilers involves susceptibility to common diseases of early age like pullorum, coccidiosis and New Castle disease etc.

5. Body Conformation

The body conformation traits include breast angle, keel length, shank length, breast meat yield, abdominal fat percentage, overall appearance etc. Conformation traits improve when the stock is selected for body weight as both are positively correlated. The ideal meat bird is having plump body with, a long, broad and heavily fleshed breast. The back must be broad and heavily fleshed with minimum abdominal fat. Breast is low in fat therefore fetches high price than other retail cuts; therefore the parents are selected for higher percentage of breast muscle yield. Sib selection is followed for carcass traits because sacrifice and measurement of these characters is not possible in the selected birds.

6. Skin Colour

The skin colour is inherited by complete dominance where, white colour is dominant to yellow. The common breeds used in evolving commercial broilers such as Cornish, Plymouth Rock and New Hampshire are yellow skinned. Therefore developing a yellow skinned broiler is practically simple. For developing a white skinned broiler, Sussex, an English breed with white skin can be included in the breeding programme as a female line.

7. Plumage Colour

Although both melanins and carotenoid pigments contribute to the feather color of certain avian species, it is the melanins that determine the plumage color and patterns of the domestic fowl. Each plumage color and pattern is the result of a series of genetically determined events, and an awareness of these facilities understanding its inheritance. Coloured plumage has the disadvantage since the coloured pin feathers and filoplumes give unpleasing appearance to the dressed carcass. But the pin feathers of white plumage blend well with the skin colour of the carcass. Pin feathers are the feathers at their very early stage of growth which are still to erupt out of their follicles.

8. Rate of Feathering

Slow feathering birds have a large number of pin feathers. Early feathering is one of the desirable characteristics in broilers avoiding the problem of pin feathers at the time of processing. Rate of feathering is inherited by sex-linked dominance, in which, slow feathering is dominant to fast feathering. Making all the lines involved in crossing as homozygous recessive for rate of feathering (kk) can ensure this character in all the progenies.

9. Fertility and Hatchability

All the reproductive characters including fertility and hatchability are lowly heritable. The fertility and hatchability rates are very less in broilers compared to layers as these traits are negatively correlated with body size. English breed Cornish is the common male line in broiler breeding. Though this breed is good in conformation characters, the reproductive traits are at the lowest among the poultry breeds. Therefore special attention has to be given to improve the fertility in breeding programmes.

Question Bank

I. Choose the Correct Answer

1.Which of the following is measured taking into account the mortality of hens ?

a. Hen housed egg production
b. Hen day egg production
c. Part-term egg production
d. none of these

Ans (b)

2. Which among the following is a highly heritable trait ?

a. Egg number
b. Broodiness
c. ASM
d. Rate of lay

Ans (b)

3. The foundation breed in layer breeding is

a. RIR
b. Plymouth Rock
c. New Hampshire
d. White Leghorn

Ans (d)

4. The foundation breed in broiler breeding is

a. RIR
b. White Leghorn
c. White Cornish
d. Plymonth Rock

Ans (d)

5. Multicoloured plumage is preferred for

a. Commercial layers
b. Commercial broilers
c. Backyard poultry strains
d. None of these

Ans (c)

6. Fertility and hatchability are

a. Highly heritable
b. Moderately heritable
c. Lowly heritable
d. Not heritable

Ans (c)

7. Selection for egg mass improves

a. Egg number
b. Egg weight
c. Both of these
d. None of these

Ans (c)

II . Fill in the blanks

1. The primary selection criterion for a female parental line (dam line) in poultry breeding is .... (egg number)
2. Very early maturing birds lay .... sized eggs. (small)
3. The ideal full record egg production in layers is upto ....weeks of age. (72)
4. Selection for juvenile body weight in broilers is done at .... weeks of age. (6)
5. .... and .... are negatively correlated traits in layers.

   (egg number and egg weight)
6. The two most important economic traits in broiler breeding are

   ....and .... (juvenile body weight and feed efficiency)
7. Dressing % in broiler is ....% (70)
8 Restricted. ....is the method of selection employed for the simultaneous improvement of egg number and egg weight. (selection index)
9. ....rate of feathering is desirable in broilers. (high)

10. The economic trait most influenced by restriction in feed and light is ....(ASM)

11. Good layers exhibit .... moulting, and .... pause, but ....clutch size with a .... inter clutch interval and will be .... broody. (late and rapid moulting, no pause, big clutch size, short inter-clutch interval and less broody)

III . True / False

1. Age at sexual maturity in poultry is a sex linked trait - True
2. Rate of lay and egg numbers are inversely proportional - False
3. Broodiness in poultry is autosomal in origin - True
4. Broodiness is a desirable trait in backyard poultry production - True
5. Egg quality traits are highly heritable - False
6. Feed efficiency can be improved by selecting egg weight (or egg production) as a correlated response - True
7. Body weight and egg weight are positively correlated traits - True
8. Selection for body weight can improve egg weight - True

7

Backyard, Scavenging and Semi-intensive Systems of Management

A. Bhattacharyya

Importance of Backyard Poultry Farming in India

Commercial chicken production in India has undergone a remarkable change in the last three decades. While India is among the top five chicken producing and top seven duck producing countries in the world, the gap between the demand and production is still alarming. Average per capita availability of eggs in big cities is 170 while it stands at 9 eggs per annum in the rural areas. Though the commercial poultry sector has made a stupendous progress over the years, the conventional free and backyard poultry farming remain neglected. Backyard poultry farming contributes around 11% to the national production while in certain states like U.P. around 60% of the poultry population is indigenous fowls reared under backyard system. The backyard sector contributed to 23 per cent of the total egg production in 2005-06.

Commercial chicken production is capital intensive and is generally concentrated in and around urban areas. There is a wide disparity in consumption of the poultry products between urban and rural population. Around 75% of country's population living in the rural areas has limited access to the protein rich poultry products. Protein deficiency is quite common in the diets of rural people. Adoption of rural poultry farming may ameliorate the high incidence of protein hunger in growing children and pregnant women.

It has been seen that the commercial birds have poor immunity against common poultry diseases. As production is inversely proportional to the viability traits, the nutrients absorbed are mostly diverted for growth in commercial chicken. On the other hand, indigenous birds reared in rural areas are resistant to many diseases and pests. Unlike the local breeds maintained in villages, the commercial breeds require high level of input pertaining to feed and health care to maintain production and check mortality.

One of the major inputs required for commercial poultry is feed. On the other hand, the birds reared under backyard system requiring low input technology, can easily sustain on kitchen wastes, insects, worms, leaves etc. Further, commercial poultry production under intensive system of production causes environmental pollution and large scale intensification of poultry rearing is often debatable from the environment point of view. Thus, the concept of backyard poultry farming or Family Poultry Farming is gaining momentum in African, Asian and Latin American countries. Around 80% of the poultry production in Africa is based on low input scavenging or backyard system.

Rearing Units for Low Input Technology Poultry Farming

Generally, three types of rearing units are used for raising poultry under low input technology. The type of unit depends upon the availability of capital and space.

Free range or extensive system: It is the oldest method of raising poultry wherein birds are allowed to roam about during the daytime; whereas night shelter is given to protect from natural enemies. The birds scavange on fallen grains, insects, herbs etc. Space provided is generally 1 acre for 100 birds. A flock of 10-20 birds may be left scavenging around the house during day time. They may be given kitchen wastes, sorghum, maize bran etc as supplementary feed. Many a times, the birds may have to move long distances for feed and water. The birds are kept in small houses or shelters at night (Fig. 19).

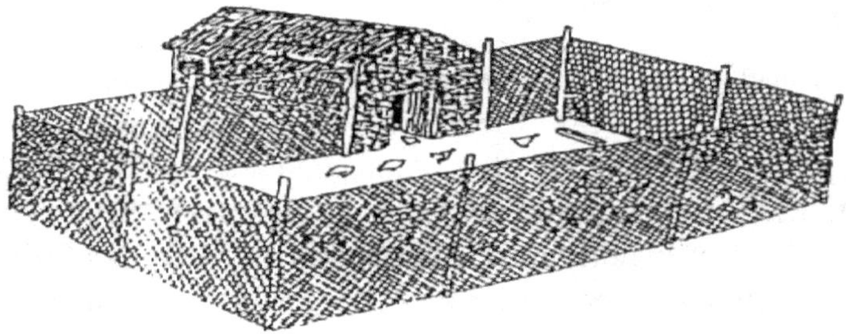

Fig 19 : An overnight shelter for chickens raised on free range

Semi intensive system: It is generally adopted where the availability of space is limited. This system was once popular for laying and breeding flocks on the assumption that it imparts physical stamina to the birds. Space provided up to 6 weeks of age is 0.09 m^2 per bird. In this system a bird is generally provided with 20-30 square yards for outside run. Sometimes, this run may be divided to provide 10-15 square yards per bird on either side of the house. Further, the size of semi intensive unit depends upon the number of birds, availability of space and capital. However, in all cases the maximum density is 500-750 birds/ha of land.

Folding unit system: In this system, recent in origin, the birds are confined to a small run and the position is changed every day. This enables the birds to avail fresh grounds. One of the major disadvantages of this system is that water and supplementary feed have to be brought by the labourer to the fresh grounds. Generally, a unit for 25 hens is most commonly used. Around 1 sq. ft./ bird of floor space and a run of 3 square feet/ bird are allowed.

Scavenger Feed Base of Village

The quantity of scavenger feed base of village varies according to seasonal rainfall, changes in the environment, agricultural practices, socio-economic status, ethnic groups etc. If the feed base is lesser than the flock biomass, there may be large scale mortality. Further, some birds may travel longer distance to scavenge while others may not. Certain birds have better scavenging ability than the others. Hence, it is important, the scavenger feed base is monitored from time to time thereby assessing the gap between the availability and requirement. During the lean period, the birds may be supplemented with different nutrients.

Generally, birds reared under scavenging system feed on maize, millets, insects, earthworms, snails, termites etc. to satisfy their nutrient needs. Many a times the household wastes are imbalanced. During lean period, the birds can develop various mineral and vitamin deficiencies for which supplemental feed may be provided. The requirement of supplemental feed may vary between 20-60 g/bird/day. During the laying period, the birds may be provided with marble chips or shell grit @ 5-7g/bird/day for better egg shell quality. In addition, the quality of scavenger feed base may be improved by including different unconventional feed ingredients viz. maggots, termites, worms etc. Another method of improving the scavenger feed base could be achieved by integrating poultry with cropping.

Management of Chicks Under Backyard System

One of the major reasons for failure in backyard programs is the early chick mortality. In the rural areas lack of scientific knowledge on poultry management gives rise to the conditions for loss in farming. Vaccination for New Castle disease may curtail this loss. Further, monitoring the scavenger feed base throughout the year will effectively optimize the egg and meat production.

Economic Achievements

Backyard poultry farming has several pivotal roles *viz.* providing high quality proteinous food in the form of eggs and meat, generating income to rural households, controlling pests with minimum labour, low input and environmental degradation. Besides, it also provides women empowerment since backyard birds are managed by them overall improving the rural economy, especially those of rual and tribal people. In fact, like many other South East Asian nations, commercial and backyard poultry farming can together fulfill the nutritional and economic requirement of rural India.

Question Bank

I. Fill in the blanks

a) The average per capita availability of eggs per annum in urban areas is ....

b) The average per capita availability of eggs per annum in rural areas is ....

c) The average pre capita availability of eggs per annum in India is ....

d) Per capita consumption of eggs as recommended by ICMR annually is ....

e) The contribution of backyard poultry farming in national production is ....

f) .... deficiency is quite common in the diets of rural people.

g) The requirement of cereals will rise to .... million tons by 2015 AD.

h) Around .... % of the poultry production in Africa is based on backyard system.

i) The type of low input rearing unit for poultry depends on .... & ....

j) Generally in a semi intensive system the birds are provided with .... square yards/bird of outside run.

Key: a) 170 b) 9 c) 45 d)180 e) 11% f) Protein g) 32 h) 80 i) capital & space j) 20-30

II. State True/ False

a) Backyard poultry farming causes more environmental pollution than commercial farming.

b) Folding unit system is cheaper than free range system.

c) The quantity and quality of scavenger feed base of a village varies according to climate and socio economic status.

d) The quality of scavenger feed base may be improved by including unconventional feed ingredients.

e) During the laying period, the birds under backyard system may be provided with shell grit.

f) Commercial poultry farming solely can ameliorate the protein hunger of rural India.

g) Vaccination against New Castle disease is advisable in backyard poultry farming to check early chick mortality.

h) One of the methods to improve the quality of scavenger feed base is integrating poultry and cropping.

i) Family poultry farming helps to improve the socio economic status of rural women.

j) With low input and minimum management, birds under backyard system are more beneficial than commercial high yielding birds.

Key: a) False b) False c) True d) True e) True f) False g) True h) True i) True j) True

8

Coloured Feathered Birds Developed for Rural Poultry

S.T. Viroji Rao

Poultry industry in India has registered a phenomenal growth during the last four decades making it one among the world leaders in poultry production. The development of organized poultry has in fact masked the contribution of backyard poultry or house-hold poultry of rural sector. Backyard poultry production in India is characterized by small flock size consisting of 5-10 predominantly non-descript birds maintained in extensive system under zero input conditions but fetch the owners much needed animal protein and supplementary income. Importance of backyard poultry is well recognized by Government of India and special programmes are formulated for its promotion.

Non-descript Chicken

Maintaining small flocks of local non-descript fowls under free range condition by landless poor, small and marginal farmers are a common sight in rural areas. These birds are very popular due to their adaptability to local agro climatic conditions and management practices with prominent brooding behaviour and mothering ability. But these birds are small in size, poor layers (40-50 eggs/ annum), with small clutch size and intense brooding behavior, thus making them not suitable for commercial exploitation.

Status of Native Breeds

Though India processes 20 well defined native chicken breeds, their proportion in the backyard chicken population is very small. Most of the indigenous chicken breeds like Kadaknath and Nicobari fowls are common in tribal areas of their origin.

Among native breeds, Aseel has special place in Indian culture. These birds are specially bred for cock fighting. It is known for heavy body size, long shanks, endurance and aggressive behaviour. It has also contributed in evolution of major broiler breeds.

Traditionally a flock of 5-10 native breed or non –descript fowls are maintained by farm families to meet their dietary needs or to meet small cash needs. They are maintained under range conditions thriving on insects, kitchen waste or grains in threshing floor during the season. But backyard poultry hardly finds a place in the transformed agriculture setup. Lack of suitable germplasm, scientific management practices, organized market channels, research priorities; policy options for backyard poultry development and change in the attitudes of rural producers are responsible for neglect of this sector which needs immediate and focused attention.

Attributes of an Ideal backyard chicken: If backyard chicken has to perform up to the expectations to meet the nutritional and livelihood security, it shall have the following attributes.

- Medium in size
- Ability for flight to avoid predation
- Egg production of about 125-150 eggs/year in free range system
- Ability to thrive in harsh climate with little supplementary feeding
- Resistance to commonly occurring poultry diseases.

Improved Backyard Poultry Varieties

Release of *Giriraja* chicken by University of Agricultural Sciences, Karnataka in the year 1989 can be viewed as the first initiative by poultry breeders to develop varieties suitable for backyard rearing. The breeds viz. White Plymouth rock, Red Cornish and New Hampshire available at broiler breeding project were utilized to bring out a bird with colour plumage, high egg production and body weight compared to local non- descript fowls and instantly became popular.

Recently Karnataka Veterinary Animal and Fishery Sciences University released "*Swarnadhara*" chicken suitable for backyard production system which is smaller than *Giriraja* chicken but produce more eggs. Taking cue from the success of *Giriraja* birds, Project Directorate on Poultry (PDP Now: Directorate of Poultry Research), Hyderabad has evolved *Vanaraja* chicken utilizing the Red Cornish as male line and random bred meat control population as dam line which was released in the year 1998. *Krishibro* is another meat type genotype released by the PDP using broiler germplasm. Subsequently, *Gramapriya* chicken was also developed by PDP on the specific request from Kerala farmers using Random bred meat control population as male line and a White Leghorn selected population as female line. These birds have more white plumage, medium in size and good egg laying capacity. Cockerels are better suited for tandoory chicken preparation. During the same period CARI, Izatnagar produced CARI-gold using RIR as male line and WLH as female line which is comparable to *Gramapriya* in its performance. Though they became popular among farming community, many have opined that most of these improved varieties are prone for predation, require supplementary feeding to perform at optimum level and the farmers are dependent on breeders for replacements. In subsequent years poultry breeders tried to overcome the above shortcomings by manipulating the breeds which can be viewed as second phase in backyard poultry breeding initiatives. JNKVV, Jabalpur evolved *Krishna* – J variety using dwarf gene population.

Central Avian Research Institute, Izatnagar released CARI – *Nirbheek*, CARI – *Shyama*, UPCARI, HITCARI by crossing Aseel, Kadaknath, Frizzle and Naked neck chicken with Dahlem Red breed, with an aim to incorporate desirable traits of native chicken breeds in new genotypes. Several private agencies also developed their own coloured chicken like *Kuroiler* and *Indbro* suitable for backyard or small scale production system. However, most of them are strain crosses of indigenous and exotic breeds and cannot breed true in farmer's field.

After reviewing the above poultry breeding initiatives in backyard production system, a need was felt to develop designer birds having the attributes such as medium body size, long shanks, better flight , egg production ranging between 125-150 eggs, ability to resist common diseases, able to withstand adverse climatic conditions and suitable for regeneration in backyard. AICRP on Poultry Breeding, Sri Venkateswara Veterinary University, Hyderabad took the initiative by developing a cocktail genotype with three exotic breeds viz. RIR, Delham WLH and also incorporating local fowls' inheritance at 25% level. This synthetic variety was named as *Rajasri* capable of producing about 150 – 170 eggs per year.

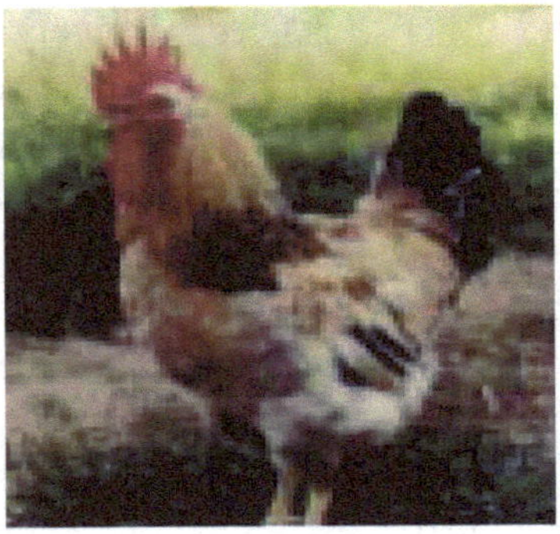
Giriraja male.

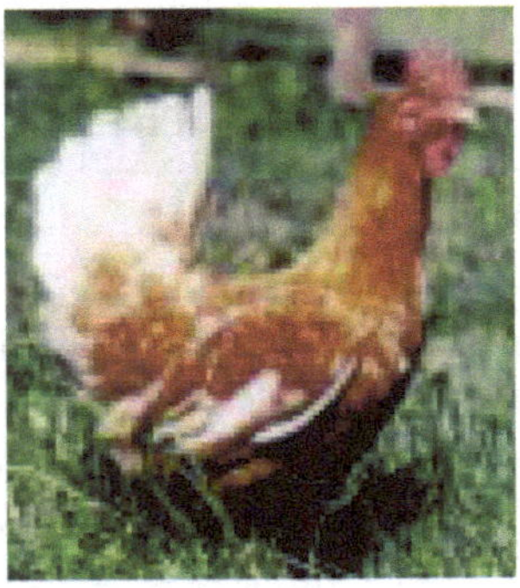
Giriraja female.

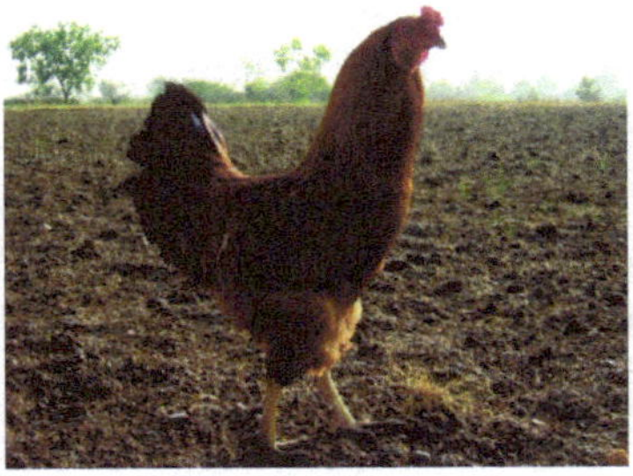
Vanaraja male.

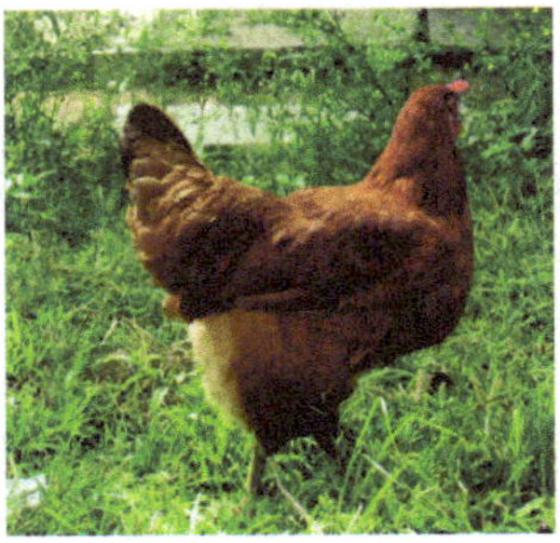
Vanaraja female.

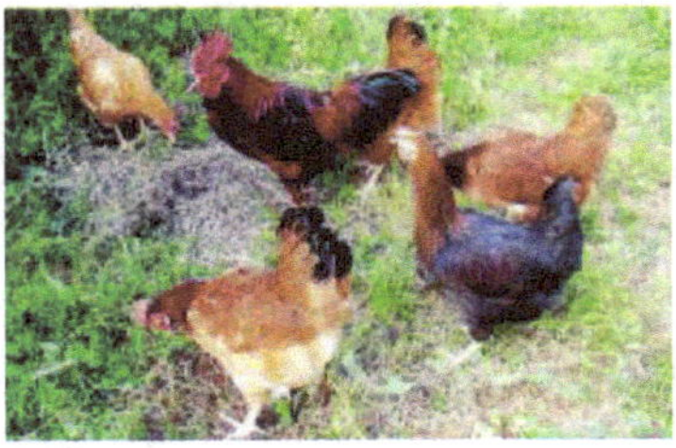
Gramapriya

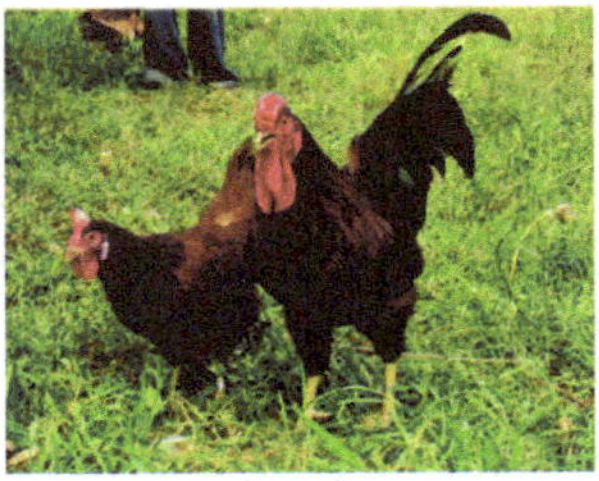
Rajashri.

Future Needs

Most of the work in backyard poultry breeding was carried out at ICAR /SAU research institutes and the genetic material is available only in limited quantity. In future, when scaling up is planned, research institutes may not be able to meet the demand. Hence public and private partnership (PPP) initiatives need to be planned for future. Improved varieties so far available also need supplementary diet, health care and prophylactic measures for optimum performance. Hence developing location specific package of practices for each of the varieties need of the hour.

Question Bank

Q. 1. What is backyard / free range poultry production system? Briefly explain about the same in Indian context.

Q. 2. What are ideal attributes of backyard chicken?

Q. 3. Name some chicken bred for backyard production system by public sector organizations and give their genetic constitutions.

Q. 4. Fill in the blanks

a) University of Agricultural Sciences, Bangalore released .... a coloured bird suitable for backyard production in the year 1989.

b) .... is the egg type coloured chicken developed by Project Director on Poultry, Hyderabad.

c) .... is a synthetic variety having 25% non-descript fowl inheritance.

d) .... and .... are colour feathered chicken developed by private agencies.

e) .... colour feathered chicken was developed by crossing RIR x WLH at Central Avian Research Institute.

Keys: (a) Giriraja, (b) Gramapriya, (c) Rajasri, (d) Kuroiler and Inbro, (e) CARI-Gold

Q. 5. Match the following

Krishibro	(E)	(A) Frizzle bird x Dahlem Red
UPCARI	(A)	(B) 25% non-descript fowl inheritance
Rajasri	(B)	(C) Necked neck x Dahlem Red
HITCARI	(C)	(D) Kadaknath x Dahlem Red
CARI Shyama	(D)	E) Developed from colour broiler germplasm.

9

Mixed Farming

M.V. Dhumal

Mixed farming exists in many forms depending on external and internal factors. External factors are weather patterns, market prices, technological developments, etc. Internal factors relate to local soil characteristics, composition of the family and farmers' ingenuity. Farmers can decide to opt for mixed enterprises when they want to save resources by interchanging them on the farm - because these permit wider crop rotations and thus reduce dependence on chemicals, because they consider mixed systems closer to nature, or because they allow diversification for better risk management. There is wide variation in mixed systems. Even pastoralists practice a form of mixed farming since their livelihood depends on the management of different feed resources and animal species. Mixed farms are systems that consist of different parts, which together should act as a whole. They thus need to be studied in their entirety and not as separate parts in order to understand the system and the factors that drive farmers and influence their decisions. It may be the most important principle to achieve increased production in mixed systems, together with the awareness that crops and animals have multiple functions.

Classification of Mixed Farming

Mixed farming systems can be classified in many ways - based on land size, type of crops and animals, geographical distribution, market orientation, etc. Three major categories, in four different modes of farming are distinguished as:

1. On-farm *versus* between-farm mixing
2. Mixing within crops and/or animal systems
3. Diversified versus integrated systems

Role of Mixed Farming in Poultry

Poultry includes a variety of species such as ducks, geese, chickens and turkeys etc. They often provide a living for the family by scavenging (chickens and turkeys) or by grazing on harvesting rice fields (ducks and geese). The particular features of these birds in mixed systems are that they are in small units, reproduce easily, do not need large investments and thrive well on kitchen waste, fallen grains, worms, snails or insects. However, the common problems encountered are, like other birds, they are susceptible to diseases, theft or to predators.

Ducks and Geese

Ducks and geese are basically waterfowls, but they can be raised without water and, except in some rare cases, the keeping of these birds does not develop into large-scale, high-input production. Rare cases of specialized production of these birds are, for example, geese for "foie gras" (French for 'fat liver') or ducks for meat in countries such as France and China. More typical for mixed farming systems is duck keeping for eggs in harvested rice fields, wherein fallen grains, weeds, snails and worms provide free feed for large flocks.. The occasional use of geese as "watchdogs" is worth mentioning as an indigenous way to fend off thieves.

Fish-cum-Chicken

The droppings of birds in this system are utilized to fertilize the pond. Poultry litter recycled into fish pond produces 4500-5000 kg fish per hectare per year. Broiler production provides good and immediate return to the farmers. Success in production depends mainly on the efficiency of the farmer, experience, aptitude and ability, in the management of the flock. This involves procurement of better brood stock, housing, brooding equipment, feeders, water trays and management practices, which also include prevention and control of diseases. The poultry litter is applied to the pond in daily doses at a rate of 40-50 kg per hectare. The application of litter may be deferred during the days when algal blooms appear in the ponds. One adult chicken produces about 25 kg of compost poultry manure in one year. 500-600 birds would provide sufficient manure for fertilization of one hectare of fish pond. Farmer can get a net income of

Rs.137157/- from one hectare of pond in one year. Govt. provides financial assistance to the farmers for promoting this system.

Economics of Fish-cum-Chicken

A) Expenditure	**Amount Rs.**
1. Construction of Pond, Water Supply Channel, Installation of Tube well/ Renovation/ Lease	20,000/-
2. Electricity & Water Charges	10,000/-
3. Construction of Poultry Shed (Rs. 80,000/- for 10 Years)	8,000/-
4. 550 NOs Chicks	2,750/-
5. 22500 Kg Poultry Feed	90,000/-
6. Medicines for Fish and Poultry	5,000/-
7. Fishing and Labour Cost	20,000/-
Total Expenditure	1,57,250/-
A) Expenditure	**Amount Rs.**
Sale of 4200 Kg Fish	1,26,000/-
Sale of 118750 Eggs	1,48,437/-
Sale of 500 Kg Birds	20,000/-
Total Income	2,94,437/-
C) Net Income (B-A)	**1, 37, 157/-**

Note: The Income may vary based on the productivity, market price of a pond and locality.

Fish-cum-Duck Farming

Fish-cum-duck integration is most common in the developing countries and NE parts of India. However this type of mixed farming is not popular in northern states of India. Fish pond being a semi-closed biological system with several aquatic animals and plants provides an excellent disease-free environment for the ducks. In turn, ducks consume juvenile frogs, tadpoles, dragonfly etc. thereby making a safe environment for fish. Duck droppings go directly into the pond, which in turn provide essential nutrients such as carbon, nitrogen and phosphorus those stimulate growth of natural food organisms. Ducks also help in aerating the pond water, along with bottom racking. About 300 ducks are enough to fertilize a pond of one hectare. The system results in a net income of Rs. 77500/- per year per hectare. However, due to difficulty in marketing of duck eggs and meat, the system is not very common in all the states.

Question Bank

Q. Choose appropriate word (s).

i) Farmers can decide to opt for mixed enterprises because

a) Save resources, b) Maximum Production,

c) Intensive Management, d) None of above

ii) The most important principle to achieve increased production in mixed systems is:

a) Crop and Bird multiple function, b) Symbiotic relationship,

c) Utilization of better natural resources d) All of above

iii) Mixed farming systems can be classified as

a) On-farm versus between-farm mixing, b) Mixing within crops and/or animal systems,

c) Diversified versus integrated systems d) All of above

iv) Mixed farming systems can base on

a) Land, b) Species of birds,

c) Family size, d) All of above

v) Kinds of poultry function in mixed farming are

a) Watchdogs, b) As a social activity,

c) Commercial production, d) a & b

vi) Common problem of mixed farming is:

a) Intensive management, b) Intensive feeding,

c) Intensive breeding, d) Predator

vii) In mixed farming systems (duck keeping) the feeding system adapted is:

a) All mash method, b) Pellet

c) Crumble, d) Feeding of harvested grains in field

viii) Major problem in chicken keeping in mixed farming is

a) Occurrence of infection, b) Higher cost of production,

c) Low cost of production, d) a & c

ix) Success in production during mixed farming depends mainly on

a) Efficiency of the farmer, b) experience,

c) aptitude and ability, d) All of above

Key: i) a; ii) d; iii) d; iv) d; v) d; vi) d; vii) d; viii) a; ix) d

Q. 2. What is mixed farming? Classify its different types.

10

Brooding and Rearing of Poultry

D. Sapcota

Brooding and Rearing Practices Used for Chicken

What is Brooding?

Rearing of young ones immediately after hatching for at least 2-3 weeks, either by natural means or by artificial method is called brooding. Brooding is done by two ways i.e., Natural or Artificial ways.

Natural Brooding

In the natural method a *desi* fowl which acts both as incubator and brooder is used to raise only a small number of chicks. She sits on eggs (chicken) for 21 days to produce chicks from fertile eggs and broods thereafter.

Artificial Brooding

In the artificial brooding auxiliary or supplementary heat is provided to the chicks through some sources of heat. With the rapid growth of poultry industry brooding of chicks by artificial method has largely replaced the natural method. The artificial brooding has several advantages such as: (i) chicks can be brooded at any time of the year, (ii) brooding can be done in large numbers and (iii) the sanitary conditions can be controlled.

Brooding Equipment

Brooder is a device of providing auxiliary or supplementary heat to chicks. These are of several types depending upon the size and the nature of fuel used. Examples: hover (canopy) brooders, infra red brooders, gas (LPG) brooders etc.

General Procedure for Brooding and Rearing

1. To provide warmth, hover brooders (umbrella type with electrical or tungsten bulbs), infra-red bulbs, coal stoves or gas brooders may be employed. The common practice is to use hover with electrical bulbs under deep litter system.
2. About 24 hours before the anticipated time of arrival of the chicks, the brooder arrangements are made and kept ready. Plan the requirements of chicks, book in advance with hatchery or local agent and confirm the exact date and time of arrival of chicks.
3. Spread the litter materials like paddy husk, groundnut hulls, wood shavings or saw dust etc. to about 5cm height. Spread some old newspapers on it to prevent young chicks eating the litter.
4. Arrange chick guards of about 30-35 cm height in a circular fashion.
5. The height of the hover may be adjusted to be at one foot above the floor level, initially.
6. The required number of feeders and waterers are arranged alternate to each other on the newspaper area in cart-wheel fashion. Two linear feeders of 60 cm size and two chick waterers may be used for every 100 chicks. Allow free moving space on the sides of waterers and feeders.
7. Switch on the bulbs 1-2 hours before the arrival of the chicks to keep the environment warm.
8. Keep boiled and cooled drinking water ready. Add 8 g of glucose per litre, electrolytes and vitamin mixture at recommended dosage in water for the first 3-5 days.
9. Spread a little feed on the newspapers also.

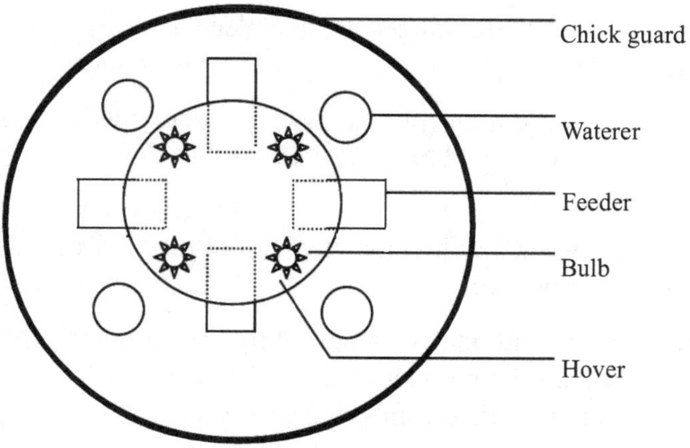

Fig. 20: Arrangement of brooder to brood chicks

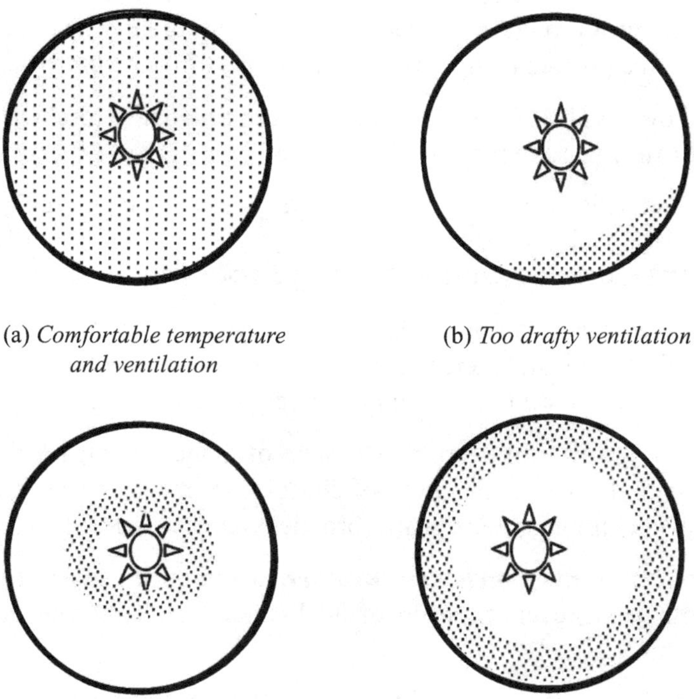

(a) *Comfortable temperature and ventilation*

(b) *Too drafty ventilation*

(c) *Low brooder temperature*

(d) *High brooder temperature*

Fig. 21: Behaviour of chicks under the brooder indicates the correct brooding temperature

10. Count the chicks which should be healthy (40-48 g, each), dip the beak of few chicks in the drinking water and place it gently into the brooder arrangement. Fellow chicks will follow the trained ones.

11. Heater coils in severe cold places may also be provided if warranted as a source of heat but should be hanged above the reach of the chicks.

12. °C warmth which may be reduced by 3°C every week. A thermometer kept at the bird's head-level will indicate the temperature.

13. Adequacy of warmth may be assessed by watching the distribution of the chicks within the brooder guard. If they crowd under or near the source of heat, then the warmth given is not sufficient. Then, bulb may be added to the hover brooder, wattage increased or the height of the hover may be brought down. If chicks have moved to the periphery and are reluctant to come to the centre under heat source, then temperature in the environment is higher than required. The hover may be pushed up or a bulb removed or wattage reduced. If the chicks feel comfortable at the given temperature, they walk actively throughout the area unmindful of the heat provided and some take rest setting their head down on the side, the posture being given the name as "*Chick comfort*".

14. A hover with 150 cm diameter will accommodate 225 chicks; whereas 180 cm will have room for 300 chicks.

15. Soiled news papers may be removed after day one and replaced.

Important Considerations During Brooding

i) ***Temperature:*** Starting chicks immediately after hatch require 35°C during the first week and thereafter temperature requirement decreases by 3°C every week until the temperature reaches around 21.1°C.

ii) ***Chick guards:*** In deep litter system of management, for the first 6-7 days to avoid straying away of chicks from the source of heat so as to prevent chilling, chick guard (brooder guard) is used.

iii) ***Protection from inclement weather:*** Cover open sides of sheds with curtains to prevent exposure of chicks to drafts of cold wind and to warm the house.

iv) ***Ventilation:*** It is required to provide fresh air by removing obnoxious gases like carbon monoxide, carbon dioxide and ammonia from the house for healthy respiration and dryness in shed. Therefore, opening and covering of curtains need to be done correctly depending on the weather condition.

v) ***Feeding and watering:*** Feeding of balanced ration and ensuring supply of fresh potable water at all times are very important for optimum growth and development of chicks.

Table 9: Floor space, feeder space and drinker space requirement for chicken in deep litter system.

Age (week)	Floor space (sq.ft)	Feeder space (in)		Drinker space (in)	
		Linear	Circular	Linear	Circular
0 – 3	0.0 – 0.5	1	¼	0.5	⅛
4 – 6	0.5 – 0.75	2	½	1.0	¼
6 – 8	0.75 – 1.0	3	¾	1.5	½

vi) ***Debeaking :*** 7th to 10th day of age.

vii) ***Health and immunity:*** To grow healthy, vigorous and viable chicks, adopt only essential and correct medication along with effective vaccination programme.

Brooding and Rearing Practices Used for Ducklings

Brooding can be done either on floor or in battery as that of chicken. The starting temperature is 35°C which is reduced by 2.5°C, each week. The floor space requirement on wire floor is 0.045 m^2 and that on litter is 0.093 m^2 up to three weeks. The depth of waterers should be 12.5 to 15 cms, sufficient for immersion of heads failing which eyes become scaly, crusty or blind in extreme cases.

Vaccination schedule for ducks

Age	Disease	Vaccine
Day old	Duck viral hepatitis	DVH (Only used in prevalent areas)
4 and 16 weeks	Duck cholera (*Pasteurella*)	DCV
8 weeks	Duck plague (Duck viral enteritis)	DPV

Brooding and Rearing Practices Used for Turkeys

Turkeys are brooded with additional heat up to 8 to 10 weeks of age. Early mortality may be more in turkey poults than chicks and ducklings, which is often due to lack of drinking, feeding facilities or inadequate light. Therefore, adequate feed, water and light must be provided to avoid initial mortality. The brooding temperature in 1st week should be at least 35°C which should be gradually reduced by 2°C, each week till it reaches to room temperature. The diseases encountered are Newcastle disease, turkey rhino-tracheitis, pox, pasteurellosis and erysipelas for which protective vaccination should be given. Adequate floor space of 0.08 to 0.24m^2/ turkey is given up to 14 weeks on litter, better ventilation and fresh litter are basic essentialities of brooding.

Brooding and Rearing Practices Used for Quail

Japanese quail chicks are small in size, hence cannot adjust themselves to a cold weather. Therefore, adequate warmth must be provided by using electric bulbs, coal-stove heating or gas brooding. In a brooder guard circle of 3 feet diameter (90 cm), about 150 chicks can be accommodated. It is not advisable to allow more than 300 chicks inside one circle. An electric bulb with a hood cover can be provided at 15 cm height at the centre of the circle, providing approximately 1 watt per chick. The heating arrangement has to be continued day and night during the first week, but only during the night from the second week onwards. The brooder house temperature at the level of the birds has to be about 36.7°C, which may be reduced by about 3°C every 3 days till it reaches around 21°C. The chicks should feel comfort during brooding period, which may be assessed by observing their movement. The pattern of spread of faeces will indicate as to how the chicks spent the previous night. Drinkers and feeders should not be kept under the source of heat inside the brooder circle. A watering space of about 0.3 cm, and a feeder space of 0.6 cm per bird, must be provided during 0-2 weeks, and this has to be increased to 0.6 and 1.2 cm respectively from 3-5 weeks of age.

Brooding and Rearing Practices Used for Guinea Fowl

Guinea chicks (keet) are subject to chilling during the first few weeks. The brooder house should be completely cleaned prior to each new brood; the floor should be covered with clean, fresh litter at least 3 inch deep. The litter inside the brooder should be covered with rough surface paper/gunny bag for firm footing and to prevent young keets from eating litter materials. The keets should be placed in the brooding quarters and given feed and water within 24 hours after hatching. All types of chicken brooders are suitable for keets; which should operate at 37°C from day-old stage and reduce the temperature by 4°C, each week. In the first 4 weeks it is important to prevent chilling of the keets. Keet mash should contain 24% crude protein. Adequate cool, clean water is essential at all times. Twenty keets with a stocking density of 1 m^2 is optimum at day-old. Young keets will perch from 6 weeks of age. Reduce stocking density to eight birds per square meter by 10 weeks of age.

Question Bank

I . Choose the Correct Answer

1. While initiating the brooding litter material is spread to about 5/10/15 cm height. (5).
2. For brooding, the chick guard is arranged to about 30-35/35-40/45-50 cm height in a circular fashion. (30-35).
3. The feeder space (linear) provided to chick during 4-6 weeks is 2/3/4 inch. (2).
4. It is ideal to program the first debeaking to layer chicken at the age of 4th -7th / 7th -10th / 10th – 13th day of age.(7th -10th).
5. The floor space requirement for ducklings under deep litter system is 0.093/0.096/0.099 m^2 up to three weeks.(0.093).
6. The turkeys are given a floor space of 0.04 - 0.08/0.08 - 0.24/0.24 - 0.34m^2 up to 14 weeks of age under deep litter system. (0.08 - 0.24).
7. A brooder guard circle of 3/6/9 feet diameter is recommended for 150 quail chicks. (3).
8. An electric bulb with a hood cover can be provided at 15/20/25 cm height at the centre of the circle, providing approximately 1/2/3 watt per quail chick. (15 and 1).
9. Keet mash should contain 22/24/26% crude protein. (24).

II . Fill in the blanks

1. Rearing of young ones immediately after hatching for at least 2-3 weeks is called ....(brooding).
2. In natural method a *desi* fowl acts both as .... and .... (Incubator and brooder)
3. For brooding the required number of feeders and waterers are arranged alternate to each other on the newspaper area in .... fashion in deep better system. (cart-wheel).
4. Beginning first week the brooding chicks require .... °C warmth which may be reduced by .... °C every week till reaches ambient temperature. (35 and 3)
5. In deep litter system of management, ... is used for the first

6-7 days to avoid straying away of chicks from the source of heat (chick guards/brooder guard).

6. Ventilation is required to provide fresh air by removing obnoxious gases like .... , ... and .... from the house for healthy respiration and dryness in poultry shed. (Carbon monoxide, carbon dioxide and ammonia).
7. A watering space of about .... cm and a feeder space of .... cm must be provided during 0-2 weeks per quail chick. (0.3 and 0.6).
8. For keet the brooders should operate from 37°C which should be reduced by .... °C, each week.(4).
9. Young keets will perch from .... weeks of age. (6).

III . True / False

1. For proper brooding, height of the hover may be adjusted to at one foot above the floor level, initially. (True).
2. It is not advisable to allow more than 300 quail chicks inside one brooder guard circle. (True).
3. All types of poultry brooders are not suitable for keets. (False).
4. Twenty keets with a stocking density of 1 m^2 is optimum at day-old stage for rearing. (True).
5. The floor space provided to chick during 4-6 week is 0.5-0.75 sq. ft. (True).
6. Among all types of brooders hover brooder is most common. (True).

11

Economic Production of Poultry

M.T. Banday

Among various animal husbandry enterprises, poultry production has emerged as number one position and attained industrial status in many countries, including India.

This tremendous growth in poultry production is due to the following reasons:

1. There is no religious taboo towards poultry and poultry products.
2. Egg is the most nutritious, natural, unadulterated and easily digestible food with the highest biological value.
3. Eggs can be consumed by all age groups and economic classes, since it is the cheapest among all the nutritious natural foods on the earth.
4. Among various meats, poultry meat has the highest protein, lowest fat and cholesterol content.
5. Poultry is the best converter of feed into meat and eggs. A hen needs only 1.5 kg feed to produce 1 dozen eggs. Similarly a broiler needs less than 2 kg of feed to produce one kg broiler meat whereas other species need more than 3 kg of feed to produce 1kg of meat.
6. Poultry has the shortest generation interval among various livestocks.
7. Poultry produces the largest number of offsprings per dam exceeding other livestocks.

8. The requirement of space for poultry farming is much lesser when compared to other livestock. In one sq metre of floor space about 150 kg of broilers can be produced per annum whereas only 50kg of beef or 60 kg of pork can be produced in the same area.
9. Poultry has the highest dressing yield ranging from 70 to 80%with less offals. On the other hand, many livestock will give only 45-65% dressing yield with a higher percentage of offals.
10. The newly emerging speices of poultry such as Ostrich and Emu can live for more than 50 years with a reproductive period of more than 40 years.
11. Poultry can be reared successfully under wide agro climatic conditions in any type of soil.
12. Poultry are highly adaptable for intensive system with more automation leading to lesser labour cost.
13. Poultry processing and marketing are well organized in many countries. This will create more demand for poultry products.
14. With the introduction of many feed additives, less nutritious unconventional feedstuffs can be better utilized by poultry leading to reduction in feed cost and environment pollution.

Like any other animal enterprise, the ultimate aim of poultry farmer is to maximize or optimize the returns. Several factors contribute to his efficiency; they include the quality of stock, feeding, management and marketing efficiency.

Factors Affecting Gross Output in Egg Production Units

1. **Strain of bird:** The strain of bird is highly decisive influencing gross output in a layer farm.

The following level of egg output provides guidance to average levels of performance that may be expected:

Strain	No of eggs produced/year
Light	240
Medium	228
Heavy	216

Various other factors also influence the egg production, i.e., light pattern, stresses; low or high house temperature, level of nutrition, season of the year etc.

2. **The size of the egg:** A premium price is obtained for larger eggs and this may influence gross output. Heavy strains tend to produce larger eggs.
3. **Incidence of diseases:** Proper medication and preventive measures will have to be taken to minimize production loss through diseases.
4. **Selling price of egg:** Eggs sold at higher price per dozen will increase the gross output of the farm.
5. **Feed**: Feed is a major item of expenditure in poultry production accounting for more than 70% of total recurring cost. Spiraling of prices of each of the feed ingredients especially fishmeal, ground nut cake, maize and rice polish has caused an acute increase in feed cost.
6. **Good management:** Efficient and good management will help in minimizing the percentage of mortality. Similarly efficient culling program would help in removing unproductive birds. Proper culling of pullets and poor /non-layers will save feed and other expenses.
7. **Size of flock:** Large flocks have better utilization of labour, house, equipments than smaller units and hence, it will help in reducing the production cost.
8. **Mortality:** Mortality of birds causes direct economic losses. The most costly age at which mortality occurs is the sexual maturity. Proper management with better biosecurity measures will help in reducing the percent mortality.

Factors Influencing Price of Eggs are

1. **Time of the year when birds are hatched:** Eggs prices follow a definite pattern through out the year. It will be desirable to have flocks hatched in the late summer/early autumn, so that birds come to lay between November and February i.e. when the price for egg is highest. As the birds get older larger eggs are produced which command the highest price per dozen.
2. **Size and grade of eggs:** The proportion of large and standard eggs produced will influence the overall price.
3. **Method of selling**: Considerably highest prices can be obtained by selling eggs at the farm gate than by selling to the packing stations.
4. **Shell color**: Brown shelled eggs fetch a better price than white eggs.
5. **External and internal qualities:** Different strains of hybrid layers vary considerably in respect of the internal quality of eggs produced by them,

although much emphasis is placed on this aspect in the selection of breeding stock. Further, the external quality of eggs can be influenced considerably by the way in which eggs are handled, cleaned, collected and stored.

6. **Replacement costs:** While calculating the gross output of a laying flock, flock depreciation must be included as well as output and prices of eggs. Depreciation covers the prices of culled birds obtained for hens at the end of their production period as well as cost of replacements purchased to replace them in flock. Heavier strains fetch better cull values.

Economic traits which can be adopted as Technical coefficients in layer and broiler farms are given below:

A- Egg production

Parameter		**Economic traits**
1. Hatch weight	:	Weight in gm of chick at hatch
2. Weight at 20th week.	:	Weight of growers alive at 20th week of age
3. Livability (0-20 weeks)`	:	Percentage of chicks alive at 20 weeks of age
4 Age at maturity	:	Age on the date of first egg.
5 Age at first egg	:	Age in days from the date of hatch to the date of first egg.
6. Age at first egg where there is no trap nesting	:	Age in days of a flock when- a) the first egg was received. b) 30 percent produced (on hen day basis) c) 50 percent produced (on hen day basis)
7. 36 weeks production	:	Egg yield of a pullet from the date of first egg to the date on which it will complete 36 weeks of age.
8. 72 weeks production	:	Egg yield of a pullet from the date of first egg to the date on which it will complete 72 weeks of age.

9. a) Hen day production to 36 weeks(%)	:	$\frac{\text{Total no of eggs received to the end of 36 weeks x 100}}{\text{Hen days}}$
b) Hen housed production to 36	:	$\frac{\text{Total no eggs laid by a flock to the end of 36 weeks x 100}}{\text{No of Hens housed at 20 weeks}}$
10. a) Hen day production to 72 weeks (%)	:	$\frac{\text{Total no eggs laid by a flock to the end of 72 weeks x 100}}{\text{Hen days}}$
b) Hen housed production to 72 weeks (%)	:	$\frac{\text{Total No. eggs laid by a flock up to 72 weeks x 100}}{\text{No .of Hens housed at 20 weeks}}$
11. Livability (20-72 weeks)	:	$\frac{\text{No of hens alive at 72 weeks x 100}}{\text{No of Hens started at 20 weeks}}$
12. Feed efficiency	:	kg of feed consumed to produce a dozen eggs
13. Egg weight (or egg size) eggs laid	:	Average weight of 3 consecutive during 36 weeks of age
14. Fertility/ hatchability		
a) Fertility	:	Percentage of fertile eggs to the total eggs set.
b) Hatchability percent of fertile egg set	:	Percentage of chicks hatched to the fertile eggs
c) Hatchability percent of total eggs set	:	Percentage of chicks hatched to the total eggs set.

B- Meat production

1. Hatch weight	:	Weight in g at hatch
2. Body weight	:	Weight in g on weekly basis
3. Feed consumption	:	Weekly cumulative feed consumption in grams
4. Feed conversion ratio	:	kg of feed consumed to produce one kg of live weight.

5. Livability till 6 weeks : Percentage of chicks alive at 6 weeks to the number of chicks started.

Methods to Reduce the Wasteful Expenditure in A Farm

The cost-benefit ratio in poultry farm is lowest compared to other enterprises. The farmers have to identify the area; where they can further reduce the expenditure without affecting the production and performance of farm. Here an attempt has been made to identify few such areas.

1. Farm Building

- On square metre basis, bigger and wider houses are cheaper than smaller and narrower houses. Bigger houses also reduce the cost of labour and the requirements for lighting.
- Increasing the stock density of birds by using multi tier cages and mechanical ventilation will reduce the housing and equipment costs per bird leading to lesser interest and depreciation on the capital.

2. Management

- The fuel cost for brooding and warming the shed will be cheaper with the use of coal followed by charcoal, kerosene, LPG and electricity. Nowadays the electricity tariffs are very high and its supply is erroneous in many places. Hence the economics of the farm enterprise is related to the type of fuel used for brooding of chicks.
- Larger broiler farms with weekly capacity of 5,000 chicks and above can significantly reduce the chick cost by hatching their own chicks either by maintaining a small breeding flock or purchasing hatching eggs.
- Reduction of floor space up to 50% per bird up to 25 days of age and increasing it later will reduce the housing requirement and rearing cost by nearly 25%.
- Using locally available cheaper litter materials can reduce expenses on rearing of chicks.
- Entry of rodents, wild birds, squirrels etc. must be prevented into feed stores and poultry sheds to prevent wastage of feed and the breakage of eggs.
- Since the cost of culled hens has reduced tremendously, the pullet cost depreciation per egg will be higher, if the culled hens are kept up to 72-76 weeks of age. On the other hand, if the hens are force moulted around

75-80 weeks of age and maintained up to 100-110 weeks of age, the cost of production of eggs will be lower, due to lesser pullet cost of depreciation.

3. Equipment

- Use a required number of feeders in the shed as per the number of birds.
- Well designed feeders and waterers with proper height or automatic equipment will reduce the feed wastage. It will also save the labour.
- Use of compact fluorescent lights in place of ordinary fluorescent lights or incandescent bulbs will reduce the electricity bills considerably.

4. Health Care and Medication

- Carry out proper vaccination programmes based on the diseases prevailing in a particular area. Avoid unwanted vaccination. Thus, unnecessary cost on vaccination can be avoided.
- Maintain good health of birds by good management, vaccination, sanitation and feeding a balanced diet rather than medication and treatment.

Factors affecting profitability of layer farm

Output of eggs	→	Housing conditions
		Strain of birds
		Type of feed used
		Number of eggs laid
		Size of eggs
		Time of year when hens hatched
		Size and grade of eggs
		Method of sale
Price of eggs	→	Colour of eggs
		Percentage of cracks
Price of culls	→	Strain of bird
		Age of bird
Gross output	→	Manure sales
		Cost of replacement
		Mortality
		Feed
		Bird replacement
		Vet and Medicine
Less variable cost (Gross margin)		
Less fixed cost		
Enterprise profit		

Measures for Estimating the Performance of Broiler Chicken

The farmer will be interested in knowing at what position his farm stands on economic grounds and the efficiency of his farm operation. The following methods and formulae may be used as tools to measure the performance of the birds.

1. Feed Conversion Ratio

This is the most important and commonly used efficiency measure in a broiler farm. It is calculated by using the formula:

$$\text{FCR} = \frac{\text{Total feed consumed in kg}}{\text{Total body weight in kg}}$$

A value of less than 2 .00 at 6 weeks of age is preferable. Lower the value, better will be the efficiency.

2. Performance Index (P.I)

$$\text{P.I} = \frac{\text{Live weight in Ibs x 100}}{\text{Feed conversion ratio}}$$

Higher the value, better will be the index. A value of 200 or more is desirable.

3. Broiler Performance Efficiency Factor (BPEF)

$$\text{BPEF} = \frac{\text{Live weight in kg x 100}}{\text{Feed conversion ratio}}$$

Higher the value better will be the index. A value of 100 and above is desirable.

4. Construction Coefficient (CC)

$$\text{CC} = \frac{\text{Total constructed area x 100}}{\text{Total farm land area}}$$

Construction coefficient should be 25 to 35 for an ideal farm. A higher value indicates congestion, overcrowding, poor ventilation and more disease problem. Lower values are suggestive of poor utilization of land which means higher investment on land per bird.

5. Gross Margin Per Unit Floor Area

Gross margin per unit floor area depends upon the stocking density, growth rate, mortality and the market prices for the outputs.

$$\text{Gross margin/m}^2 = \frac{\text{Total receipts / year}}{\text{Total floor area (m}^2\text{)}}$$

Higher the value better will be the efficiency.

6. Point Spread (PS)

PS = (Live weight in lbs - Feed conversion ratio) $\times 100$

A value of 200 or more is considered to be more economical. If the live weight is expressed in kgs, the PS will be near to zero or even a negative value; hence, it is not advised to calculate PS with metric units.

7. Benefit- Cost Ratio (BCR)

It is the ratio between the total gross receipts and the total expenditure incurred by the farm.

$$\text{BCR} = \frac{\text{Gross receipts}}{\text{Total cost of inputs}}$$

A value of one BCR indicates no profit or loss, more than one indicates profits and less than one indicates losses to farm. Values of 1.20 and above are desirable.

8. Broiler Feed Price Ratio (BFPR)

$$\text{BFPR} = \frac{\text{Total value of meat or live chicken produced}}{\text{Total value of feed}}$$

Higher body weight gain, lower mortality, better feed efficiency, lower feed cost and higher selling price results in a favourable BFPR value; A value of more than two is desirable.

9. Broiler Performance Efficiency Index (BPEI) :

$$\text{BPEI} = \frac{\text{Total saleable live weight (kg)}}{\text{No of chicks purchased} \times \text{Feed efficiency}} \times 100$$

A BPEI value of 100 or higher is desirable.

10. Formula for Calculating Cost of Production / Kg Live Broiler

i. Chick cost = $0.55 \times$ Cost of one day-old chick = A

ii. Feed cost = Feed efficiency $\times$ cost /kg of feed = B

iii. Miscellaneous expenditure = Add 12% of A+ B = C

iv. Therefore, production cost/kg live broiler = A+ B + C

11. Formula for Calculating Cost of Production / Broiler

i. Chick cost = 1.05 × Cost of one day old chick = A

ii. Feed cost = Live weight (kg) × Feed efficiency × cost /kg of feed = B

iii. Miscellaneous expenditure = Add 15% of A+ B = C

iv. Therefore, production cost per broiler = A+ B + C

12. Formula for Calculating Cost of Production/Kg Ready to Cook Broiler

$$\text{Cost of 1 kg RTC} = \frac{1 + \text{Cost of one Live chicken}}{\text{Live weight (kg)} \times 0.73}$$

13. Broiler Farm Economy Index (BFEI):

$$\text{BFEI} = \frac{\text{Average Live weight (kg)} \times \text{Percent livability}}{\text{Feed efficiency} \times \text{Growing period (days)}}$$

A BFEI value of 2 and above indicates better management.

Value of less than 1.3 indicates poor performance.

Layer Farm Efficiency Measuring Parameters

1. Feed Efficiency/kg Egg Mass

It is the ratio between the feed consumed and the egg mass (kg)

$$= \frac{\text{kg of feed consumed}}{\text{kg of eggs produced}}$$

A value of 2.4 or less is advantageous.

2. Feed Efficiency / Dozen Eggs

It is the feed consumed per dozen of eggs.

$$= \frac{\text{kg of feed consumed}}{\text{12 eggs produced}}$$

A value of 1.6 or less is desirable.

3. Hen Day Egg Production

$$\text{HDEP} = \frac{\text{No of eggs produced}}{\text{Total no of live hens}} \times 100$$

For a long period of time, it is calculated as :

$$\text{HDEP} = \frac{\text{Total number of eggs produced during a period}}{\text{Total number of hen days during that period}} \times 100$$

A farm or flock average of 85% or 310 eggs per year or above is desirable.

4. Hen Housed Egg Production

It is the egg production based on the initial number of hens housed in the flock.

$$\text{HHEP} = \frac{\text{No of eggs produced on a given day}}{\text{Total number of hens housed at the beginning}} \times 100$$

For a longer period of time it will be calculated as :

$$\text{HHEP} = \frac{\text{Average daily No of eggs produced on a given day}}{\text{Total number of hens housed initially}} \times 100$$

A value of 295 or 80% or higher is desirable.

5. Net Feed Efficiency Index

$$\text{NFEI} = \frac{\text{Mean egg mass (g)} + \text{Mean body weight}}{\text{Average feed consumption}} \times 100$$

NFEI value of 45 and above is desirable.

6. Performance Efficiency Index

This is based on the data on egg weight, body weight, egg production and feed consumption.

$$\text{PEI} = \frac{30\,(\text{EW})^2\,\text{P}}{\text{BW} \times \text{F}}$$

EW = Average egg weight in g.

BW = Average body weight in g.

P = Percentage hen-day egg production.

F = Average feed consumed /day in g.

7. Egg: Feed Price Ratio

$$\text{EFPR} = \frac{\text{Total value of eggs produced}}{\text{Total value of feed consumed}}$$

8. Egg Mass / Hen Housed

Kilograms of eggs produced / hen housed.

9. Formula For Calculating Production Cost of Egg:

$$\text{Production cost of one egg} = \frac{\text{Total feed consumption in the laying year X feed cost/kg+total of other inputs (25 \% of feed cost)}}{\text{Total Nos of egg produced.}}$$

Question Bank

State whether True or False

1. Heavy breeds produce about 216 eggs in a year. (True)
2. Quality of eggs influences the gross returns of a layer farm. (True)
3. Farm capacity will not influence the cost of chicks. (False)
4. Layers maintained beyond 100 weeks of age will not influence the cost of production of eggs. (False)
5. A value of 100 and above indicates better performance index of a farm. (False)
6. Cost of construction is the largest single item of expenditure in poultry production. (False)
7. About 25% expenditure can be saved if own feed is self manufactured. (True)
8. Fixed cost remains constant irrespective of value of production. (True)
9. A good commercial layer is capable of producing more than 300 eggs on hen-day egg production basis. (False)

Fill in the blanks

1. A value of less than .... at 6 weeks of age in broiler chicken is desirable. (Two)
2. A lower construction coefficient is suggestive of .... (poor utilization of land)
3. A value of.................. or less is advantageous feed efficiency for a good Layer.(2.4)
4. A value of one BCR indicates .... (No loss or profit)
5. A farm with .... percentage is desirable for hen-day egg production on long term basis.(85%)

6. The most costly age at which mortality can occur is .... (sexual maturity)
7. Grading helps to get .... % more profit .(15)
8. Higher egg production .... cost per egg. (reduces)
9. .... is the most important and commonly used measure for estimating the efficiency of a farm.(FCR)
10. .... kgs of broilers can be produced in one square meter area.(150)
11. .... cost is the decisive factor for optimum performance of broiler.(Feed)
12. Mortality in a broiler flock should never exceed .... percent.(5)
13. For a given flock , hen-day and hen-housed production will be .... when all birds survive.(same)
14. .... is the popularly used index for estimating the performance of layers.(Hen –day production)
15. The permissible mortality percent per month is .... in case of layers.(1%)

Tick the right choice

1. The depreciation percentage on buildings is estimated at

   (a) 5% (b) 10% (c) 15% (d) 20%

   Ans: (a)

2. Rate of interest on term loan is:

   (a) 5% (b) 10% (c) 15% (d) 20%

   Ans: (c)

3. A value of one BCR indicates :

   (a) No loss (b) Loss (c) Profit (d) No profit

   Ans: (a) & (d).

4. Average number of eggs produced by a Light breed hen is:

   (a) 200 (b) 216 (c) 228 (d) 240

   Ans: (d)

5. The most economical point spread is :

   (a) 50 (b) 100 (c) 150 (d) 200

   Ans: (d)

6. The most desirable BFPR value is :

   (a) more than 1 (b) Less than 1

   (c) More than 2 (d) Two

   Ans: (c)

7. Most desirable feed efficiency in a layer farm is:

   (a) 4 (b) 3 (c) 2 (d) 1

   Ans: (d)

8. Net feed efficiency index in a layer flock should be:

   (a) 25 (b) 30 (c) 45 (d) None

   Ans: (c)

9. Performance efficiency index in a layer is related to:

   (a) Egg weight (b) Feed intake

   (c) Body weight (d) All of them

   Ans: (d)

Define the following

1. Performance efficiency index.
2. Hen-housed egg production.
3. Net feed efficiency index.
4. Broiler farm economy index.
5. Broiler performance efficiency index.

Write short notes on

1. Methods to reduce wasteful farm expenditure.
2. Factors affecting profitability of a broiler farm.

12

Marketing of Poultry Products

Ashok Kumar and Jyoti Palod

Poultry meat and eggs have high nutritive value. Egg is used as a standard for measuring the quality of other food proteins. It is a well balanced source of nutrients. Similarly poultry meat is easily digestible, high in protein and low in fat content. It contains all the essential amino acids. Though the poultry meat and egg production have tremendously increased in India during last few decades however due to lack of organized marketing channels poultry producers are not getting reasonable returns. Indian broiler and egg markets are in a disorganized state. In last few decades various efforts have been made so as to organize and co-ordinate marketing channel of poultry meat and eggs. Through these efforts producers are also benefited but only in some particular areas. Therefore, there is need to expand it further covering the country.

What is Marketing?

Marketing may be defined as exchange of a produce for an agreed sum of money. It is a commercial process involved in promoting, selling and distributing a product. In simple words marketing is finding out what customers want and supplying it at a profit. Marketing is a business in terms of customer needs and their satisfaction. As per P. Taylor, marketing is not simply providing products or services; it is essentially about providing changing benefits to the changing needs and demands of the customer.

Marketing Activities

Various activities involved in marketing include the collection, evaluation and dissemination of marketing information; planning and scheduling of production; forming contracts between buyers and sellers; constant improvement of all post-harvest activities and co-coordinating inputs viz. transport, processing, storage, credit, health-care etc. A complete and continuous flow of products from the producers to the consumers contributes to the maintenance of high level of economic activity. Efficient marketing of poultry products is a strong bridge between production and consumption and is essential to provide reasonable returns to rural small poultry producers, for whom it becomes extremely difficult.

India's share of the world trade in poultry and poultry products is very small, however India tops in dried eggs exports (FAO, 2007). India ranks 8th in duck exports, but for other products like chicken, chicken meat and liquid egg, India does not rank in top 20 countries. The major products exported by India are live poultry, hatching and table eggs, egg powder, frozen eggs, poultry meat and specific pathogen free eggs (SPF eggs). The exports of poultry and poultry products from India have a great potentiality due to competitive production costs and nearness to major export markets.

Objectives of Poultry Marketing

i) It provides gainful employment to millions of people and thereby increases income of the people.

ii) It enhances the demand for poultry products, thereby creating employment opportunities to rural masses for producing different poultry products.

iii) It also improves the income level, standard of living and health status of poultry farmers by providing essential amino acids, fatty acids, vitamins, minerals etc. in the form of poultry products which are essential for their health.

iv) Marketing of poultry products makes available of the same at the right time, place, quantity and price.

v) Organized marketing system contributes to the rise in the standard of living of the society by identifying the needs of the society, which would ensure required supply of poultry products.

Marketing of Eggs

Marketing of eggs includes movement of eggs from producer to the consumer. Eggs are marketed in various forms. Development of Indian egg market is not in pace with the increased egg production. Egg price vary from town to town and season to season. Egg marketing involves physical movement and distribution of eggs from place of production to place of consumers and type of package in which it is offered for sale. Between producers to consumer, there are many details of collections, grading, transportation and storage, financing and selling. The main objective of marketing of the whole eggs is to put the eggs in the hands of the consumer with good quality.

Organizational Structure of Egg Marketing

There are mainly two organizations related to egg marketing.

These organizations are:

1. National Egg Co-ordination Committee (NECC)
2. Agro-corpex India Limited

National Egg Coordination Committee (NECC)

In India National Egg Co-ordination Committee (NECC) was formed on 14th May 1982 by Dr.B.V.Rao with a membership of more than 25,000 poultry farmers. It is the largest single association of the poultry farmers in the world. It is a unique institution where irrespective of size or location, the farmer for his entire production, at his farm-gate gets the official notified price (as decided by elected farmer representatives of NECC every day and is published in local leading dailies).

NECC has role in market intervention, price support operations, egg promotion campaigns, consumer education, market research, rural market development and liaisons with the government on vital issues concerning the industry. It is based on co-operative spirits and right to determine their own selling price. It takes no profits and subsists on voluntary contribution from members of layer farmers.

NECC is the only agency, well recognized by policy makers in State and Centre as representative body of poultry industry to represent the interests of poultry. Two strategies are taken by NECC to declare and maintain the prices of eggs: (i) Egg promotion campaigns to increase the market size and demand for eggs (ii) Market intervention to stabilize egg prices. To ensure that traders do not exploit farmers, NECC undertakes Market Intervention Scheme as and when necessary by extension of subsidy or directly procuring eggs for cold storage in the domestic market. NECC also has Agrocorpex India Limited (ACIL), a Public Limited Company, entirely owned and managed by poultry farmers. NECC has also been instrumental, at the instance of poultry farmers, in incorporating Bharat Egg Producer's Association (BEPA), which encourages export of shell eggs, promotion of eggs in electronic and print media and sponsors sports and related activities to promote consumption of poultry products. However marketing on the basis of NECC has some practical problems like limited operational area and lack of resources to undertake a total programme of procurement, storage, transportation and retailing of eggs.

AgroCorpex India Limited (ACIL)

ACIL was started in the year 1982 by the farmers in Andhra Pradesh; however it became operational in April, 1987 at Vijayawada. Now ACIL has operations at Hyderabad, Ajmer, Ludhiana, Ambala, Delhi, Kolkata, Chennai and Hospet. It procures eggs from its farmer members only. As a result, the farmers are assured of marketing of their egg produce. It lifts eggs on its own and also with the help of NAFED, NECC and BEPA. It keeps surplus stocks in cold storages and helps farmers getting over the crisis. Therefore, ACIL helps farmers in marketing of their eggs without loss.

ACIL has been successful by regular procurement of eggs from its farmers and market their eggs, thereby improving marketing of poultry products. It initiated export of eggs in the year 1990 and in the year 1999-2000 it had exported about 18.6 million eggs and earned foreign exchange of 28.97 million. Streamlining the domestic markets it has made a place in international markets and brings the Indian poultry on the global map.

National Agricultural Cooperative Marketing Federation of India

The National Agricultural Cooperative marketing Federation of India (NAFED) has taken up egg – marketing in Delhi and other big cities. It has also announced support price for eggs during slum periods to help small poultry farmers. It has its own cold storage facility to store surplus eggs received during peak season. NAFED performs these duties on the recommendation of NECC, the losses if any due to this intervention are shared by the government and NECC.

Marketing Channels for Eggs

Broadly, there are 4 channels of marketing:-

a. **Direct marketing**: Producer to Consumer

b. **Indirect marketing**: Producer to Consumer via- Retailer

c. **Integrated marketing**: Producer to Consumers via some Collectors or Commission agents.

d. **Co-operative marketing**: Producer to Consumer via Cooperative agency.

Under direct marketing (channel a), there is benefit to both producer and consumer. However in co-operative marketing (channel d) poultry farmers receive some other benefits also from cooperative societies such as cheap and good quality feed, medicines, technical advices and some time day-old chicks at relatively cheaper price. The price spread i.e. difference between cost of production and retail price of egg tends to increase by increase in the number of intermediaries.

Challenges

In India, eggs are still transported in open condition and in un-refrigerated vehicles. The entire chain of distribution and physical handling up to consumer is in open climate exposed to varying temperatures of seasons and agro climatic conditions. Shelf life of eggs is therefore restricted to 11-14 days in summer and 18-20 days in winter. The egg is still sold as a commodity in India and purchased by consumer mostly from shop next door for daily needs i.e. *kirana* stores, bakeries etc. With a drastic increase in egg production it should be ensured that eggs for consumers must be made available in vast number of shops and stocked sufficient to meet daily needs of consumers.

Suggestions for Successful Marketing of Eggs

i) Formation of co-operative should be greatly encouraged.

ii) Grading of eggs as per BIS must be encouraged and their price should be strictly on the basis of grade.

iii) Cold storage facility should be created to overcome the spoilage of eggs due to seasonal fluctuation.

iv) Proper care must be taken during packaging & transportation of eggs.

v) Vigorous campaigns need to be done for sales promotion and consumer's education about the nutritive value of eggs.

Marketing of Poultry Meat

The production of poultry for the purpose of meat becomes very popular in recent years. In olden days most of the poultry meat marketed were by-product of egg production, but now the poultry meat marketed are produced by large farms which are well specialized in production of chickens, turkeys, ducks and Japanese quail etc. The success of the broiler industry in the last few decades leads to the change in food preferences of the consumers.

Marketing of poultry meat ranges from street corner live bird slaughter (wet market), to a highly sophisticated, fully automated and International Standards Organization (ISO) certified facilities and ready to eat convenience products.

Trading of poultry meat is very volatile where prices are determined based on demand-supply in a given market for the day. The prices of poultry meat fluctuate widely and even short surpluses result in a very wide fluctuation in market prices.

In India, there is lack of suitable coordinated channel for marketing of poultry meat. Marketing of live or dressed chickens is the major problem faced by most of the small and medium farmers. They are dependent on traditional traders. If there is overproduction compared to market demand, the farmers get great economic losses. Mostly middlemen exploit poultry farmers.

Organizational Structure of Poultry Meat Marketing

The poultry meat consumers are becoming more and more aware of quality and demanding for meat and poultry products processed in clean and sanitary environment and "convenience items" such as semi cooked, ready-to-eat, ready-to-cook products. A focused approach and intensive efforts are required to address the issues related to production of hygienic, safe and wholesome poultry meat and meat products; harmonization of domestic and international standards and also to address the arising environmental issues.

The organizations related to poultry meat marketing in India are:

1. Broiler marketing Cooperative Society (BROMARK)
2. Broiler Coordination Committee (BCC)
3. National Meat and Poultry Processing Board (NMPPB)

1. Broiler Marketing Cooperative Society

Bromark is an all India Broiler Farmers' body registered under the Multi State Cooperative Societies Act in 1994. The objective of the BROMARK is to ensure that the gap between producer's and consumer's price should be reduced and promote the consumption of chicken meat by highlighting its nutritive value. Similar to NECC, BROMARK fixes price for live broiler at all important production centers in the state by assessing the demand and supply trends and try to reduce middlemen exploitation to the maximum extent.

2. Broiler Coordination Committee

Broiler Coordination Committee (BCC) is an organization formed by leading poultry integrators in India for fixing the price of marketing broilers.

3. National Meat and Poultry Processing Board

National Meat and Poultry Processing Board is launched in the year 2009 with the aim to raise domestic standards in meat and poultry processing to international level. The board will also take market surveys and help the industry to create market intelligence, database and its dissemination on regular basis for improvement of the meat sector. It is an autonomous body and initially funded by the Government of India and later it would be managed by the industry itself.

Marketing Channels for Poultry meat

In India the prevailing marketing channels for meat are as under

1. Producer → Consumer
2. Producer → Retailer → Consumer
3. Producer → Wholesaler → Retailer → Consumer
4. Producer → Commission agent → Wholesaler → Retailer → Consumer
5. Producer → Cooperative society → Retailer → Consumer
6. Producer → Institutional market/ own retail outlets → Consumer

Direct marketing (1) is much better than all other channels, wherein, both poultry farmers and consumers are benefited. However major portion of meat is being marketed through channel no. 3.

The price spread i.e. difference between cost of production and retail price of meat tends to increase by increase in the number of intermediaries.

Challenges

In India most of the poultry meat is sold as live birds or in wet form. Under this type of marketing there is no chance for storage whatever birds produced in surplus are to be sold by producers at very low costs. But in developed countries, poultry meat is sold as ready-to-cook frozen form. In this form there is convenient transportation even to distant places as there are least chances of spoilage and deterioration of meat. Properly frozen meat is superior to chilled or fresh poultry. Though in India processed meat marketing has also been started but to a limited extent, it should be encouraged further so as to improve the potential for both export and domestic uses.

Suggestions for Successful Marketing

Integration: Integration in broiler production is recently introduced and has been gaining momentum. A bulk of production i.e. approximately 60% is under integration and the rest is held by independent and small scale producers. Now, **contract farming** under integration is assuming significance, wherein, farmers are given all the inputs and paid for growing charges based on performance. As all-in-all-out system is practiced and farm size is small with owner and family supervision of the flock, the performance is better and cost of production is lesser as compared to production by individual farmer.

Marketing of Processed chicken: The market for frozen or chilled poultry products is only limited to few institutions i.e. hotels, fast-food restaurant chains and limited urban consumers. This very small segment of consumers is served by processing sector, whose volume account for about 2% - 3% of production. However, there is scope in the coming decades for new chicken processing plants to come up and selling of processed chicken to increase to cater both domestic market as well as export markets.

Opportunities for Marketing of Poultry Products

- **Rural market:** In India poultry farms are mostly located in semi urban and urban areas therefore, availability of eggs and poultry meat are high in urban and semi urban areas, but in rural areas and rest of the country, the availability is low. Thus there is a vast scope to tap the rural markets and NE states where consumption is low because of poor availability. Along with this, sufficient number of sale outlets for eggs and poultry meat in villages will help in improving the per capita consumption of eggs.
- **Export of Eggs and Poultry meat:** India is ideally located and can fulfill the requirements of the Middle East and Far Eastern countries for shell eggs. Therefore vast scope exists for export of shell eggs and of poultry meat.
- **Eggs in Mid-day meal scheme:** Egg is a balanced food item that cannot be adulterated. The Supreme Court has advised all states to implement the midday meals scheme. This scheme is implemented in certain states only. Even if one egg per child per week is served, the egg consumption will increase enormously. This will improve the health status of the under-privileged children, and improve the attendance in schools, besides help in increasing the per capita egg consumption and maintaining remunerative price for eggs.

The future growth of poultry industry will depend on systematic planning for efficient marketing of poultry products in the country.

Question Bank

I. Fill in the blanks with word (s)

1. .... is the process of selling & distribution of a product.
2. NECC stands for..
3. NECC was established in the year ....
4. NECC strategies to declare and maintain egg prices are ....and ....
5. ACIL stands for ....
6. ACIL was incorporated in ....and started its operation in ....
7. .... are the various ways through which products flow from producer to consumer.

II. Match the following

1. Egg marketing in 1980	:	a) Dr.B.V.Rao
2. Duck export	:	b) Marketing of poultry meat
3. Father of modern Indian poultry	:	c) 8th rank
4. ACIL	:	d) Monopoly
5. BROMARK	:	e) Marketing of eggs

III. What is marketing & what are the different activities involved in marketing?

IV. What are the objectives of poultry marketing?

V. Why there is a necessity to setup an organization for egg marketing?

VI. Describe the role of NECC in egg marketing.

VII. What are the different channels for eggs and poultry meat marketing?

VIII. What are the measures to be followed for successful marketing of eggs?

IX. What is poultry integration & how it helps in commercialization of broilers?

Answers

I. (1) Marketing (2) National Egg Co-ordination Committee (3) 1982 (4) Egg promotion campaign , market intervention to stabilize egg price (5) AgroCorpex India Limited (6) 1982, April 1987 (7) Marketing channels

II. (1) d (2) c (3) a (4) e (5) b

13

Setting-Up of Farm for Different Classes of Poultry

J.D. Mahanta

Selection of site for a poultry farm: The following points should be considered while selecting site or location for a poultry farm.

- The farm should be located at an elevated area with proper facilities for drainage.
- To protect the farm against strong wind, tall trees may be planted surrounding the farm complex.
- The farm should be located not too far from city to bring in and take out materials.
- The commercial farm should be located near to marketing centres.
- The breeder farm should be located in an isolated area away from commercial farm to ensure biosecurity.
- The farm should have an easy access to connecting roads.
- The site should have provision of electricity.
- The desirable soil type for a poultry farm is loamy or sandy loam.
- There should be provision of abundant potable water at the site. The water should be tested for various impurities like total solids, microbiological contamination, high percentage of salts of Na, K and Chlorine, nitrite, nitrate etc. Total bacterial count and Coliform count should be 0/ml.

Setting-Up of Broiler Chicken Farm

Chicken in many forms has always been a dish to relish among most Indians. Widely accepted and consumed, the demand for chicken is only increasing. India ranks fourth in broiler production contributing 3.0 million tons of broiler meat in the world. In a country like India, due to lack of religious associations, the demand for broiler products is growing rapidly. Translated, this provides great potential for success and growth in the poultry industry.

Housing for Broilers

- **System of housing**: The broilers may be raised on deep litter, in cages or in batteries with slatted or wire floor systems. However, deep litter system of housing is the most widely used system for broilers.
- **System of rearing**: All-in all out system and Multiple batch systems.
- **Optimal environmental conditions for rearing broiler**: Temperature: 22-30°C (70-85°F), Relative humidity: 30-60%, Ammonia: less than 25 ppm, Litter moisture: 15-25%, Air flow: 10-30 metres per minute.

Essentials of Broiler Housing

- **Orientation**: The broiler houses should be oriented with their long axis facing East-West direction to avoid direct sunlight falling into the building.
- **Elevation**: The floor level of broiler houses should be elevated 30 cm (one foot) above the outer ground level to prevent seepage of water into the house. However, in high rainfall and flood prone areas like Assam, the floor level should be raised upto 90 cm (three feet) above the ground level.
- **Floor type**: The floor should be made of cement concrete to prevent damage by rodents and to permit easy and efficient cleaning and disinfection.
- **Width and length of broiler house**: The width of open-sided broiler houses should not be wider than 24 ft (7.2 m) or less than 16 ft (4.8 m) to permit optimal cross ventilation. However, in tunnel ventilated broiler houses fitted with automatic feeders and drinkers, the width may extend upto 12.0 m. The length of the house may vary depending on the required capacity and the length of the available land.
- **Walls:** The long walls on the sides should not be more than 35 cm high above the floor level, with the rest of the area covered with a mesh. The

top of the sidewall should be tapered sloping downwards to avoid young birds perching on the wall. The wall should be thoroughly cement plastered. The space between the top of the sidewall and the roof must be covered with wire mesh (1.25 x 1.25 cm, 20-22 gauge thick), welded mesh (2.5 x 5.0 cm, 12-14 gauge thick) or chain link (2.5 cm, 12 gauge thick). It should be durable, strong and close enough to prevent the entry of rodents and predators.

- **Doors**: The doors may be fitted with strong G.I. rod supporting frames of welded mesh at 8-10 m interval, each 1m in width and 2m high.
- **Roof**: The roof may be thatched, tiled or covered with light roof (asphalt or bitumen), asbestos sheets or C.I. sheets. Thatched roofs are cheaper, but less durable and may leak. They provide a cooler environment during the hot summer. To prevent leakage, the slope of thatched roofs must be steeper. Asbestos or C.I. sheets are durable, but more costly. Tiled roofing is good for small scale farm and asbestos roofing for larger farms. The height of the roof should preferably be 2.5 to 3.0 m at eaves. The height at ridge should be 3.5 to 4.5 m in case of deep litter house. Thatched roof may have a lower height of 1.95 m at the eaves. The roof may be painted with white aluminium paint to reflect the sun's ray and thereby reduce the heat build-up within the house. Roof overhang should be 1.0 to 1.5 m on either side to provide shade and prevent rain water. No free space be provided between roof and wall to prevent entry of sparrows and other predators. In severe summer, it is better to provide ridge ventilation at the roof.
- **Floor space allowance**: The floor space requirement per broiler depends on their body weight, housing system and climatic condition. About 0.6 sq. ft. per kg live body weight is the required floor space on floor under tropical condition. For a body weight of 1650 g, one sq. ft. of floor space is sufficient. In summer the space allowance may be increased by 20 per cent and in winter deduced by 15 per cent.
- **Footbath**: A footbath should be constructed at the entrance of the poultry house. An ideal dimensions of a foot-bath is : 90 cm X 45cm X 10cm.

Choice of Strains of Broiler

Choice of strains of broiler is one of the major factors responsible for successful broiler farming. It depends on strain of the broiler chick available in the hatchery, chick weight, distance to the farm from hatchery, vaccination programme followed in the breeding flock, vaccination given to the chicks, feed efficiency and body weight. Choice of strain is also done on the prevailing records of the products in the field or Random Sample Poultry Performance Test conducted by Central Poultry Performance Testing Centre, Ministry of Agriculture, Govt. of India. Some of the popular commercial strains of broiler are Cobb-400, Cobb-200, Hubbard, Hybro, B-77, Ross, Starbro, Charbro, IBB-83, IBB-80, IBL-80, Caribro-91, Pearlbro Samrat, Hubchix etc.

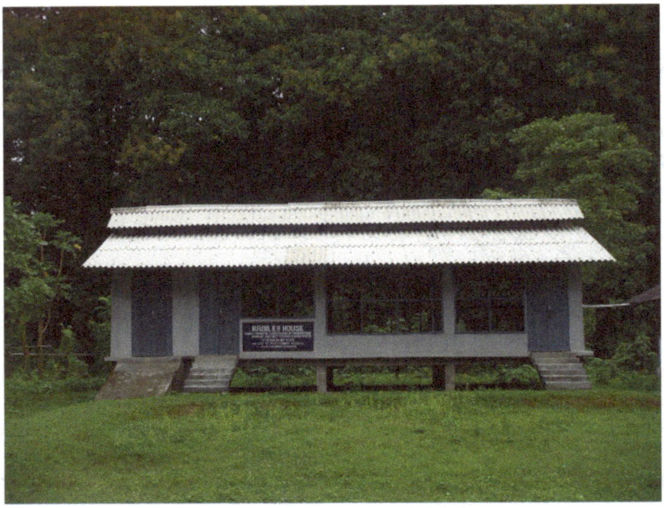

Fig. 22: Full Monitor type broiler house

Setting-Up of Layer Chicken Farm

Egg being an excellent source of proteins is fast becoming a favorite among urban Indians. India today is the third largest egg producer in the world. According to the Ministry of Agriculture, India's egg production is estimated at 59.84 billion eggs per annum. Today, with more and more 'eggitarians' on the rise, egg consumption is growing at 8 to 10 per cent annually.

Essential of a Good House

- **Proper type**- optimum width, height, roof and ventilation according to housing system.
- **Adequate floor space**- The floor space allowances depending upon breed, age, size etc. are as follows:

Age of bird	Floor space (cm^2) minimum	
	Light breed	Heavy breed
0-8 weeks	700 cm^2	700 cm^2
9-12 weeks	950 cm^2	950 cm^2
13-20 weeks	1900 cm^2	2350 cm^2
Above 20 weeks	2300-2800 cm^2	2800-3700 cm^2

In battery system the floor space required is 1/3 of the space recommended for intensive system

- **adequate ventilation**- adjustment according to season
- **sunlight**- without any glare on water and equipment
- **distribution of light in the house**- adequate
- **sanitation** in-and-around poultry house
- **dryness** in-and-around poultry house
- **protection** from predators and parasites

Number of Layer Houses

The number of buildings required for layers varies according to the length of intervals between introduction of each batch of chicks. Based on this the layer farm may be established as under:

- 1+2 pattern- One brooder cum grower house + two layer house (chicks to be received at 28- week interval).
- 1+3 pattern- One brooder cum grower house + three layer house (chicks to be received at 20- week interval).
- 1+1+5 pattern- One brooder house + one grower house + five layer house (chicks to be received at 12- week interval).

Types of Poultry Houses

According to purposes: Brooder house, grower house and layer house

According to roof style: Flat (RCC) roof, shed type, gable, full monitor, dome and half-monitor

According to construction: Deep litter and cage house

Types of Cages

Battery cages: The compartments of cages are arranged one above the other in 3 or 4 tiers on stands and dropping tray is kept underneath of each tier for collection of faeces. Dropping trays are to be cleaned daily or on alternate days. Feeders and waterers are attached to cages from outside.

Elevated platform/ Californian cages: The compartments of cages are arranged stepwise on both sides of cage row in two or three tiers on stands. Elevated cages are 3 types

(a) Brooder cage (0-6 weeks)

(b) Grower cage (7-18 weeks)

(c) Layer cage (19 weeks and above)

3-tire, M-type layer cage

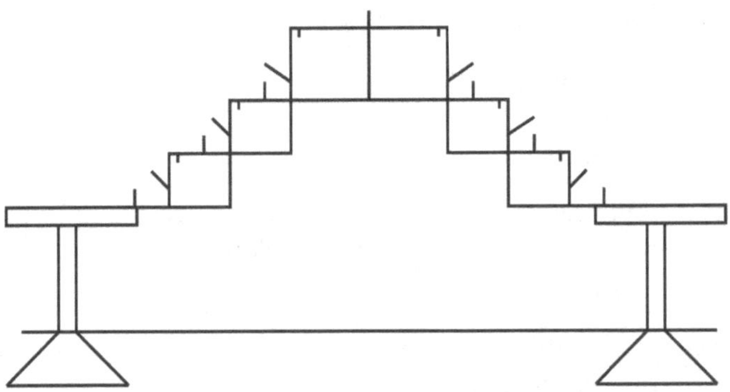

Raised Platform Broiler, Breeder Cage House

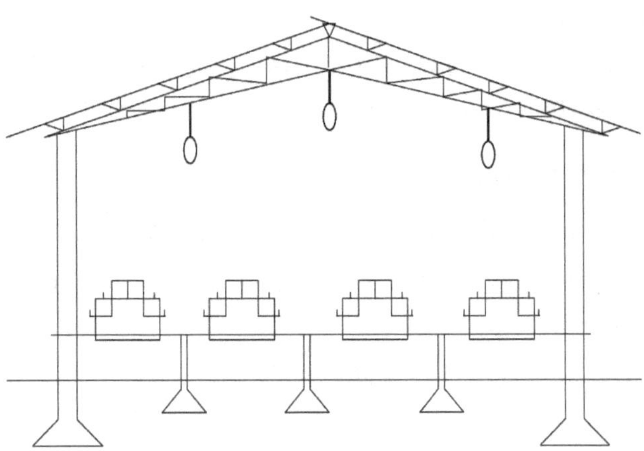

Cage house for breeders

Cage sizes depending upon the capacity of birds

- 45 x 30 cm- for 3 birds
- 45 x 40 cm- for 4 birds
- 50 x 35 cm- for 4 birds
- 50 x 45 cm- for 5 birds
- 60 x 37.5 cm- for 5 birds

Setting-Up of a Duck Farm

Systems of Rearing

- **Range system:** Under rural conditions ducks are traditionally reared in free range system of management. Generally a thatched house is provided for brooding and rearing upto one month of age. Later they will be partly fed and let out during day time for foraging and later the house is used only as a night shelter.
- **Semi-intensive system:** In semi-intensive system of rearing, the house should have easy access to outside run as the ducks prefer to come out during the day time, winter and rainy time. The run should have slope away from the house to provide drainage. In the house of semi-intensive system, a continuous water channel of size 50 cm wide and 15-20 cm depth should be constructed at the far end, on the both sides, parallel to the pen in the grower and layer houses.

Table 10: Floor space, feeder space and drinker space requirements of duck (under intensive system)

Age	Floor space (sq. ft)		Feeder space (linear inches)		Drinker space (linear inches)	
	Meat type	Egg type	Meat type	Egg type	Meat type	Egg type
0-3 weeks	1.0	0.85	2.0	2.0	1.0	1.0
4-8 weeks	2.5	1.75	4.0	3.0	2.0	1.5
9-20 weeks	4.0	3.00	5.0	3.5	2.5	1.75
Adult	5.0	4.00	6.0	4.0	3.0	2.0

- **Intensive system-** In this system ducks are fully confined inside the house with all facilities of feeding, watering, lighting etc.

Location and Layout

- A duck farm usually comprises pens, yard space for foraging and ponds / water troughs for swimming. While the later is optional because ducks can survive without water for swimming, experience has shown that the presence of ponds / troughs help to maintain ducks in healthier condition.
- Yards should slope gently away from the pens to provide good drainage. Ponds/ water troughs should be located at the end of the yard opposite the pens. Pens should be constructed in an East – West direction to protect the birds from direct sunrays and reduce the amount of rain that can be blown into the pens.
- The houses should be well ventilated, dry and rat-proof.

Setting-Up of a Turkey Farm

Systems of Rearing

- **Range system**: Turkeys are reared under range system in the backyards of rural households. For rearing a flock of 100 turkeys, the land required is 1-2 acres with good foraging or large backyard under free range village atmosphere. A thatched house is provided for brooding and rearing upto one month of age. Later they will be partly fed and let out during day time for grazing and the house will be used only as a night shelter. Turkeys are better forager than chicken and can digest fibre better than chickens.
- **Semi-intensive system**: For commercial production semi-intensive system is popular. Under this system, turkey poults are reared up to 6 weeks of age in closed, confined houses, after which they are allowed to forage for a few hours in an open yard during the day and then housed in the shelter for the rest of the day and night. Growers and breeders are reared under this type of semi-intensive system.

Table 11: Floor space allowance for turkeys under semi-intensive system

Age in week	Space per bird (m^2)	
	Shelter	Open yard
7-12 weeks	0.09	0.18
13-16 weeks	0.16	0.32
17 week to market age	0.22	0.45
Breeders	0.27	0.54

- **Intensive system:** In general the management of turkeys is similar to that of chicken. The house should be located at an elevated place and cement floors are preferred. Turkeys require warmer condition than chicken.

Table 12: Floor space allowance for turkeys under intensive system

Age (weeks)	Space per bird
0-4 weeks	900 cm^2
5-8 weeks	0.135 m^2
9-12 weeks	0.180 m^2
13-16 weeks	0.230 m^2
After 16 weeks	0.360 m^2

Setting-Up of a Guinea Fowl Farm

Systems of Rearing

- **Free range system**-In this system birds sometimes spend their nights on the trees around farmer's dwelling or a night shelter is provided
- **Semi-free range system**-For meat type guinea fowl, aviary rearing in enclosures surrounded by wire mesh and roofed over by netting is very common. For 1000 guinea fowl chicks, a starter house of 24 m^2 is required for housing during first three weeks. This communicates with the rearing house to which the chicks are then transferred. This comprises of 40 m^2 shelter equipped with perches and further leads into an aviary of 200 m^2. This accommodation should be located on a permeable soil showing slight slope for water drainage. For egg type guinea fowls, hens are made flightless by amputating extremity of wings at the most distal joint. The hens lay eggs wherever she chooses and nest need not be provided

Setting-Up of a Japanese Quail farm

Japanese quail is a small fast growing bird. Its meat is a gourmet's delight. The Indian and Chinese systems of medicine claim that the flesh of Japanese quail has varying medicinal properties. Japanese quail is the domesticated species widely reared throughout the world for meat and egg.

Systems of Rearing

- **Floor rearing-** Under floor rearing system , the roofing can be made of thatch or tiles, while the floor has to be made of concrete to facilitate easy cleaning and disinfection. When Japanese quails are reared for table purpose, about 5 quails per square feet area (floor space per bird: 180 cm^2) can be raised. In a 10' x 10' (0.9 m^2) room, about 500 Japanese quails can be reared up to market age (5 weeks). Alternatively, after two weeks of rearing on the floor, quails can be reared in cages up to market age. Brooding of chicks is done in brooder house having litter materials like paddy husk or groundnut hulls upto the depth of 2.5 cm. In a brooder guard circle of 3 feet diameter (90 cm), about 150 chicks can be accommodated.

Table 13: Feeder and drinker space requirements for Japanese quail

Age in weeks	Feeder space per bird (cm)	Drinker space per bird (cm)
0-2 weeks	0.6	0.3
3-5 weeks	1.2	0.6

Up to 2 weeks, two chick drinkers of 10 cm diameter and 1.5 cm high on the sides, each of 500 ml capacity and two feeder plates of 22 cm diameter and 2 cm high will be sufficient for 150 chicks in each brooder circle. From the third week, a linear feeder 45 cm long, 2.5 cm height and 10 cm wide and a drinker of 15 cm diameter and 2.5 cm high at the brim and 1200 ml capacity will be sufficient for 75 quail chicks.

- **Cage rearing**: Two different types of cages are required to rear Japanese quail chicks upto market age.

i) **Brooder quail cage rearing**: In brooder cage, chicks are reared from day-old to 17-18 days of age. The cages are designed as multi-tier cages (four to five tiers arranged one over the other) with about a 10 cm gap between each tier, and a dropping tray fitted into the gap. The size of a brooder cage of 4 to 5 tier is 180 x 120 x 25 cm and each tier can be divided into four compartments of 90 x 60 cm size each. About 100 chicks can be reared in each compartment, and 400 chicks in each tier, Provisions must be made for heating bulbs in the centre of each compartment.

ii) **Grower quail cage rearing**: The size of a grower cage is 240 x 120 x 25 cm and each tier is divided into four compartments of 120 x 60 cm size each. About 60 quails can be reared in each compartment up to market size. Feeders and waterers are fixed outside the cage unit. Japanese quail chicks should not be left without feed or water at any time. This will affect their growth rate and increase the mortality rate.

Question Bank

I. Fill in the blanks

1. Desirable soil type for a poultry farm is .... or ....
2. The optimum ammonia level in a broiler house should be less than ....ppm.
3. The floor level of broiler houses should be elevated .... above the outer ground level.
4. The width of open-sided broiler houses should not be wider than .... feet
5. Height of the roof of broiler house should preferably be .... to .... metre at eaves.
6. For a body weight of 1650 g, of broiler .... sq. ft. of floor space is sufficient.
7. For rearing a flock of 100 turkeys, the land required is .... acres
8. In a brooder guard circle of 3 feet diameter, about.........quail chicks can be accommodated.
9. For commercial turkey production .... system is popular.

II. What are the criteria for selection of site for a poultry farm ?

IV. Write down the optimal environmental conditions for rearing of broiler chicken.

V. Describe the essentials of broiler housing.

VI. Write short notes on the following

a. Semi-free range system of guinea fowl
b. Essentials of a good chicken layer house
c. Semi-intensive system of duck rearing
d. Setting up of a turkey farm
e. Cage rearing of Japanese quail

Answers

(1) loamy, sandy loam (2) 25 (3) 30 cm (4) 24 (5) 2.5, 3.0 (6) one (7) 1-2 (8) 5 (9) semi-intensive

14

Organic and Hill Farmings

Ranjana Goswami and M Sarma

Organic Farming

The FAO/WHO Codex Alimentarius Commission defines organic farming as "*a unique production management system which promotes and enhances agro-ecosystem health, including biodiversity, biological cycles and soil biological activity, and this is accomplished by using on-farm agronomic, biological and mechanical methods in exclusion of all synthetic off-farm inputs*". It is a certification of a production system as opposed to the certification of a product. For a product to be certified organic, all operators in the product chain, including farmers, processors, manufacturers, exporters, importers, wholesalers and retailers must be certified organic. The establishment of organic animal/poultry husbandry requires a specific period called as "conversion period". This period is the time taken between the start of the organic management on farm and certification of livestock farm and its product. Changing from conventional to organic management system for livestock enterprises requires a careful and gradual approach. It is learnt that global organic product has increased 20% annually over the past 10 years. Though Australia, European Union and USA are leading organic producers, a recent study indicated that developing countries including India are also adopting the system and marching ahead.

Why Organic Poultry

In the last few decades poultry industry has transformed from mere backyard poultry to industrial status, but the issues of food safety and quality remained unaddressed. Today, consumers are increasingly concerned about the quality, source and conditions under which their food is grown. Hence, organic poultry farming has become an approach to address these issues. Organic products can help the consumers to limit exposure to pesticides and chemical based fertilizers. Organic chicken farming is cleaner and more environmental-friendly. In organic production, the chicken is treated in a most humane manner throughout its life. Consumers may also prefer the flavour of organic chicken or its products.

Certain Key Characteristic of Organic Poultry Production

- Preference for the use of natural rather than artificial processes
- Limits on unit sizes and stocking density, avoid intensive housing conditions
- Slower growing breeds encouraged
- No routine prophylactic drug treatments-usually only individual animals which are actually ill are treated
- Homeopathic and/or Ayurvedic treatments are preferred to Allopathic
- Breeding strategies are being developed to improve health, including fertility
- Considers the wider social and ecological impact of the organic production processing system
- Encourages and enhances biological cycles within the farming system involving micro-organisms, soil flora, plants and animals
- Maintains and increases the long-term fertility of soil
- Maintains genetic diversity of the production system and its surroundings, including the protection of plant and wildlife habitats
- Uses as far as possible renewable resources in locally organised production systems
- Creates a harmonious balance between crop production and animal husbandry
- Minimises all forms of pollution.

Guidelines for Producing Certified Organic Eggs

1. To produce a certified organic egg, the layer chicken itself must be certified organic or if from a conventional source, the layers must be fed with certified organic feed for at least six months prior to laying. No herbicides, fungicides, insecticides or chemical fertilizers are used.
2. Housing must allow for "reasonable liberty, normal socialization, maximum fresh air, day light and shelter from inclement weather conditions". The birds must have access to free range or large open air runs and has contact with the earth.
3. No antibiotics, prohibited parasiticides or coccidiostats are allowed to feed the layers; however, in the event of treatment, birds must be withdrawn from organic production for a period of 90 days or twice the official waiting period, whichever is later.
4. The minimum floor space for each layer be given 1.75 sq.ft. inside and 5 sq.ft., outside the shed.
5. The temperature in egg holding area be maintained at 60^0F.
6. *Nest:* At least one per 20 layers, which must be kept at least 20 inch above the ground.
7. *Temperature and Humidity:* 40 - 80^0 F and 60 - 80%.
8. *Waterers:* At least one bell drinker per 75-100 birds, or one nipple per 10-15 birds on line waterers.
9. *Feed:* All laying hens must be fed 100% certified organic feed from day one. Kitchen scraps feeding should be avoided. Organic standards prohibit the inclusion of genetically modified materials and products produced using genetically modified organisms. The vegetable origin feed resources and their by-products, include cereals, oil and legume seeds, tuber roots and forages. However, the by-products prepared using chemical solvents are not permitted. Animal products permitted for inclusion under the regulations include milk and fish or other marine animals, plus by-products.
10. *Roost Area:* Six inches per bird is allowed.
11. *Dust bath:* Should be provided, filled with materials like, dry sand, lime, earth etc.
12. *Litter:* Materials like sawdust, shavings, hay or straw, or ground cobs can be used.

13. *Floor:* The litter must be dry and microbially alive, and turned periodically sometimes mixing with lime to disinfect.

14. *Transportation and Transition:* Down time of two weeks between batches is encouraged to break parasite cycle. Clean house thoroughly, lime heavily, or spray a mild bleach solution to disinfect.

15. *Ventilation:* Should maintain proper air movement to avoid an overwhelming ammonia smell. *Ammonia levels in house should be less than 20 ppm.* Ridge ventilation is recommended to remove ammonia and moisture.

16. *Lighting:* Supplemental lighting is not mandatory but encouraged. A photoperiod of not more than 16 h. is recommended. Never decrease for hens once they are laying.

Guidelines for Producing Certified Organic Meat

- Chosen breed should be adaptable to local conditions; genetically engineered species or breeds are not allowed.
- Feed should contain 75% cereal and remaining 25% is composed of vegetable based protein.
- Stocking density requirement in France is 11 birds/m^2.
- Slaughter age – minimum 81 days
- Minimum free range – 2 m^2/bird.
- Birds must not be transported for more than 100 kms or 2 hours by road.
- Feed is intended to ensure quality production rather than maximizing production.
- Disease prevention is by the use of high quality feed, together with regular exercises and access to pasturage, having the effect of encouraging the natural immunological defence of the animal.
- Generally it is accepted that mortality rates are likely to be higher in birds kept under range.
- The estimated mortality rate is 10% for organic table birds.
- The development of an animal health plan is an essential part of any organic farming system. It takes account of all aspects of the individual including stress, general well being as well as physical symptoms.

Main Issues to be Considered for Organic Poultry Farming

1. **Soil type:** The soil needs to be relatively free draining. Heavy, wet land not only makes access difficult, but also creates more challenges for the birds.
2. **Shelter:** Poultry need a sheltered environment. If possible, exposed locations should be avoided.
3. **Feed:** Emphasis should be given to get 100% organic ration. It is important to maintain organic principles on home grown feed. Increasing feed prices and the emphasis organic principles place on home grown feed mean that feed is a major consideration for setting up an organic poultry production unit.
4. **Labour cost:** As compared to conventional system of rearing, organic poultry production is more labour intensive. The birds are housed in smaller groups, often in mobile housing.
5. **Infrastructure requirement:** Water should be available in the house and preferably also on the free range area. Organic feed ingredients should be available round the year. If there is no existing slaughter facility available, a processing unit should be set up on the farm.
6. **Capital investment:** To establish a successful and efficient organic poultry production unit, a considerable amount of capital investment is required.

Key Management Practices for Organic Poultry Production

1. **Selection of Breeds:** While selecting breeds emphasis be given on certain qualities like, disease resistance, productivity, hardiness and suitability for ranging. Organic poultry may be grown starting from conventional day-old chicks. Parent stock need not be an organically produced; conventional hatcheries may be utilized. Organic meat producers usually need meat-specific breeds that have been developed to finish in 12-14 weeks. There are no organic pullet rearing enterprises to supply layers for organic egg production, other than those who breed their own stock requirements. Under Soil Association standards, layers may be bought in from conventional sources up to 16 weeks of age and undergo a six weeks conversion period-the preferred option for large scale producers.
2. **Housing:** Housing must allow exercise, freedom of movement and reduction of stresses. Organic standards aim to provide an environment for poultry in which all normal behavior patterns can occur as this will

minimize the stress to the birds. Low stress levels are likely to have a positive effect upon both the health and production capacity of the flock. To protect poultry from predators, well designed housing system is important.

3. **Litter material:** Typical bedding may be dust-free wood shavings (not from treated wood), organic hay or straw etc.

Poultry Houses May be 2 Types: Static or Mobile

Static house: The main advantage of static housing is that it is easier to modify for atomization or semi- atomization for supply of feedstuffs, water and for the collection of eggs and droppings. One disadvantage of static housing system is the management of the outside area, where some rotational grazing needs to be implemented to reduce the risk of soil borne parasites and diseases and to maintain vegetation cover.

Mobile house: The main advantage of mobile housing is that the birds can be moved to fresh grass areas so that the risk of soil borne parasites in the outside area can be kept low. However, the disadvantage is that all other production system (feed, bedding/litter material and water) need to be transported to and from the houses, which increases the labour requirements, considerably. The cost of production is higher as compared to static housing system.

Free Range area: Organic poultry must have access to the outdoors, as seasonally appropriate. Any land the bird has access to must be certified organic.

Brooding: The aim during the brooding period is to create a comfort zone where the chick has the ideal temperature.

4. **Feeding:** Feed must be either purchased as certified organic or produced at the farm as per guidelines. Any agricultural product in feed or feed supplements must be organic and must be free of genetically modified organisms. Non-agricultural, natural ingredients, such as calcium or fish meal must be approved for use in organic operation. No animal by-products should be incorporated in organic poultry feed.

5. **Health management**:Proper biosecurity measures must be followed. Conventional veterinary medicines are allowed to treat the bird when no other suitable alternatives are available, but in all such cases the withholding period should be double the legal period. Uses of substances of synthetic origin including antibiotics are strictly prohibited. Vaccination should be used when diseases are established. As per National Standard for Organic Production in India, natural medicines including homeopathy and ayurvedic medicines shall be emphasized for treatment of diseases

in poultry. **Beak trimming** and **forced moulting** are not allowed in organic poultry production system. Poisons are not allowed for **predator** control.

6. **Slaughter Ages:** Slaughter ages depends upon the nature of birds used. All *converted birds* must undergo a 10 week conversion period. Fast growing and slow growing chicks (one-day-old) of non organic parent must be kept for at least 80 and 70 days respectively under organic standards. Poultry are regarded as slow growing if live weight gain is less than 45 g per day on standard feed ration. For egg production, if stock is usually purchased at about 12-14 weeks of age, then requires a conversion period of 6 weeks.
7. **Record keeping:** Records must be maintained on: the source of poultry, feed and supplements, source of any health products, vaccination, mortalities, outside access, house sanitation practices between flocks, and sale of finished products.

Advantages of Organic Poultry Farming

1. Products are safe and of good quality for human consumption.
2. It ensures to keep poultry in comfortable housing and environment and provides better welfare measures so that productive performance is better.
3. The production system is sustainable and scientific.
4. It generally avoids the use of antibiotics/drugs etc. for the treatment of sick animals, so that there is less chances of residual effect of drugs on animal products.
5. The organic chicken is only about 20% higher priced than conventional, compared to 30-40% price premiums for other organic meats.

Disadvantages of Organic Poultry Farming

1. It is generally difficult to spare more housing space as per standard.
2. The conversion period is very long.
3. Prolonged withdrawal period is required after any treatment with antibiotic or other drugs.
4. Due to strict adherence of various rules and regulations for organic poultry farming the products become costlier.

Hill Farming

1. Since time immemorial chickens are traditionally associated with tribal people with their religious rituals or sports. In hilly areas chickens are traditionally reared by tribal people to support their livelihood. Mostly the rearing is integrated with other animal husbandry practices. In the villages almost every household rears chicken, predominantly with *desi* or indigenous breed under scavenging system. The farmers spent very little time, money or rearing them. However, now-a-days exotic breeds like RIR, WLH, NH etc and improvised indigenous chicken breeds like Giriraja, Vanaraja, Athulya, Kuroiler etc. have found place in their sheds. As a result development of crossbred from these stocks due to indiscriminate mating in not uncommon.
2. The chickens are let loose in day-time for scavenging. During evening they are shut in and supplemented with extra feed.
3. Eggs produced from hill farming have good demand in local markets for their brown shell and yellow yolk. Both eggs and chicken meat are preferred by the consumers for delicacy and characteristic flavour as compared to that of exotic birds/eggs.
4. No elaborate housing is required for hilly chickens. Housing system allows the birds to be protected from inclement weather as well as from predators. Looking into smaller flock sizes the chicken sheds are erected smaller. In the hilly tracts where extreme weather is prevalent special type of housing is recommended. It should have double wall with some insulating space in between. The outer surface be painted with black to trap solar radiation. The roof should be double layered. Large glass walls or glass windows can be provided to trap the solar heat during the day. Double layered curtains made up of HDPE (High Density Polyethylene) can be used as double doors to prevent incoming chill air while opening and closing of the door. A false ceiling will make the shed cosy. Smaller houses are better, which should face South or South-East to get maximum Sun light. Proper ventilators should be constructed for oxygen supply to the birds and drive away litter ammonia. The bottom one-third of walls should be cemented. During night, curtains can be used to cover glass windows to avoid chilling.
5. **Rearing of egg laying chickens under intensive system:** Egg laying birds can also be raised under intensive system. Birds have to be fed with balanced diet. Special type of feeding with high energy has to be provided in winter. However, the feed cost will be increased due to the addition of transportation cost.

6. In certain areas where electricity is a problem brooding can be accomplished by using LPG (liquefied petroleum gas).
7. During cold season the birds have to be protected from chill wind. For this purpose the shed is to be arranged in such a way that the open sides are closed with HDPE sheet. Utmost care should be maintained while opening or closing the curtain since long time closing may pile up ammonia concentration; while frequent opening may lead to wind –chill.
8. **Feeding**: When the environmental temperature is low chicken eats; more feed to maintain its body temperature. As a rule of thumb 1% more feed should be provided for each 1^{0}C decrease of house temperature of 18-20^{0}C. To prevent feather loss, as this could lead to chilling of birds, extra fish meal or methionine should be provided.
9. **Commercial hill farming**: In high altitude of hill areas, the prevailing low oxygen concentration has detrimental effects on the embryonic development of chicken. A decrease in 10% hatchability has been observed for every 300 meter increase in altitude. Therefore, even if commercial breeding farms are maintained at high altitude their hatchery unit should be built at low altitude.
10. **Health care management**: High altitude may lead to respiratory problem of the flock due to lower atmospheric oxygen and chilling. Improper ventilation may complicate the situation. Cold air in the shed has lower water holding capacity; as a result the litter cacking may result. Improper ventilation may also lead to high ammonia concentration inside the shed associated with coccidiosis and ascaridiosis.
11. **Farmers training**: Exposure poultry farm training programme should be organized to the interested folks followed by periodical trainings to upgrade their knowledge on poultry husbandry.

Question Bank

I. True/False

1. Beak trimming is allowed in organic poultry farming.
2. Force moulting is not allowed in organic poultry farming.
3. In organic poultry farming vaccination against prevalent diseases may be allowed.
4. In organic poultry farming synthetic growth promoters or substances of synthetic origin for production are strictly prohibited.

5. For predator control, poisons are allowed in organic poultry farming.
6. Animal byproduct may be incorporated in organic poultry feed.
7. In organic poultry farming antibiotics are used to treat a specific problem, but can't be used routinely.
8. In high altitude of hill area, the low oxygen concentration has detrimental effects on the embryonic development of chicken.
9. At increasing altitude, hatchability generally increases.
10. In emergencies if antibiotics are used in organic poultry farming, in such cases the withholding period should be double the legal period.

II. What are organic egg and meat?

III. What is organic feed ?

IV. Write the difference between free range poultry and organic poultry.

V. What are the characteristics of organic poultry?

VI. Write the advantages and disadvantages of organic poultry farming.

Answers

I. 1.F 2.T 3.T 4.T 5.F 6.F 7.T 8.T 9.F 10.T

15

Conservation of Indigenous Germplasm

P.K. Shukla and Sujit Nayak

Conservation Biology emerged as the scientific study of the nature and status of Earth's biodiversity with the aim of protecting species, their habitats, and ecosystems from excessive rates of extinction. Biodiversity itself has a wider meaning unifying and taking into account species, within species breeds/ varieties, ecosystem, genetic and molecular diversity.

Need for Conservation

The progenitor of modern-day chicken has been the Red Jungle Fowl and over the years breeds have been developed slowly for commercial purpose as layers and broilers. However we still have lot of indigenous birds which cannot be defined in either category.

Breeding capabilities *Vs* biodiversity erosion: Presently only about 3-4 poultry breeding companies provide meat stocks for farms around the world. A similar number of companies supply birds for commercial egg production. As a result modern animal industry now uses only a few breeds of any species. Of the many breeds once commonly seen on farms, many have declined sharply in numbers and others have disappeared almost completely.

Productivity *Vs* Conservation: On one hand, to increase productivity we want certain natural characters to be eliminated and on the other we talk of conserving the indigenous varieties, which sounds contradictory.

Disease Resistance and Consumer Preferences

We have evidence in certain cases that indigenous breeds may have resistance to certain diseases, or are simply liked by local population for taste, look etc. For example research is underway for developing/ finding avian influenza resistant variety of poultry and may be some indigenous characters at genetic or molecular level come to the rescue in not only cases of avian influenza but other economically important diseases as well. Some characters of flavour or juiciness found in indigenous varieties may also be exploited for commercial purpose, later. For example, today tinted eggs, which have always been favoured in rural areas, are fetching a higher market value in urban areas also.

Food Security

The poorest of the poor in rural areas keep indigenous poultry for subsistence and nutrition. The commercial variety cannot survive as they require higher inputs and management as compared to that of indigenous varieties. Therefore, it is all the more necessary to establish the indigenous breeds and varieties and conserve them with an eye on posterity not only for commercial gains but possibly also as a potent tool for addressing livelihood.

Reasons for conservation can be summarized:

a) Economic potential

b) For research

c) To overcome selection plateaus which occur when genetic variation is lost

d) To take advantage of heterosis (hybrid vigour)

e) For cultural and organoleptic reasons

f) To provide a possible alternative for circumventing problems of:

- spread of disease
- climate change
- changing availability of feedstuffs
- social change, such as issues of animal welfare and environmental sustainability
- selection errors

Evolutionary and Domestication History

Systematics is the science of constructing an evolutionary history or phylogeny of a group of species. The following are the four major approaches:

a) Classical evolutionary taxonomy used to be done based on physical observation like Darwin did by grouping and classifying animals as per similarities and dissimilarities.

b) Phenetics is more like numerical taxonomy using multivariate statistical methods.

c) Cladistics focuses on shared derived characters and prepares a cladogram showing the lineage with specific breaks showing special acquisition of shared derived characters.

d) Cytogenetic and molecular techniques to assess chromosomal and molecular homologies and rearrangements, using techniques like karyotyping, Fluorescent *in-situ* Hybridisation (FISH), specific molecular probing, mitochondrial DNA sequencing etc.

Origin of Domestic Fowl

The present-day domesticated fowl is believed to have descended from the Red Jungle Fowl (*Gallus gallus domesticus*). Evolution of genus *Gallus* probably dates back 8 million years ago.

Red Jungle Fowl is similar to modern day chicken but characterized by some notable differences like moulting into eclipse plumage visible in male hackles, dusky blackish legs, females lack comb completely, horizontal carrying of tail, proportionately longer beaks and long prominent spur.

Domestication of Fowls

Domestic fowl occurred about 6000 BC in India, South-East Asia and China. The earliest evidence of domestication of chicken in Indian subcontinent is from Mohenjo-Daro. Malay Fowl or *Aseel* is reported to have evolved into our indigenous varieties. It is generally accepted that the keeping of chickens was for cock-fighting, later assuming religious significance and subsequently used for eggs and meat.

Emergence of Breeds

Natural selection and mutations within the species bestowed advantage to birds in certain environmental conditions leading to stable populations. Man influenced the evolutionary process by altering the rate of reproduction and production by selectively choosing favourable characteristics etc. This resulted in evolution of new types of birds within species having distinct characters. The geographically isolated groups ultimately formed breeds.

Definition of breeds varied and has been debated extensively. Largely we adopt the following version:

Breeds are Either

(a) A sub-specific group of domestic birds with definable and identifiable external characteristics that enable it to be separated by visual appraisal from other similarly-defined groups within same species; or

(b) A group for which geographical and/or cultural separation from phenotypically similar groups has led to acceptance of its separate identity.

Table 14: Some registered chicken breeds of India

S.N.	Breed	Home Tract
1.	Ankaleshwar	Gujarat
2.	Aseel	Chhattisgarh, Orissa and Andhra Pradesh
3.	Busra	Gujarat and Maharashtra
4.	Chittagong	Meghalaya and Tripura
5.	Danki	Andhra Pradesh
6.	Daothaigir	Assam
7.	Ghagus	Andhra Pradesh and Karnataka
8.	Harringhata Black	West Bengal
9.	Kadaknath	Madhya Pradesh
10.	Kalasthi	Andhra Pradesh
11.	Kashmir Faverolla	Jammu and Kashmir
12.	Miri	Assam
13.	Nicobari	Andaman & Nicobar
14.	Punjab Brown	Punjab and Haryana
15.	Tellichery	Kerala

Modern-day Chicken: Most of the present day populations are commercial hybrids involving WLH, Cornish, Barred Plymouth Rock, Rhode Island and Black Australorp. Presently we broadly categorize the birds under the following categories for census purpose:

Desi birds- Birds with production as low as 30-50 eggs per year and broody in nature; they include indigenous varieties but most are not well defined. However, most of the poultry population we refer to as '*desi*' are not defined under any breeds but are largely non-descript.

Improved birds- Synthetic and commercial varieties with higher yield and production.

Indigenous ducks mostly include, Nageswari, Sylhetmete, Chara and Chemballi and Muscovy varieties have been introduced to increase egg and meat production.

Steps Necessary for Conservation

***Inventory* and *Recording*:** Definition of a breed using breed descriptor and its level of risk has to be assessed for which factors such as the number of breeding males and females, overall numbers, number of sub-populations, and trends in population size need to be considered. It is thus important to monitor numbers and change in numbers on an on-going basis.

***Evaluation*:** Stocks must be characterized for phenotype and genotype, using new technology as appropriate. Gene mapping approaches such as testing for Single Nucleotide Polymorphisms (SNP's) help to track ancestry and to determine the genetic distance of one group from another. Phenotypic performance evaluation must be standardized, and carried out in the environment in which the stocks might be used.

Choice: Choice of breeds for conservation must include cultural reasons, potential value and threat of extinction. New mathematical techniques and economic theories assist in assessing risk of loss and potential benefits. Saving pure breeds preserves that breed's characteristics and makes a readily identifiable animal. Crossing several breeds to produce composites has the advantage of saving the genetic material from all while reducing upkeep costs. However the total genotype of each breed is lost.

Note: Conservation and Preservation are considered synonyms by many. However, rescuing and restoration of breeds which have reached a critical level may be more appropriately called preservation. Cryogenic storage of germplasm may also be termed as preservation. Conservation is management for a sustainable use and further enhancement of potential.

Methods of Conservation

Ex situ preservation involves the conservation of poultry away from its normal habitat. It is used to refer to the collection and freezing in liquid nitrogen of animal genetic resources in the form of living semen, ova or embryos. It may also be the preservation of DNA segments in frozen blood or other tissues. The potentiality exists to use DNA and cloning to re-develop breeds, but the technology is still new and costs are high.

In situ conservation is the maintenance of live poultry in their adaptive environment or natural habitat, as close to it as is practically possible.

The relative advantages and disadvantages of the major systems are summarized below:

Table 15: Comparing *Ex situ* and *In situ* merits

Parameters	*Ex Situ*	*In situ*
Cost		
initial set up cost	Relatively high	Low to high
maintenance cost	Low	Relatively low to high
GENETIC DRIFT		
Initial	Relatively high	Low
Annual	None	Moderate to high
Applied to all species	No	Yes
Safety/Reliability	Good to bad	Moderate
Local access	Moderate to poor	Moderate to good
International access	Good	Not good
Population monitoring	None	Good
Environmental adaptation	None	Good
Selection for use	None	Good

(*Source*: FAO)

Who are doing or can do it?

Individuals: Private producers keep stocks of minor breeds, as a hobby or as part of a farm enterprise. Emphasis may be on phenotype and small populations may lead to reduced genetic diversity. Stocks are subject to loss as a producer's situation changes.

Commercial poultry industry: Commercial industry must emphasize traits of economic value now and in the short-term future. Industrial breeders keep genetic stocks as necessary to satisfy that need. Increased globalization and vertical integration of companies puts such genetic reserves at risk around the world. So far in India however there is no such instance where any indigenous breed has been taken up by industry but attempts at organic production have been there.

Conservation groups: Non-Governmental Organizations and Breed Societies may assist in conservation of minor breeds. Information on management methods, breeds at risk, and exchange of genetic material is facilitated through meetings, a newsletter and website etc. Rare Breeds International is an umbrella organization for such groups around the world. The establishment of the Society for Conservation of Domestic Animal Biodiversity (SOCDAB) with its headquarter at National Bureau of Animal Genetic Resources (NBAGR) in June, 1998 is the culmination of dedicated efforts of such professionals.

Organisations: *The* Government research institutes and Universities are major sources where breeds are kept and maintained *in situ*. The NBAGR is mandated with identification, evaluation, characterization, conservation and utilization of livestock and poultry genetic resources. Examples, e.g. *Aseel* breed is characterized at Indira Gandhi Krishi Viswa-Vidyalaya, Raipur, M.P; *Ankaleshwar* breed at State Animal Husbandry farm and Gujarat Agril University, Junagadh; *Kadaknath* at J. N. Krishi Vishwa Vidyalaya, Jabalpur and State Poultry Farm, Jhabua; *Miri* breed at Assam Agril University, Khanapara; Kashmir Faverolla at Shere-Kashmir University of Agri-Technology, Srinagar; *Nicobari* fowl at Central Agricultural Research Institute, Port Blair.

International: The Food and Agriculture Organization (FAO) plays a major role in assisting individual countries with conservation programs and provides a forum for international consultation and planning.

Question Bank

Q. 1. Fill in the blanks

i) The present-day domesticated fowl is believed to have descended from the..............................

ii) Presently only about .... poultry breeding companies provide broiler stocks and layer stocks around the world.

iii) Domestic fowl occurred about .... in ...., ... and South East Asia.

iv) Breed: A sub-specific group of domestic poultry with definable and identifiable .... characteristics that enable it to be separated by .... appraisal from other similarly-defined groups within same species

v) .... preservation involves the conservation of poultry away from their normal habitat.

vi) .... conservation is the maintenance of live populations of poultry in their adaptive environment or natural habitat, as close to it as is practically possible.

Answers (i)- Red jungle fowl; (ii)- three to four; (iii)- 6000 BC, India, China; (iv)- external, visual (v)- *ex-situ*; (vi)- *in situ*;

Q. No. 2. Multiple choice Questions

i) National Bureau of Animal Genetic Resources is responsible for conservation of

  a) Exotic breeds in India
  b) Indigenous breeds of India
  c) None of the above
  d) Both (a) & (b)

ii) *In situ* conservation can be applied to

  a) all species
  b) most of the species
  c) very few species
  d) only rare species

iii) The following are indigenous duck breeds

  a) Indian Runner, Muscovy, Khaki Campbell,
  b) Nageswari, Sylhetmete and Muscovy ducks
  c) Khaki Campbell, Chara and Chemballi ducks
  d) Nageswari, Sylhetmete, Chara and Chemballi ducks

iv) *Ex- situ* conservation is commonly collection and freezing in liquid nitrogen of animal genetic resources in the form of

  a) Tissues and organs
  b) Blood and serum
  c) living semen, ova or embryos
  d) All of the above

v) Evolutionary biology uses following cytogenetic and molecular techniques

  a) Karyotyping, Fluorescent *in-situ* Hybridisation (FISH)
  b) specific molecular probing and mitochondrial DNA sequencing
  c) Both (a) & (b)
  d) None of the above

vi) Some reasons for conservation are

a) to maintain genetic variation

b) to take advantage of heterosis

c) economic potential

d) all of above

vii) Indigenous poultry may be more disease resistant than exotic breeds because of

a) adaptation to local environment

b) inherent genetic capability

c) both (a) and (b)

d) none of the above

viii) Conservation may help circumvent problems of

a) spread of disease and climate change

b) changing availability of feedstuffs and selection errors

c) none of the above

d) both (a) and (b)

Answers: (i)-b; (ii)-a; (iii)-d; (iv)-c; (v)-c; (vi)-d; (vii)-c; (viii)- d

Q. 3. True or False

i) Conservation is keeping genetic variation as gene combinations, in an easily recoverable form. (T/F)

ii) Domesticated chickens were first used as pets. (T/F)

iii) Man did not influence the evolutionary process of domestic animals. (T/F)

iv) A group for which geographical and/or cultural separation from genotypically similar groups has led to acceptance of its separate identity (T/F)

v) Population monitoring, environmental adoption and selection for use is good in ex situ conservation. (T/F)

vi) Evolution of genus *Gallus* probably dates back 8 million years ago. (T/F)

vii) Eclipse plumage is visible in male hackles of modern-day chicken. (T/F)

viii) International access to in situ conserved animals is good. (T/F)

ix) Natural selection and mutations within the species bestowed advantage to animals in certain environmental conditions leading to stable populations. (T/F)

Answers: (i)-T, (ii)-F, (iii)-F, (iv)-F, (v)-F, (vi)-T, (vii)-F, (viii)-T, (ix)-T.

Q. 4. Objective type short questions

i) Summarise the major reasons for conservation

ii) Enumerate the steps necessary for conservation

iii) Describe two major differences between in *situ* and *ex situ* conservation.

iv) Name five registered chicken breeds of India.

16

Project Preparation for Rural People

J.D. Mahanta

Project for Rural People on Chicken

For rural people *Desi* (indigenous) chicken plays an important role. Family poultry farming is a part and parcel of a typical rural household in India touching social, cultural and economic aspects. People residing in rural areas primarily maintain their indigenous chicken under backyard farming. With the same management system the rural people can rear improved varieties of chicken instead of their traditional counterpart. The improved varieties being *Giriraja*, *Vanaraja*, *Kuroiler*, *Gramapriya*, *Gramalaxmi, Swarnadhara*, *Krishna J etc*. A model project on improved chicken is given herewith:

A unit consisting of 100 number *Vanaraja* or *Giriraja* is economical and remunerative to the farmers whose family labour will be utilized for rearing these chickens. Initially, the farmer will buy about 225 straight-run day- old chicks. The males will be sold at 20 weeks of age. The females will be maintained for 1.5 years. In order to have continuous operation, next batch of 225 chicks have to be procured 6 months before disposal of the old batch. Birds will collect their feed through foraging or scavenging in the field. Supplementary feeding will be provided to meet their requirements.

Technical Standards

Space requirement	=	2.5 sq. ft./bird
Cost of day-old chick	=	Rs. 25/- each
Run area	=	30 sq. ft./ bird
Feed requirement		
a. 0-8 weeks	=	40 g/chick/day
b. 9-20 weeks	=	20g/chick/day
c. 21 weeks and above	=	40g/layer/day
Cost of vaccine		
a. R.D. LaSota/ F(200 dose)	=	Rs.40/-
b. IBD vaccine (200 dose)	=	Rs 188/-
c. Fowl pox (200 dose)	=	Rs.100/-
Cost of electricity, litter, medicine, vaccine	=	Rs.10/- layer
Cost of equipment	=	Rs 10/- bird
Number of eggs produced	=	140/ layer/ year
Body weight at 20 weeks of age	=	1.5 Kg
Bank share	=	75%
Promoter's share	=	25%
Mortality	=	10%
Interest rate on bank loan	=	15%

(Contd.....)

	Particulars	Amount in Rs.
A Capital investment		
1.	Construction of one poultry shed: 250 sq. ft. @ Rs. 300/ sq.ft.	Rs. 75,000.00
2.	Cost of equipment for 200 birds @ Rs. 10/- per bird	Rs. 2,000.00
3.	Stock : (Working capital)Cost of rearing 200 chicks from one-day old to the point of lay (20 weeks):	
(a)	Cost of 225 day-old unsexed chicks @ Rs. 25/- per chick	Rs. 5,625.00
(b)	(i) Cost of feeding 225 chicks upto 8 weeks of age @ 40g /day/chick= 9.0 Kg per day x Rs.15/- kg feed x 56 days= Rs.5625 (ii) Cost of feeding from 9-20 weeks @ 20g /day/chick = 4.5 Kg per day x Rs.15/- Kg feed x 84 days= Rs.5670/-	Rs. 11,295.00
(c)	Cost of electricity, litter medicine, vaccine etc L.S. Rs. 18,420.00	Rs. 1,500.00
	Total	**Rs. 95,840.00**
	Entrepreneur's share (Margin money 25%)	Rs. 23,855.00
	Bank loan (75%)	Rs. 71,985.00
B.Operational/Recurring expenditure for 21-72 weeks of age		
1.	Cost of feeding 100 layers for one year @ 40 g/layer/ day =4 kg x Rs.15/- Kg feed x 365 days	Rs. 21,900.00
2.	Cost of litter, electricity, medicine, vaccines etc. @ Rs. 10/- per layer for 100 layers.	Rs. 1,000.00
3.	Miscellaneous expenditure	Rs. 2000.00
	Total	Rs. 24,900.00
C.	Receipts	
1.	Sale of 100 male chicken at 20 weeks of age @ Rs. 225/- per chicken	Rs. 22,500.00
2.	Sale of 14000 eggs @ Rs. 4.00 each egg (egg production @ 140 eggs per bird per year)	Rs. 56,000.00
3.	Sale of 90 numbers of spent hen @ Rs. 200/- per hen	Rs. 18000.00
	Total	**Rs. 96,500.00**
GROSS PROFIT		
Total Receipts		**Rs. 96,500.00**

(Contd.....)

Particulars	Amount in Rs.
Expenditure	
Operational/ Recurring Expenditure	Rs. 24,900.00
Expenditure on replacement flock :Cost of rearing 225 layers from day-old to point of lay (20 wks)	Rs. 18,420.00 Rs. 43,320.00
GROSS PROFIT	**Rs. 53,180.00**
Less : a) Depreciation on building and equipments L.S.	Rs. 1,000.00
b) Interest on bank loan @ 15% annually	Rs. 10,798.00
Net Profit	**Rs. 41,382.00**

Net profit : Thus, rearing of 100 *Giriraja/ Vanaraja* chickens and adopting improved management, feeding and disease prevention practices will generate a net income of Rs.3449/ - per month by selling of eggs and chicken.

N.B. : All rates and values varies from place to place and fromtime to time. L.S= Lump sum.

Project Report for a Duck Farm

A 200 duck (eggers) unit is economical and remunerative to the farmers, whose family labour will be utilized for rearing the ducks. There will be no elaborate housing, except a bamboo and thatch- made enclosure for night shelter. Initially the farmer will buy about 450 straight-run day-old ducklings, preferably *Chara-Chemballi* or *Khaki Campbell* X *desi* cross, which will have better laying potential. The males will be sold at about 8 to 10 weeks of age; whereas, the females will be maintained for at least two laying years. They will be mostly fed in the range by allowing them to graze from 9 am. to 5 pm., daily.

Only during the brooding period and during the scarcity months of December to February they will be given supplementary feed. At 8 weeks of age they will be vaccinated against duck plague and the same will be repeated during the subsequent years. In order to have continuous operation the next batch of 450 ducklings have to be purchased 6 months before the disposal of the old batch. The income and expenditure of this operation are as shown below:

I. Expenditure per batch (2.5 yrs.)

a)	Cost of feeders, waterers, bamboo, thatch, egg filler flats etc	=	Rs. 4000.00
b)	Cost of 450 day-old straight- run ducklings @ Rs. 30/ each	=	Rs. 13500.00
c)	Cost of feeding up to one month of age with grains, rice bran and fish meal mixture @ 1.5 kg/ bird = 675 kg x Rs. 15/- kg	=	Rs. 10125.00
d)	Cost of vaccination, medication and other miscellaneous items	=	Rs. 2000.00
e)	Cost of feeding during dry months partly for 6 months in 2 years for 200 birds @ 2kg per bird/ month (part feeding only) 200 birds x 6 months x 2Kg x Rs.15/- kg.	=	Rs. 36000.00
f)	Total expenditure for 2.5 years	=	Rs.65625.00
g)	Bank finance needed = 75% of items (a) to (d) above	=	Rs.49219.00
h)	Interest per batch	=	Rs.18457.00

II. Gross and net income per batch

a)	By selling of 200 drakes (males) at 2 months of age @ Rs.60/- bird	=	Rs. 12000.00
b)	By sale of 180 eggs during first year and 150 eggs during second year of lay per dam at Rs.4.50 each (200 ducks x 1 80 eggs = 36000 + 180 ducks x 150 eggs = 27000 @ 4.50 each x 63000 eggs)	=	Rs 283500.00
c)	By sale of 170 ducks at the end of second year @ Rs.120/ each	=	Rs.20400.00
d)	Gross receipt	=	Rs.315900.00
e)	Less expenditure including interest	=	Rs. 84082.00
(f)	Net return in 2.5 years	=	Rs. 231818.00
g)	**Net profit per month = Rs. 231818.00/ 30 months**	=	**Rs. 7727.00**

The above capacity of duck farm can be maintained by a single person with his family and can earn Rs 258 per day approximately. If eggs are sold in retail market still higher profit could be earned.

Project Report for a Japanese Quail Farm

Japanese quail is a small fast growing bird. Its meat is a gourmet's delight. The Indian and Chinese system of medicine claims that the flesh of Japanese quail has varying medicinal properties. It is good tonic for tuberculosis and other convalescent patient and also act as 'Aphrodisiac'. The taste of urban consumers has become more selective for culinary delights. With the buying power of the consumer ever increasing this would be the ideal time for people with less land area and having a keen eye on good profits to go in for Japanese quail farming. A project report for Japanese quail is give herewith as model farming.

Technical Standards

Cost of day-old Japanese quail chick	= Rs. 5/- each
Cost of medicine, electricity, labour and other miscellaneous expenditure.	= Rs. 2/- bird
Cost of feed	= Rs. 15/- kg
Cost of cage 4-tier brooder-cum-grower cages to accommodate 100 birds	= Rs.4000/-
Cost of rat-proof quail house with asbestos roof	= Rs.500/- sq.ft.
Total feed consumption from 0 to 5 weeks of age	= 400 g/ bird
Feed efficiency (feed/ kg body weight)	= 3.0
Growing period (marketing age)	= 5 weeks
Livability	= 90%
Average body weight at 5 weeks of age	= 30g
Manure production by 1000 birds	= 25 kg.
Cost of manure tonne	= Rs. 400/-
Cost of empty feed bags of 75 kg capacity	= Rs. 10/- bag

I. Fixed cost

a)	Cost of cage grower house for 6 batches of Japanese quail = 100 sq. ft. @ 500/- sq. ft.	= Rs. 50000.00
b)	Cost of 6 cage unit for 6 batches of 100, each @ Rs. 40/- bird	= Rs. 24000.00
c)	Cost of a well; pipelines, pump-set etc	= Rs. 15000.00
d)	**Total**	**= Rs. 89000.00**
e)	Annual depreciation (10%)	= Rs. 8900.00

II. Working capital (2 months)

a)	Cost of Japanese quail chicks (8 batchesx100 chicks x Rs. 5/-chick)	= Rs. 4000.00
b)	Feed cost for different period average 0.3kg/ birdxRs.15/-kg x 800	= Rs. 3600.00
c)	Miscellaneous expenditure @ Rs. 2/- bird	= Rs. 1600.00
d)	**Total**	**= Rs. 9200.00**

III. Capital Investment

a)	Fixed cost + working capital	= Rs 98200.00
b)	Bank loan (75% approx)	= Rs. 73650.00
c)	Promoter's share (25%)	= Rs. 24550.00

d)	Annual bank interest on capital (@12.5%)	=	Rs. 9206.00

IV. Annual Recurring Expenditure

a)	Cost of Japanese quail chicks (Rs.5/- x 100 x 52 batches)	=	Rs. 26000.00
b)	Cost of feed 0.4 Kg x 52 batches x 100 chicks/ batch x Rs.15/- kg.	=	Rs. 31200.00
c)	Miscellaneous expenditure @ Rs. 2/- chick	=	Rs. 10400.00
d)	**Total**	**=**	**Rs. 67600.00**
e)	Annual depreciation	=	Rs. 8900.00
f)	Interest on capital	=	Rs. 9206.00
g)	**Total annual expenditure**	**=**	**Rs. 85706.00**

V. Annual Returns and Profits

a)	By sale of 52 batches of 90 Japanese quails/ batch at Rs.20/-each	=	Rs. 93600.00
b)	By sale of manure at Rs. 400/- tonne x 25 kg/ batch x 52 batches	=	Rs. 520.00
c)	By selling of empty feed bags 28 bags at Rs. 10/- each	=	Rs. 280.00
d)	Total gross receipts	=	Rs. 94400.00
e)	Less total annual expenditure including interest and depreciation	=	Rs. 85706.00
e)	**Annual net profit**	**=**	**Rs. 8694.00**

The annual net profit will be less during the first 5 years due to bank loan repayment, thereafter it will go up.

Project Report for a Guinea Fowl Farm

Under rural condition, a farm can be started under backyard venture with sufficient area for foraging with 20 numbers of two- months old unsexed keets as a foundation stock. The stock could be multiplied through hatching of fertile eggs under broody hen. Nest box should be provided to encourage the birds to lay in the nest. As a supplementary feeding, kitchen waste and other agro-waste may be provided to the birds. No medication and vaccination are carried out routinely as the birds are very hardy. The annual egg production is about 50 eggs per hen.

I. Capital expenditure

a)	Cost of night shelter, nest boxes, water tub etc	=	Rs. 2000.00
b)	Cost of 20 numbers of two months old keets @ Rs. 30/- each	=	Rs. 600.00
c)	Cost of supplemental feed for 3 months with grains for 20 birds X 90 days x 25 g/bird x Rs.15/- kg	=	Rs. 675.00

d)	**Total capital expenditure**	=	**Rs. 3275.00**

II. Annual recurring expenditure

a)	Cost of supplemental feed for 3 dry months/ year with grains for 20 adult birds X 90 days x 25 g/bird x Rs.15/- kg	=	Rs.675.00
b)	Cost of supplemental feed for about 200 brooding keets for 2 months @ 500 g/bird x Rs.15/- kg	=	Rs. 1500.00
c)	**Total annual expenditure**	=	**Rs. 2175.00**

III. Annual gross and net profit:

a)	Sale of about 200 eggs for hatching or table purpose @Rs. 5/- each	=	Rs. 1000.00
b)	Sale of about 100 keets of 2 months of age for breeding @ Rs. 30/- each	=	Rs. 3000.00
c)	Sale of about 50 adult birds for table or breeding purpose @ Rs. 100/- each	=	Rs. 5000.00
d)	Total annual gross receipts	=	Rs. 9000.00
e)	Less annual expenditure	=	Rs. 2175.00
f)	**Net profit/ annum**	=	**Rs. 6825.00**

Thus, this type of rural backyard guinea fowl farm will provide a subsidiary side income to a household family besides providing needed protein for the family.

Project Report for a Turkey Farm

Unlike in western countries, turkey farms are not popular in India due to the following reasons:

- Hybrid turkeys are not available.
- The day-old poult cost is higher due to lesser number of poults per hen and higher cost of maintenance.
- The feed cost is very high due to higher nutrient requirement and poorer feed efficiency (> 2.5).
- Growing period is longer (13-20 weeks); hence lesser number of crops per year.
- All the above factors have increased the cost of production of turkeys.
- Lesser or only seasonal demand for turkey meat.

- Limited purchasing power of consumers.

However, small flocks of non-descript turkeys can be reared in the backyard to meet the seasonal demand. The economics of a 50 turkey flock under semi-intensive system is discussed below:

Technical Details

Land required = 1-2 acres with good foraging or large backyard under free range village atmosphere

Housing = A thatched house of 150 sq. ft. will be provided for brooding and rearing up to one month of age. Later they will be partly fed and let out during day time for grazing and the house will be used only as a night shelter.

Poults = Day-old poults will be purchased from reputed sources at Rs. 35/- poult, growing period = 6 months i.e. 2 batches/ year. Expected body weight at 6 months = 4 kg.

Feeding = Broiler starter or chick mash supplemented with kitchen waste will be up to one month of age. Later they will be let out for grazing in the backyard in search of kitchen waste, insects, seeds, greens, grains etc. During scarcity some grains may be fed. If possible waste vegetables may be collected in the market and fed to reduce the feed cost.

Management = In general, the management of turkeys will be similar to that of backyard chicken.

I. Fixed capital

e)	Cost of 150 sq. ft. thatched house for brooding and night shelter	= Rs. 9000.00
f)	Cost of feeder, waterer, bulb and other equipment	= Rs. 1000.00
g)	Total fixed capital	= Rs. 10000.00
h)	Depreciation on fixed capital at 25% per annum (including repair)	= Rs. 2500.00

II. Working capital

a)	Cost of 50 day-old poults @ Rs. 35/- each	= Rs. 1750.00
b)	Broiler starter feed* for one month at 1.5 Kg / bird = 75 kg @ Rs.15/kg	= Rs. 1125.00
c)	Grains and other purchased feed items to feed during scarcity period at 10 kg/ bird = 500 kg x @ Rs. 12/- kg	= Rs. 6000.00
d)	Total working capital	= Rs. 8875.00

III. Total project cost= 10000 + 8875 = Rs. 18875.00

IV. Share of the promoter (25%)		= Rs 4719.00
V. Bank finance needed (75%)		= Rs.14156.00
VI. Annual interest on capital @ 12.5%		= Rs. 1770.00
VII. Annual repayment of capital (Rs.14156/ 5 yrs)		= Rs. 2831.00
VIII. Annual recurring expenditure		
g)	Cost of 50 x 2 batches of poults @ Rs. 35/- each	= Rs. 3500.00
h)	Broiler starter feed* = 150 kg x Rs. 21/- kg	= Rs. 3150.00
i)	Misc. feed items and other expenses @10kg/bird x 100 x Rs.12	= Rs.12000.00
j)	Bank interest	= Rs. 1770.00
k)	Total annual expenditure	= Rs.20420.00
IX. Annual gross returns and net profits		
a)	By selling of 47 turkeys (5% mortality) x 2 batches = 94 turkeys each weighing 4 kg at Rs. 140/- kg	= Rs. 52640.00
b)	Other receipts are insignificant and hence Annual gross returns	= Rs. 52640.00
c)	Less annual recurring expenditure	= Rs. 20420.00
d)	Annual gross profit	= Rs. 32220.00
e)	Less repayment of bank loan (-) Rs. 2831.00	= Rs. 29389.00
f)	Less depreciation (-) Rs. 2500.00	= Rs. 26889.00
g)	Annual net profit**	= Rs. 26889.00
h)	Profit/ bird = 26889/ 94	= Rs. 286.00
i)	Benefit : cost ratio = 52640/ 20420	= Rs. 2.57

* Broiler starter feed may be used for poultry.

** The net profit will go up further, after the bank loan repayment. The number of turkeys reared depends upon the land availability.

Question Bank

Q. 1. Prepare a project report for rural people on

i. 50 numbers of improved variety of chicken

ii. 50 numbers of improved variety of ducks

iii. 20 number of turkey

iv. 10 number of guinea fowl

17

Poultry Housing

S.S. Nagra

Housing constitutes the second largest component of cost of poultry production. An ideally located and well planned poultry farm is an essential requirement for efficient egg and meat production. Poultry housing normally serves the following major functions:

a. Provides shelter and protection to the birds

b. Provides comfort to the birds.

c. Helps in organization of large flock into a manageable unit.

Poultry housing must suit to the climatic conditions of the geographical area. Accordingly, the house design may differ distinctly between temperate and the tropical regions.

Planning a Poultry Farm

Before planning to start a poultry farm, one must consider the following factors for trouble-free long operations:

1. Selection of the site.
2. Orientation of houses.
3. Lay-out of operations.
4. Design and construction.

Selection of the Site

While selecting a site for the poultry farm, the factors that require proper attention will include:

- The farm should be located on a high level and porous land to facilitate natural drainage and protection from flood. It should be away from residential areas to avoid any public objections concerning environmental pollution and housefly problems.
- Good quality drinking water should be available at the site.
- It should be connected with a good linkroad to facilitate easy transportation. But should be located reasonably away from the main public roads to avoid unnecessary disturbance to the birds from vehicular noise.
- It should have access to good electricity and telephone connections.
- The land area should be large enough to provide space for future expansions.

Orientation of Poultry Houses

The direction of poultry houses in the tropical areas should be placed with their long axis facing east to west. This will facilitate proper use of sun light and keeps the house warm during winter. Whereas during summer, it will prevent the entry of direct sun rays into the house, thus helps in keeping the house temperature low. But for the environmentally controlled poultry houses, the direction of the house may not be of much significance.

Layout of Operations

The layout plan will vary with the size and type (egg or meat) of operation, the management system followed and the flow of materials (manual/ automated). Following points must be given due consideration for layout of poultry operations:

- The brooding house should be isolated from the growing and adult bird houses to avoid cross infections.
- The poultry houses should be located approximately 100 feet away from each other to facilitate proper air circulation and to avoid the risk of fire spread. This also provides space for plantation of trees in between the houses.

- The feed/egg store and day- old chick delivery points at the farm should be located such that the delivery vehicles do not require to enter the main farm premises.
- The reception office should be located near the main gate so that the visitors do not enter the rearing areas.
- The entire farm complex should be secured by constructing a boundary wall with only one main gate for entry.

Design and Construction

Poultry are most comfortable when the temperature varies between 10 to 24^{0}C and the relative humidity between 50 to 75%. Proper ventilation of the house is important for flow of fresh air into the house and for removal of moisture, carbon dioxide, ammonia and other harmful gases from the house. The general considerations in construction of the poultry houses are as under:

- The foundation should be strong enough to support the weight of the structure and it should be rodent-proof.
- The floor should be smooth, preferably concrete made, impervious to moisture with a reasonable slope for easy cleaning and washing.
- The walls should be smooth finished and water-proof for easy cleaning and disinfection. The long axis walls in the open sided houses have window openings for proper ventilation with wire mash security. The wire mash netting may cover up to 90% of wall area with only concrete column supports in the northern planes for cage housing.
- The doors should be large enough to allow free to-and-fro flow of materials into the house. It should be minimum 4' x 7'size.
- The width of poultry house should not be more than 30 to 32 ft. to allow movement of natural air through the house. Assisted air movement with provision of inlet/outlet fans will be required in houses which are wider than this.
- The length can be adjusted to any size depending upon the availability of space. Too long sheds may be partitioned into pens of convenient size for better management.
- The height of the poultry house should be enough for proper ventilation and convenience of the workers (minimum 9 ft. for deep litter house). The height, however, depends upon the roof-type used.

- The roof should be water-proof with proper slope. The roof type may be plain concrete laid or made of asbestos sheets in monitor, shed, gable and other forms as shown in Fig.23. A roof extension of one meter beyond the walls should be provided as overhang to prevent the entry of rain water into the shed.
- Economy in construction should be given due consideration with the use of locally available materials.

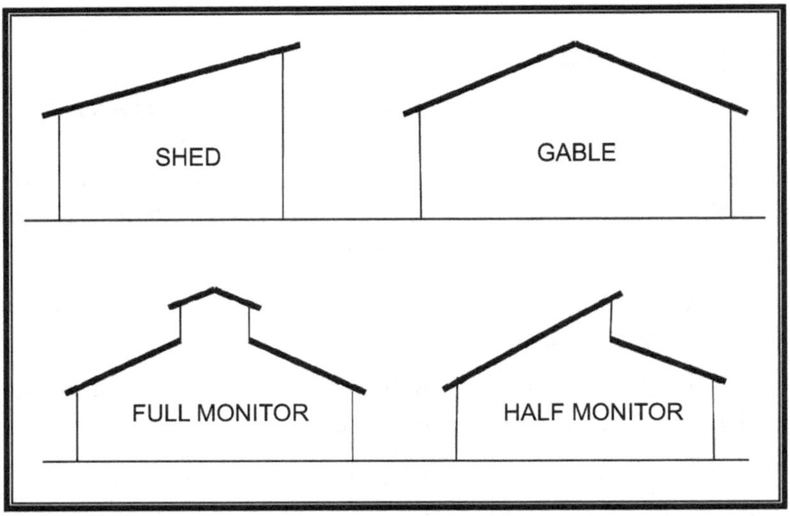

Fig. 23: Different roof types for poultry houses

Types of Poultry Structures

There are two types of poultry structures related with poultry operations.

1. Hatchery.
2. Poultry Farm Facilities.

Hatchery

Hatchery is a place where artificial hatching of chicks is carried out. The hatchery is preferably located away from the commercial poultry farms to check the cross infections from farms to the hatchery. A well designed hatchery has two divisions:

1. The administrative wing.
2. The operational wing.

The administrative wing consists of the offices for keeping all records of the hatchery, enquiry office, waiting room for visitors and customers.

The operational wing is the actual workplace for hatching operations. The hatchery operation facilities are arranged in a manner which provides efficient work flow through the hatchery in the order of egg room, setter room, hatcher room, chick room and bus bay. The auxiliary rooms such as tray wash, clean room, disposal area, box storage and utility should be strategically located to support the main work effort. The offices, lunch room and reception or lobby areas are located such that they do not interrupt the workflow. Proper layout helps to maintain a high level of bio-security. The layout plan of a modern hatchery is shown in Fig. 24.

Smaller hatcheries usually hatch two days a week, while larger hatcheries may hatch four or even seven days a week. The following information can be used to establish actual room sizes and layout of the hatchery.

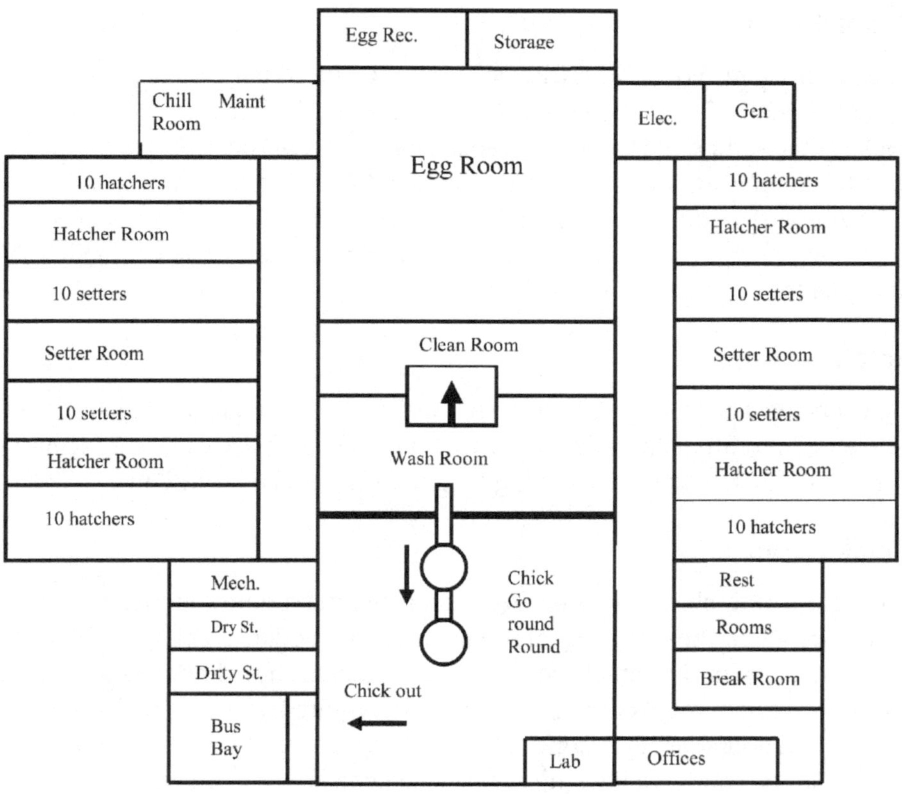

Fig 24: Floor plan of a modern hatchery (*Source*: Bell and Weaver, Jr., 2007)

Egg Room

Design the egg room to be large enough to provide space for storing, traying and grading of eggs. A ceiling height of 12ft (3.65 m) is ideal. The layout of this room depends on how many eggs are received. For calculating egg room size, provide 4 square feet of floor space for each 1,000 eggs to be stored. The minimum egg room size should not be less than 600 sq ft (55.74 sq. m)

Fumigation Room

The fumigation room should be large enough to accommodate one-half of the cases and buggies used in a single day.

Pre Warming Room

Pre warming room is located next to the egg room. Provide 15 sq ft (1.4 sq. m) floor area per egg buggy. It is important to provide airspace around all buggies and good air circulation around all eggs to maintain an even temperature.

Setter Room

The setter room should be sufficiently large to permit easy access around the setters. Usually 24 to 30 inches (60 to 75cm) space between the ends and backs of the setters and the walls is adequate for this purpose. At least 10 to 12 ft (3.05 to 3.65 m) wide space from the front of setter to a facing wall or a facing row of setters should be available free, to allow temporary storage of loaded egg buggies without interfering with normal work. The ceiling height of the setter room should be 14 ft (4.27 m).

Hatcher Room

Hatchers must have at least 10 to 12 ft. (3.05 to 3.65m) wide front aisle. Place hatchers 24 to 30 inches (60 to 75 cm) from end and back walls for cleaning purposes. The hatcher room ceiling height should be 14 ft (4.27 m).

Chick Room

The size of the chick room depends upon the maximum number of chicks processed daily. Provide adequate space to accommodate all chicks of a hatch in the chick room. The chick storage or holding area should be separated from the chick service area. Additional space will be required if sexing, beak trimming and vaccination(s) are also done at the hatchery. Generally 12 to 20 sq ft (1.12 to 1.86 sq m) floor area is required per 1,000 chicks stored in the chick room.

Washroom

The room size for this area depends upon the maximum number of hatcher buggies that will be stored in it at any one time. Space should be sufficient for the tray washer, buggy washer, vacuum waste system, and any automation equipment.

Clean Tray Room

This room is placed adjacent to the tray wash room. It should be of sufficient size to hold all the clean trays and buggies for one day's hatch. 15 sq ft (1.4 sq m) area for each buggy stored should be allowed in this room.

Poultry Farm Facilities

The general rearing facilities required at the poultry farms are as under:

- Brooder house.
- Broiler house.
- Grower house.
- Laying hen house.

Brooder House

Brooder house may not be an essential requirement for small poultry farms. A portion of the broiler/layer house may be used for brooding purpose and then extended for further rearing. However, for big poultry farms, a separate brooder house must be constructed because of continuous brooding of chicks required in different batches almost throughout the year.

The brooder house is a compact unit with little side wall surface openings. It may be divided into different compartments depending upon the needs of the farm. The chicks may be reared on floor, in batteries or in cages for brooding.

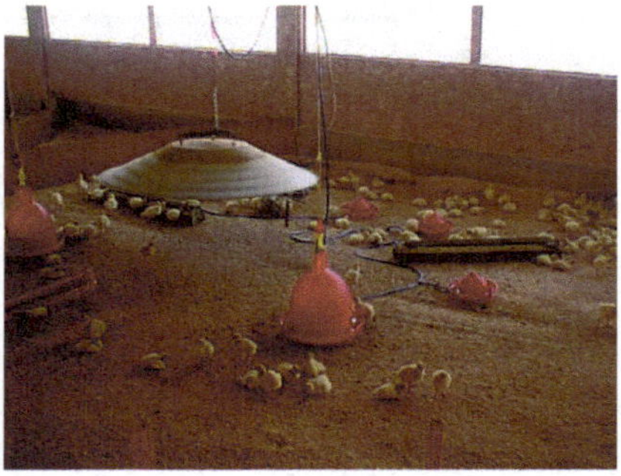

Fig 25: Inside view of the brooder house.

Two types of heating systems are employed in the brooder: cold room and hot room brooding systems. In the cold room brooding system, various types of brooders are used to keep the chicks warm, whereas, in the hot room brooding system, the entire brooder house gets heated and the temperature is thermostatically regulated. An inside view of a cold room brooder house is shown in Fig.25.

Broiler House

A broiler house should provide clean, dry and comfortable surroundings for the birds throughout the year. It must meet the following requisites:-

1. The house should be kept enough warm.
2. The litter should be kept reasonably dry.
3. There should be circulation of fresh air.
4. The house should be free from drafts.

Raising broilers in the tunnel ventilated houses is becoming more and more popular and is the most preferred broiler rearing system in many countries. In this type of system, the poultry house is converted into a wind tunnel. In the tunnel ventilation system, all exhaust fans are placed at one end of the house and all air inlets at the other end. Ventilating air is drawn uniformly through the length of the house at a velocity of 350 to 400 feet per minute (4 to 4.5 mph). This provides significant cooling for the birds. This system is most suited for warm weather. The combination of tunnel ventilation and evaporative cooling can be very effective in reducing hot weather heat stress. The fan and inlet arrangement for a tunnel ventilation system has been shown in Fig. 26. An external view of such houses is shown in Fig.27.

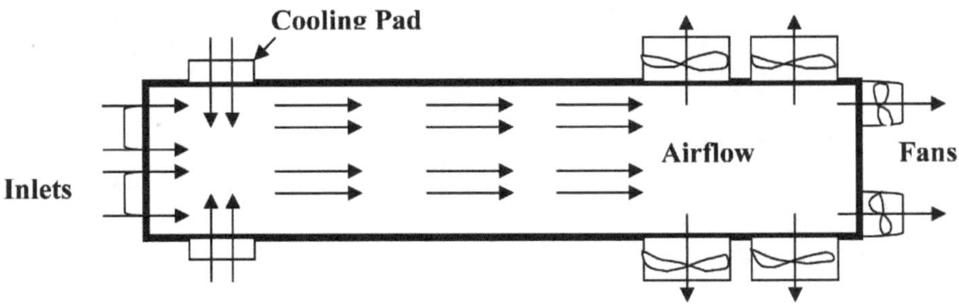

Fig. 26: Fan and ventilation arrangement for a tunnel ventilation system

Growing Pullet House

Large poultry operations require effective isolation of growing flocks from the older ones for disease prevention. Generally, the pullets are shifted at 6-8 weeks of age from the brooder house to the grower house where they are kept up to 16-18 weeks of age for rearing and then shifted to the layer house.

With better disease control programs, more and more growing birds are reared in a *'brood-grow'* house arrangement due to economic reasons. The commercial egg –type pullets are kept in the same house from day-old until 16 weeks of age when they are moved to laying house. This system is favoured because majority of pullets are moved to cages than the deep litter laying houses.

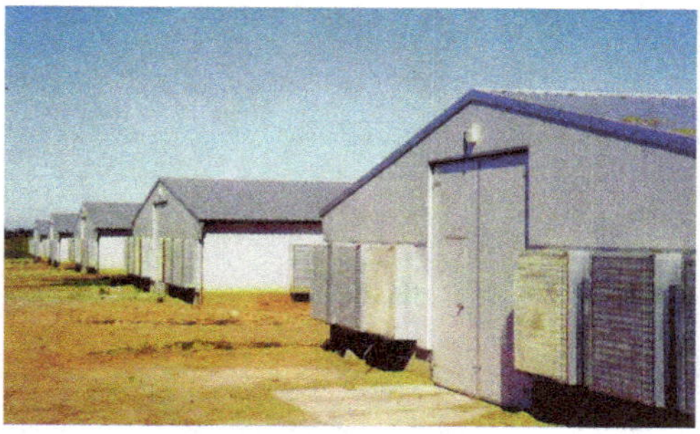

Fig. 27: Outside view of tunnel ventilated house

Layer House

Most of the large commercial egg laying flocks are kept in cages. Deep litter system is common for small size laying flocks. Laying hens perform well at any temperature up to 30^{0}C in a dry, well ventilated house free from ammonia, dust and air-borne pathogens. Confining the breeding birds in the same house from day-old until the end of laying year is also a common practice. This is called *'brood-grow-lay'* house arrangement. Necessary equipment in the house is changed according to age and requirement of the birds. However, the space remains underutilized during brood-grow stage.

Rearing Systems

There are three types of poultry rearing systems:

- Extensive or Free Range System.
- Semi-Intensive System.
- Intensive System.

Extensive or Free Range System

Before commercial poultry production, all poultry birds were reared by this system. This system permits the birds to roam freely over a large area (Fig.28) where they can find their own food from scavenging. Only a small movable shelter may be provided for protection of birds from rains etc. Only 100 to 120 birds can be kept in one acre of land in this system thus providing approximately 34-41m^2 of space per bird. However, the birds need protection from natural enemies and parasitic infestations. This system is most suited for organic poultry production, being advocated forcefully in many countries.

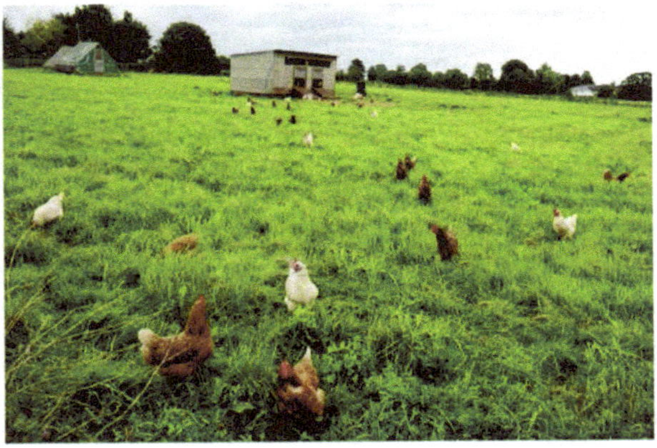

Fig 28: View of free range system (courtesy: fotosearch.com)

Advantages

- Birds are able to express their natural behaviours.
- Birds remain free and comfortable.
- Birds are exposed to natural sunlight.
- The bone development of birds is relatively better.
- Birds remain stronger and hardier.
- Labour requirement is less.
- Investment on equipments is less.
- Good system for organic poultry production.

Disadvantages

- Large land area is required per bird which is generally not available.
- Egg production is lower.
- Eggs may get soiled in bad weather.
- Birds lose more energy in activities.
- Risk of egg theft and damage by snakes and predators.

Semi-intensive System

This system can be adopted where limited free space is available. A permanent shelter is provided to the birds with a floor space of 1 sq. ft. per bird. In addition they are allowed outside run of 16-24 m^2 per hen. Preferably, the run out should be divided equally on both sides of the house to permit the bird to avail fresh ground.

Advantages

- Space requirement is less than free range system.
- Family labour can be utilized to cut labour cost.
- Investment is less on equipments and building than the intensive system.
- Birds and eggs are more secured than free range system.
- Birds can express their normal behavior.
- Birds are exposed to natural sunlight.

Disadvantages

- More land area required than the intensive system.
- Problem of bad smell and flies in rainy season.
- Birds and eggs get dirty in rainy season
- Higher risk of diseases.

Intensive System

In the intensive rearing system the birds always remain confined to the house. They have no direct access to the outside environment. All commercial flocks in large units are reared under this system due to economic considerations. Different intensive rearing systems are as under:

- Cage system
- Deep litter system
- Slat floor system
- Slat and litter systems

Cage System

The cage system of rearing (Fig.29) is most popular for laying birds, wherein the birds are kept in small wire cages placed side by side. The cages in the house are arranged in 3 rows in open sided

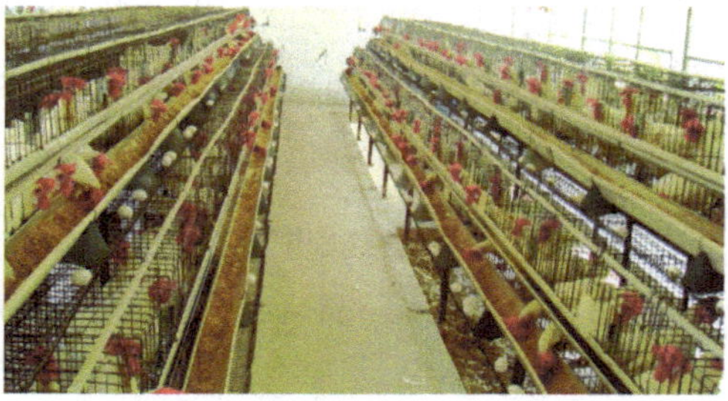

Fig 29: Inside view of a cage layer house.

houses. The cage rows are arranged on each side of an aisle which is 30 to 36 inches wide. The cages are placed at a convenient working height. The cage arrangement may range from single deck to five decks. The floor area allowance per bird in cages may vary depending upon the cage size and stocking density.

Advantages

- Accommodates more no. of birds in a given floor area than the deep litter system
- Problem of internal parasites is eliminated.
- Facilitates better maintenance of farm records.
- Broodiness is eliminated.
- Higher egg production is achieved.
- Eggs are clean.
- Better feed efficiency is obtained.
- Culling is easier.
- Vices like cannibalism and egg eating are controlled.
- Feed wastage is avoided.
- Labour requirement is reduced.
- Automation is easier.

Disadvantages

- Initial investment is very high.
- Birds are unable to express their normal behavior.
- There is a higher incidence of leg problem, osteoporosis and cage layer fatigue.
- There is a problem of flies and obnoxious gases.
- Birds require perfectly balanced feed.
- Natural ventilation is a problem.
- Manure handling is a problem.

The use of conventional layer cages has become a controversial issue with the animal welfare groups raising their voice against cage rearing in many countries like European Union, Switzerland, USA and Australia etc. Keeping in view these sentiments, the cage design and size have been modified in these countries. Under the EU directive, the enriched cage must be at least 45 cm high and must provide 750 cm^2 of space per hen.

Deep Litter System

In this system a 3-4 inch (7.5-10 cm) deep layer of a good litter material which should be dry, absorbent, free from mould growth and cheap, is spread on the floor. The feeders and waterers are placed on the litter and the nests are lined on one or both sides of the house. The dropping of birds go on mixing with the litter material and pile up to a depth of 1 to 1.5 feet in a year. The litter must be replaced after every batch. A view of the inside of deep litter house is depicted in Fig.30.

Advantages

- The birds are free and are able to express their natural behaviours such as scratching and dust bathing.
- Investment per bird is less than the cage system.
- Fly control is easier.
- Manure is of good quality.
- The litter provides warmth in winter and keeps the house cool in summer.
- Deep litter is a source of certain vitamins e.g. B_2, B_{12}, for the birds.

Disadvantages

- Vices like cannibalism and egg eating may be problems.
- More chances of diseases.
- Manure management is a problem particularly in humid season and extreme winter.
- Deworming of birds is required at regular intervals.
- There is a problem of floor and soiled eggs.
- More floor space is required per bird than cage system.

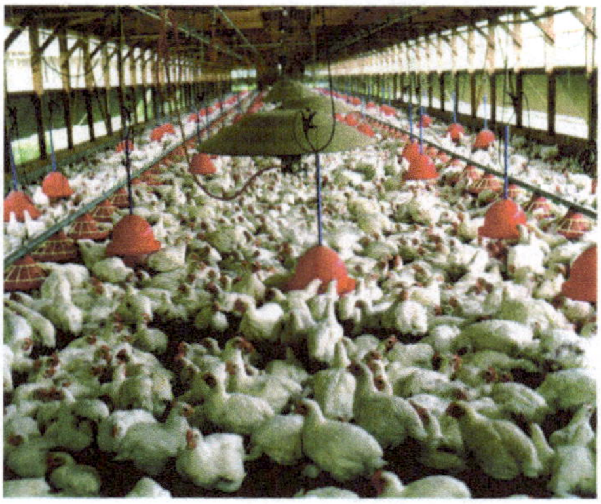

Fig. 30: Inside view of the deep litter house.

Slatted Floor System

Wire, wooden or plastic slats are used in this system instead of deep litter. The slats are about 1 to 2 in. (2.5 to 5cm) wide and spaced 1 in. (2.5cm) apart and run lengthwise of the building. The slats are made in sections so that they can be removed when necessary for removal of droppings. The slats are fixed with their top 27 inches above the floor. The space between the slats and floor provides room for the storage of dropping over a long period of time, generally one year. This system can be used both for commercial broilers and layers.

Advantages

- Birds require less floor space than the deep litter system
- No litter is needed.
- The birds have freedom of movement.
- There is a better control of bacterial diseases.
- Frequent manure removal is not required.

Disadvantages

- There is a problem of high humidity in the house.
- Birds have no place to relax.
- Feather condition becomes rough.
- There is a higher incidence of egg breakage.
- Birds cannot express their natural behavior.

Slat and Litter System

This system (Fig. 31) is popular for breeding birds particularly meat-type breeders. In this system the wooden plastic slats are placed over 60% of the floor and the remaining 40% area is covered with litter.

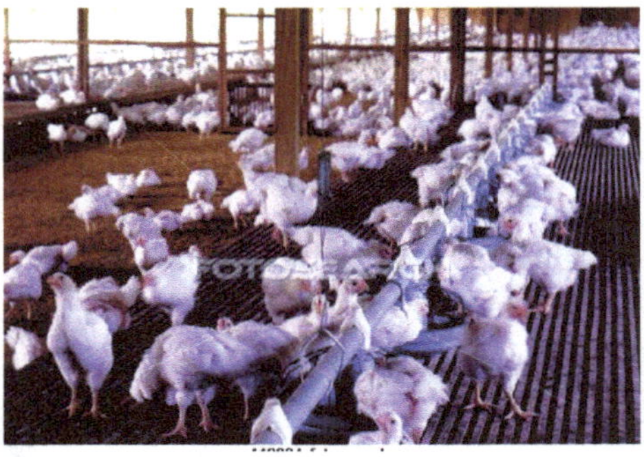

Fig. 31: A view of slat and litter broiler house. (Courtesy: fotosearch.com)

Advantages

- The birds can express their scratching and dust bathing behaviour which is not possible on all slat floor.
- The fertility of eggs is higher than in all slat system.
- Stocking density can be increased than the deep litter system.
- Litter quality remains better even at higher density than deep litter system.

Disadvantages

- The litter area of the slat and litter house is more difficult to ventilate.
- Egg production is slightly less than the deep litter system.

Environmentally Controlled Housing (EC Housing)

Optimum environmental conditions must be provided for realizing the maximum genetic potential and feed conversion efficiency. The heat production through digestion and metabolism should be equal to the heat lost by the bird through conduction, convection, radiation and evaporation to maintain their thermal balance. The temperature at which the birds achieve the thermal balance is called *critical temperature*. The laying hens perform with little or no discomfort within a temperature range of 50-75^{0}F (10-24^{0}C). It is called the *comfort zone*. Additional nutrients are required to produce heat to keep the body warm at the temperatures below the comfort zone. Also more nutrients are needed to keep the body cool through panting when temperature is above the comfort zone. The temperature range in which the birds have maximum rate of egg production and feed efficiency is called the *optimum temperature*. This range is 55-70^{0}F (13-21^{0}C) for layers. The critical temperature and comfort zone vary with different species, age, breed and physiological and productive status. The variation with age is large in chickens. The comfort zone for baby chicks is 92-95^{0}F (33-35^{0}C), whereas for adult layers it is 50 to 75^{0}F (10-24^{0}C). The optimum relative humidity for poultry house ranges between 50-75%. Air movement removes the body heat at a rapid rate. In warm weather, it makes the birds comfortable, but in cold weather, it adds to the low temperature stress. The confinement system with high density production operations is associated with problems such as wet litter, ammonia and carbon dioxide build up, odours and manure disposal.

Environmentally controlled poultry houses are designed to operate such that the environmental conditions of temperature, relative humidity, ammonia, carbon dioxide, wind velocity, light etc. are automatically maintained as near as possible to the optimum range required by the birds. These are windowless, completely enclosed and insulated structures. Air is removed from the house through exhaust fans and fresh air enters through intake openings. Natural day light is not available, so the house is illuminated using artificial light. In extreme hot conditions, inside temperature control devices have to be used. The houses do not require any heating except for brooding. The heat produced by the birds is used to maintain inside temperature within the comfortable range for the birds. The ideal environmental conditions maintained in these houses and insulation of ceiling and walls of the house are shown in Fig 32. The structural details of these houses are similar as discussed earlier in this chapter, except that it should have a gable roof and insulation of both sides and top. The overhang of the roof can be reduced to 0.25 m. The width of the environmentally controlled house can be increased up to 50 ft (15.5 m) as the air is mechanically exhausted. Mechanical air movement through the environmentally controlled house is a must to supply oxygen and to remove moisture, ammonia and carbon dioxide and to maintain optimum temperature. Typical ventilating fans of 36 in (0.9 m) to 54 in (1.4m) diameter are used for ventilation depending upon the size of the house. The ventilation system in the environmentally controlled house must ensure that the air movement in the house is uniform from top to bottom and from side to side. In modern environmentally controlled house, all the environmental requirements are controlled through various computerized sensing devices and operate automatically. These houses are most common in temperate regions where power supply is not a problem.

Advantages

- Birds are most comfortable and remain healthy.
- Feed efficiency is better.
- Growth/egg production is higher.
- Feeding, watering, egg collections, egg grading and packing operations can be automated thus saves on labour cost.
- More birds can be kept per unit land area.
- There is no seasonal influence on the performance of birds.

Disadvantages

- Initial cost is high.
- Uninterrupted power supply is needed.
- Huge losses may occur in case of power failure.

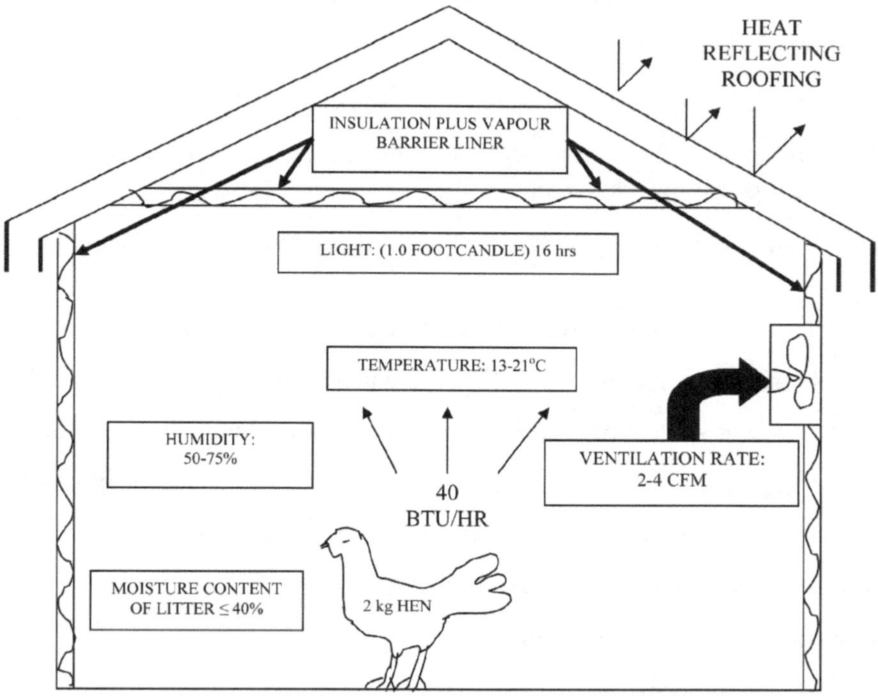

Fig 32: Environmental conditions for laying hens in the environmentally controlled house.

Question Bank

I . Fill in the Blanks

1. Housing constitutes the .... largest component of cost of poultry production (second)
2. The width of poultry house should not be more than ....feet (30 to 32.)
3. .... is a place where artificial hatching of chicks is carried out. (Hatchery)
4. A brooder house is a place where .... of chicks is carried out. (brooding)
5. The ceiling height of the setter room should be ....feet (14)
6. Poultry birds are most comfortable when the temperature varies between .... to ....^{0}C and the relative humidity between ...... to ....per cent. (10, 24, 50, 75)

7. The optimum temperature range for layers is ...... to .... ^{0}C (13, 21)

II. True / False

1. Pre warming room is located next to the egg room.- True
2. Poultry houses in tropical areas should be placed with their long axis facing east to west - True
3. Poultry housing need not suit to the climatic conditions of the geographical area. - False
4. The roof of poultry house should be water proof with proper slope - True
5. In free range system 200 to 220 birds can be kept in one acre of land - False
6. The cage system of rearing is most popular for laying birds - True
7. Deep litter is a source of certain vitamins e.g. B_2, B_{12}, for the birds - True
8. Intensive system of rearing is good for organic poultry production – False

III. Draw a floor plan of a modern hatchery.

IV. Write short notes on the following

(a) EC housing

(b) Tunnel ventilation system

(c) Planning of a poultry farm

(d) Selection of site for a poultry farm

V. What are the different systems of rearing poultry? Briefly describe about the systems with their advantages and disadvantages.

18

Brooding (Chick) Management

D. Sapcota

Types of Brooders

Brooding is a mechanism of providing auxiliary or supplementary heat to chicks through artificial heat using brooders. Brooders are of several types depending upon the size and the nature of fuel used. These are individual, multiple units or central heating systems run by coal, wood, oil, gas or electricity. The essentialities of a good brooder are i) a dependable mechanism, ii) supply of fresh air, iii) dryness, iv) adequate space, v) easy for cleaning and disinfection, vi) protection against enemies, vii) safety from fire and viii) economy.

i) Hover brooders

Such brooders are more widely used in India wherever electricity is available. They maintain uniform temperature, convenient for operation and require very little attention. However, eclectic brooders do not heat house appreciably in very cold weather. Wet litter may be another problem requiring frequent stirring and renewal of litter.

ii) Infra red brooders

This is relatively a new method of brooding chicks in which infra red lamps are suspended 20-25 inches above the litter. These do not heat the room but warm the chicks and therefore, comfort of the chicks and not the thermometer is the guiding factor. A single 250 watts infra red bulb will provide warmth for 60-70 chicks. Multiple units may be used for brooding large number of chicks.

iii) Central heating system

Very large highly commercial operations require central heating system for their large scale operations. Several different systems have been developed which use coal, oil, gas or electricity as fuel. Under this system heated air or water is circulated in pipe lines underneath the building to maintain warmth inside the house.

iv) Battery brooders

It is another type of confinement brooding provided with thermostat for easy control of temperature. It will have usually 4 tires provided with feeders and waterers. The battery brooders must be kept within a room preferably at a temperature of 21- 24^{0}C. Battery brooders are being extensively used for experimental purpose. Heated batteries (chick batteries) are used for brooding chicks up to 4 weeks; whereas unheated batteries (grower batteries) meant for chicks after 4 weeks.

v) Gas brooding

Commonly, Liquefied petroleum gas is used in producing heat. The gas is connected to heating element which is hung 3-4 ft above the chick level. Advantage of this system is that it can be taken to any location, even where electricity is scarce.

vi) Kerosene or Charcoal stove

Ordinary kerosene or charcoal stoves are used to provide supplementary heat to chicks where electricity is not available. The stoves should he covered with plate or pans to dissipate the heat; however, care should he made that there is adequate ventilation in the shed and toxic gases produced by the stoves are not accumulated.

Arrangements to be made before the arrival of chicks

i) About ten days before clean, wash thoroughly, blow lamp and white wash the brooder house.

ii) Brooders, feeders, waterers etc. should be washed with disinfectants.

iii) Put right kind of litter over the floor up to 4 inches.

iv) Arrange the brooder one day in advance and check whether it is running properly or not.

v) Spread old news papers over litter and under the brooder to avoid chicks eating litter material by any chance.

vi) Arrange feeders in cart wheel manner with waterers alternately around the brooder.

vii) Sprinkle ground maize or starter feed on the spread news papers to facilitate chicks to pick up and eat easily.

viii) Arrange chick guards 2-3 feet around brooder to a height of about 18 inches either with card board or wire.

Arrangements to be made after the arrival of chicks

i) Depending on the necessity chicks should have been vaccinated against Marek's disease on the day of hatch in the hatchery itself.

ii) While leaving chicks under the brooder train few chicks as how to eat and drink by dipping their beaks in feeders and waterers.

iii) The chick feed should have been supplemented with coccidiostats.

iv) Follow the vaccination schedule for the chicks strictly.

v) Extend chick guards as the chicks grow but remove them ultimately by 10th day.

vi) Block the corners of the brooder room after removing chick guards.

vii) As the chicks grow change the size of feeders and waterers, accordingly.

viii) Take utmost care in not damping the litter.

ix) Maintain a photoperiod of 23 h light and one h darkness.

Importance of environment (temperature, humidity and ventilation etc.) in brooding:

i) **Temperature**: Chicks require auxiliary or supplementary heat for the first 3 to 4 weeks of age since they are unable to adjust or regulate their body temperature in tender age. Further, proper temperature is essential for normal growth. Both low and high temperature are harmful to chicks and may slow down the growth or cause mortality. The chicks feel comfortable between 16-35^0C ranges of temperature. Since it is difficult to meet individual requirements, a range of temperature between 16-35^0 C is to be provided allowing the chicks to adjust to the amount of temperature they need. Starting chicks immediately after hatching require 35^0C during 1st week and thereafter temperature requirement decreases by 2.5^0C every week until they equal with environmental temperature of 21^0C.

Brooding is done for 2-3 weeks in hot climate and for 3-4 weeks in cold climate. In very hot parts of the day the brooder can be put off and similarly in cold season brooders are kept running even in daytime. After 2-3 weeks chicks usually do not require brooding in daytime. Chilling of chicks often occurs whenever there is lacuna in brooder management. However, the effect of high temperature seldom occurs because chicks will move away from heat source if they find it uncomfortable. The high lethal temperature for chicks is 47⁰C. The movement of chicks under brooder is a very good guide about the temperature rather than thermometer. If there is overheating in the brooder the chicks will move away from the brooder heat source and if the temperature is very low the chicks crowd under the brooder. On the other hand if the temperature is properly maintained they distribute uniformly underneath the brooder.

ii) **Humidity:** Both high and low humidity conditions in the brooder house are undesirable. A relative humidity of 50-60% may be considered suitable. If the humidity is too high it leads to wet litter condition and certain diseases like parasites, coccidiosis may crop in. On the other hand low humidity may cause very dried up atmosphere and result in poor feathering.

iii) **Ventilation:** Ventilation is essential to provide fresh air which is essential for developing chicks. It is also necessary to keep poultry house dry and free from odours. Proper ventilation removes poisonous gases, if any like carbon monoxide formed due to defective combustion of fuels, like oil, gas, coal etc. A concentration of 0.01% of carbon monoxide in air can initiate a slow process of poisoning. Ammonical fumes produced under deep litter system are obnoxious and irritating to the chicks in ill ventilated houses.

iv) **Floor space:** Floor space requirements vary with the size and therefore with the age of chicks. The floor space under deep litter system is as under:

0-4 weeks	=	0.5 sq. ft. per chick
4-8 weeks	=	1.0 sq. ft. per chick
8-16 weeks	=	1.5 sq. ft. per chick
16-20 weeks	=	2.0 sq. ft. per chick
20-72 weeks	=	2.5 sq. ft. per chick

For broilers 0.75 to 1.00 sq. ft. per chick floor space is provided until market age.

v) **Cleanliness and sanitation:** Cleanliness of brooders, brooder room and rearing equipment is of paramount importance. Proper sanitation is essential to obtain success. Thorough scrubbing, cleaning, washing and disinfection of brooder and grower houses as well as equipment is necessary in order to obtain good results in brooding and to prevent occurring of diseases. Disinfections act better in the absence of dust and debris. Any commercial disinfectant can be used as per manufacturers' instructions. Lysol solution, coal tar derivatives, chlorine compounds may be used.

Feeding and Vaccination at Early Stage of Chicks

Brooder Chick mash with 22% crude protein and 2700 Kcal/kg of metabolisable energy has to be prepared and provided. Good quality, potable medicated water has to be provided in the waterers. Look for the health of the chicks at the time of delivery. Lighting for heating (brooding) has to be provided for 23 hours. Depending on seasonal requirements, adjust the length of lighting. However, layer type chicks should not be provided additional lighting for more than 12 hours after four weeks, till they start laying at 20 weeks. If day length is about 10 hours, do not give any additional lighting at all. If chicks are reared during winter and the natural day length is likely to increase as the age of the bird advances, then add giving light so as to maintain 10-12 hours per day constantly until the birds start laying. If the total length of light is allowed to increase day by day up to start of lay, such birds will start laying eggs early which will be smaller in size and will continue to remain so for longer period and thus will result in fetching lesser price and consequent loss.

The required number of feeders and waterers has to be worked out and provided. Initially, smaller size feeders and waterers with lesser depth will have to be provided which should be changed to larger size with greater depth after three weeks of age. Adjust the height of the feeders and waterers to match the height of the growing birds to avoid wastage. Feed and water the birds at least twice daily at regular intervals. Watch the growth of the birds and water and feed consumption regularly. The Table 16 gives a guideline even though feed and water consumption may vary depending on seasons.

Table 16: Feed and water intake by 1000 chicks

Age in weeks	Feed intake/week (kg)	Water intake/day (litre)	Body weight at the end of the week (g)
1	40	10	60
2	80	25	105
3	140	45	160
4	200	65	230
5	250	80	300
6	300	95	370
7	350	105	440
8	390	120	510

To avoid feed wastage, the chicks are to be debeaked first at the age of 7- 10 days. Their beaks have to be cut short by debeaking machine applying electrical cauterization. It may also be performed at the end of second week and repeated at 12-14th week. The upper beak has to be cut 2/3rd and the lower beak 1/3rd portion. The cut portion has to be cauterized by touching on the hot plate. The tongue should be carefully held back. Undertake debeaking during cooler parts of the day. Provide anti-stress B-complex vitamins and vitamin K in drinking water before, during and after the day of debeaking. Utmost care need to be taken to avoid stress during debeaking. Since layer chicks are comparatively more active, they tend to peck at each other's back (cannibalism), cause injury and death also. Debeaking helps to prevent such instances. Vaccines to be given to the birds at this brooder stage.

Take care to buy quality vaccines, kept under proper storage conditions. Ensure proper dosage as per specifications. Vaccinate the birds with minimum stress to them. Medication for layer chicks include glucose and electrolytes on the first day and a mild antibiotic/ antibacterial along with vitamin tonics for the first five days; later on, no medication is required unless warranted. Chicks can also be reared in cages from 0-8 weeks. For 100 numbers of chicks the dimension of the cage should be 180 x 90 x 30 (L x B x H) cm. which can be kept 75 cm above floor level. One 100 watt bulb is sufficient on the top of the cage for providing heat for first three weeks. For first two weeks, small feeders and waterers have to be kept inside the cage and afterwards they may be fixed outside on the sides of the cage.

Vaccination schedule during chick stage

Sl. No.	Age in days	Type of vaccine	Remarks
1.	0 day	Mareks' vaccine (Hatchery)	Ensure that the same has been given at the hatchery itself
2.	5-7th day	RDVF/ LaSota	Occulonasal
3.	14-16th day	IBD vaccine (Intermediate/ killed)	Eye drops/S/C injection
4.	20th day	IB vaccine	Optional
5.	26th day	IBD (intermediate)	Eye drops/ drinking water(avoid chlorinated water)
6.	30th day	LaSota vaccine	Drinking water/ eye drops(avoid chlorinated water)
7.	56th day	RDVK/ R2B	S/C injection

Question Bank

I . Choose the Correct Answer.

1. For infra red brooding the lamps are suspended at 20-25/30-35/40-45 inches above the litter. (20-25).
2. A single 250 watts infra red bulb will provide warmth for 60-70/10-110/ 140-150 brooding chicks. (60-70).
3. Battery brooders usually have 4/6/8 tiers. (4).
4. Chicks are debeaked at the age of 7-10/ 12-15/ 17-20 days with the help of a debeaker. (7-10).
5. A relative humidity of 40-50/50-60/60-70 % may be considered suitable in brooder house. (50-60).
6. The vaccination against Marek's disease is given in the hatchery/brooder house/layer house. (hatchery).

II . Fill in the blanks

1. Battery brooders must be kept within a room preferably at a temperature between .... °C.(21- 24).
2. The height of chick guard is about .... inches. (18).
3. The photoperiod maintained during the brooding period is ....h of light and .... h of darkness.(23 and 1).
4. The chicks feel comfortable between ....°C ranges of temperature. (35-16).

5. A concentration of .... % of carbon monoxide in air can initiate a slow process of poisoning in brooder shed. (0.01).
6. Brooder mash should contain .... % crude protein and..............Kcal/kg of ME. (22 and 2700)

III . True / False.

1. Hatching is a mechanism of providing auxiliary or supplementary heat to chicks through artificial heat using brooders. (False).
2. Electric brooders do not heat house appreciably in very cold weather. (True).
3. Infra red lamps do not heat the brooder room but warm the chicks. (True).
4. Since the heating unit is inadequate the battery brooders must be kept within a room. (True).
5. Battery brooders are being extensively used for experimental purpose. (True).
6. If the total length of light is allowed to increase day by day up to start of lay, such birds will start laying eggs early with smaller in size. (True).

19

Care and Management of Commercial Growers, Layers and Broilers

D. Sapcota

Care and Management of Commercial Growers (09-20 weeks) Under Deep Litter System

Grower management essentially remains the same as that of chick management (brooding management) except for the additional space required for floor, feeders and waterers to keep with the size of birds. The growers may be reared in separate grower-houses or continued to be reared in brooder-cum-grower houses.

- **Floor space:** 1260 cm^2 (1.4 ft^2) per bird.
- **Feeder space:** 6-8 cm per bird. One linear feeder of 120 cm length and 8 cm depth for 40 growers.
- **Waterer space:** 2 cm per bird; a circular waterer of 36 cm and 8 cm depth of 6 lit. capacity for 50 growers. Growers are to be provided with fresh, cool and potable drinking water at least twice a day. Water requirement is increased during hot days. Care must be made not to spill water on litter.
- **Lighting management:** No artificial lighting is given other than natural day light since they require only 9 hours of light per day.

Growers may be fed with mash containing 16% CP and 2600 Kcal/kg ME. A bird may take 60-80 g feed per day. The height of feeder and waterer should be adjusted at shoulder level of the bird. It is not advisable to provide *ad libitum* feeding during growing stage as the bird may put more fat affecting egg laying rate in future. Therefore, restricted feeding programme should be adopted which will delay early sexual maturity so as to improve egg quality. The litter is raked often to bring down its moisture level. If necessary, super phosphate may be mixed with litter @ 2 kg/100 ft^2 area to reduce litter ammonia level. The birds may be dewormed at 16th week of age with appropriate dewormer. For efficient use, 2 hour withdrawal period is practiced before offering medicated water. The poorly grown birds are to be culled at this stage. The mortality rate during growing period must be lower than 3 per cent.

Care and Management of Commercial Growers (09-20 weeks) Under Cage System

For caged growers the floor may be made up to welded mesh of 1.25X5.0 cm size. In a cage of 180X90 cm size, 50 growers can be reared with a space allowance of 325 cm^2/bird. Feeders /waterers can be fitted lengthwise on the outside one below the other. Nipple drinker may be fitted inside the cage. Adequate care should be made to maintain uniformity of growth in the flock. Sample weight should be taken once in week to find out the average body weight as per the breeder recommendations.

Care and Management of Commercial Layers (21-72 weeks) Under Deep Litter System

At the end of 18th week growers are transferred to layer house to take special care so that optimum numbers of eggs are produced by them. They may be reared on good quality litter (5-6 cm height) with floor space allowance of 1800 cm^2 (2 ft^2) per bird. In high humid areas like north-east India the space may be increased to 2250 cm^2 (2.5 ft^2). The feeder space and water space allowances of 10-12 cm and 2.5 cm per bird, respectively may be provided.

A liner feeder of 180 cm length and 10 cm depth will be sufficient for 35 birds; whereas, a circular waterer of 45 cm diameter and 7 cm depth will be required for 50 birds. These birds are fed with layer mash containing 18% CP, 2700 Kcal/kg ME, 2.75% calcium and 0.80% available phosphorus, all the time. Waterer guards on waterer and grill on linear feeder will prevent birds standing on the edge or on top and spoiling the contents. Provide clean, fresh water at least twice a day. During laying stage 1000 birds will consume 250 liters of water and 110-120 kg feed per day, approximately. The water consumption increased during hot days; whereas, feed consumption decreases. During cold season the feed consumption increases. The feeders and waterers are to be arranged alternatively at equal distance keeping their height at bird's shoulder level filing only to 2/3 level to avoid wastage/spillage. The wastage is about 25 to 30% when filled full and about only 10% when filled two third. The feeders should be distributed in a way that the birds do not have to walk more than 3 meters (10ft) for feed.

Usually one nest box for every 5 layers is sufficient. The boxes may be made of GI, aluminum or wood and adjusted at about 45 cm height and kept in darker part of the shed. The mouth of the box should be of 30cm width with a depth of 20 cm. Clean litter material may be spared inside the box all the time so as to obtain clean eggs. It is better to provide community nest rather than individual nest. The nest should be closed during night hours so as to prevent sitting of birds in the nest. In deep-litter system, the litter materials should be treated chemically at least once in a month so as to reduce ammonia emission; it is preferably be racked in the evening, daily after the collection of eggs. Deworming should be done regularly at an interval of 6-8 weeks.

Lighting Management for Layers

From 20th week or from the commencement of 5% egg production, whichever is earlier, artificial lighting should be commenced. For every week the lighting period should be increased by 15 minutes till a maximum of 16 hours of photoperiod per day is reached which is known as step up lighting programme. Beyond 16 hours of total photoperiod (natural + artificial) has no beneficial effect. Never decrease the photoperiod during laying period and never increase during non-laying period. One watt per 3 sq ft is recommended. Bulbs of 25 to 40 watt should be firmly attached 7 ft above the floor and 8-12 ft apart. The distance between 2 tube lights (florescent) should be 15 ft. Reflectors should be used to direct all light downward and be cleaned regularly to remove dust from bulbs. The light intensity should be uniform throughout the poultry house. A light intensity of 0.5 to 1 foot candle is sufficient for egg production but normally about 0.9 to 1.2 ft. candle is provided. Unlike incandescent bulb florescent bulbs produce a lower intensity of light as they age. The use of compact florescent lamp (CFL) not only saves electricity but also does not emit heat as comparison to its incandescent counterpart.

Cage System for Layers

Layers are invariably reared in cages. Cages of various sizes are available to house 3-5 birds in a cage. Currently, reverse cages are commonly used with their longer side being fitted to remain in the front. Further, raised platform houses are constructed, of late, to facilitate quicker drying of droppings and their easy removal.

The cage of following sizes may be made and fitted in rows

45 x 30 cm	-	for 3 birds
45 x 40 cm	-	for 4 birds
50 x 35 cm	-	for 4 birds
55 x 45 cm	-	for 5 birds
60 x 37.5 cm	-	for 5 birds

These cages are arranged in two or three rows one above the other on either side. If they are arranged in staircase manner, then they are termed as *Californian cages*. A floor space of 420 – 450 cm^2 is allowed within cages. Conventionally, the bottom of the lowermost cages is fitted at 75cm height from the floor. Now-a-days, they are fitted at 120-240 cm height above the floor level with walking platforms constructed on the sides. The layer cage will be of 40 cm height. The floor is fitted with 2.5 x 5.0 cm size weld mesh of 14 gauge thickness. On sides, 7.5 x 7.5 cm size mesh of 16 gauge thickness is fitted. The bottom floor is provided with 1/6 slope downwards to the front to facilitate rolling of the eggs to the cage front. The mesh rails on cage floor should run from back to front and not sideways; otherwise they will block free run of the eggs downwards to the front. Waterers are fitted above the feeders in the front. Automatic waterer nipples/ buttons and feeders may be provided to the cages.

Cages are fitted in two or three tiers on either side of the row under Californian system of arrangement. Two to three such rows of cages are arranged in a caged layer house. Depending on the number of rows, and number of tiers in each row, the breadth of caged layer house ranges from 15-17' (5-8 m). There is no stipulation for length of such houses which can be adjusted as per the number of birds to be housed. No side walls are required for cage houses with the mesh being stretched down to the floor level to facilitate better ventilation for drying up the moisture in the droppings. Cage rearing facilitates easy management, lesser space requirement, and easier collection of eggs, less percentage of broken eggs, better egg weight, clean egg production, easy culling and reduced mortality levels.

Egg laying starts at 21st week and the rate of laying (percentage production) increases every week to reach a level of 90% and above after 28 weeks of age which is maintained well beyond 36 weeks of age even up to 40-42 weeks. Afterwards, it slumps down slowly to reach 70% or below by 72 weeks of age. When the egg production goes below 65%, it is uneconomical to retain them unless the egg price is exceptionally high. Egg production may be calculated as percentage on total number of birds available at 21st week (hen-housed egg production) or on number of birds available on each day (hen day egg production).Satisfactory egg production levels at different ages during laying stage are given in Table 17 to serve as a guide to verify whether the birds are producing at the optimal level.

Table 17: Layer performance under optimal conditions

Age in weeks	Hen-day egg production (%)	Feed intake /1000 birds (kg)	Water intake/1000 birds (litre)
21	10	75	160
22	18	85	180
23	34	96	210
24	55	105	240
25	68	109	260
26	76	113	280
27	84	115	290
28	88	115	300
29	90	115	310
30	92	115	320
31	94	115	320
32-39	92	110	310
40-47	86	107	290
48-59	82	105	270
60-64	76	103	260
65-70	70	101	240
71-76	65	96	240

The layer type chicken lay their eggs mostly during forenoon. Eggs may be collected twice in the morning and once in the afternoon. The frequency of egg collection has to be increased to four to five times during peak summer. In large layer farms, it is preferable to have air-cooled room for storage of eggs. Specially designed plastic/ cardboard trays have to be used to collect eggs. Usually 30 egg capacity collecting trays (filler flat) are used. It is not advisable to collect eggs in baskets.

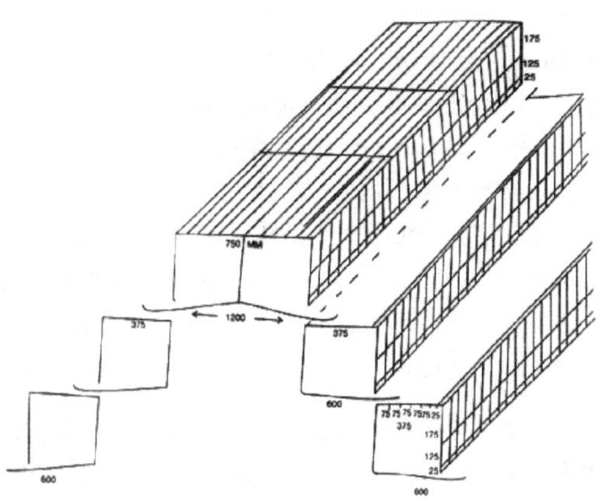

Fig. 33: A sketch of Californian cage. Courtesy: http://www.omegaweldmesh.com/commercial_layer_cages.html

A front view of Californian cage system

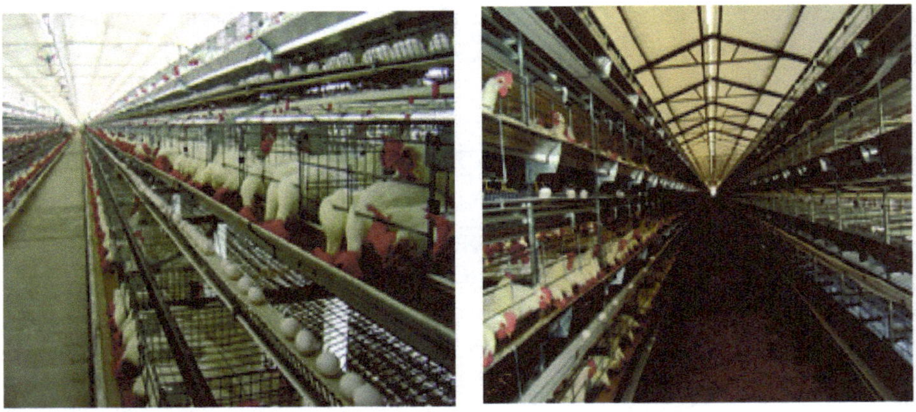

Fig. 34: Front views of battery cage.
Courtesy: http://www.gartech.co.in/images/ge-royal/pic4.jpg

Care and Management of Commercial Broilers

The brooding may be carried out on floor (using hover brooder or with infra red bulb) or on cages (battery brooder). The hover brooder may be made of galvanized iron sheet, wood or bamboo. The brooding management for straight-run (unsexed) day-old broiler chicks is similar to that of layer chicks, described earlier. The newspaper which was spread on litter under brooder may be removed after 3-4 days. Chick guard is removed after 9-10 days; however, the corners of the room may be covered with pieces of dismantled chick guard so that during dark night in inclement weather the chicks are not frighten, piled up and died in the corners. After 15 days the pieces of chick guard are may be removed and the corners are opened up. For each broiler chick the floor space allowance is 450 cm^2 (0.5 ft^2) up to 18 days and 1000 cm^2 (1 ft^2) afterwards till market age. Feeder space allowance is 3 cm and 6-7 cm per broiler and waterer space allowance is 1.5 and 3 cm per broiler for the above mentioned period, respectively. As the chick grows the smaller feeders and waterers are replaced with bigger ones.

Early in the morning each waterer should be cleaned, filled with fresh, clear and potable drinking water. Watering may be done twice a day but feeding at least four times in a day. The feeders and waterers are filed to only their 2/3 capacity so as to prevent spillage. Feeding of broilers may be done in 2 phases. During the 1st four weeks broiler starter mash/pellet/crumble containing 21%

CP and 2900 Kcal/kg of ME has to be fed and thereafter till market age broiler finisher mash/pellet/crumble containing 21% CP and 2900-3000 Kcal/kg of ME has to be given. Alternately, broiler may also be fed in 3 phases: 0-2 weeks (pre starter), 3-5 weeks (broiler starter) and above 5 weeks (broiler finisher). Feeding and watering may be done at the same time, every day. During summer feed consumption decreases and water consumption increases; whereas, during winter or rainy season the water consumption deceases and feed consumption increases.

Feeders and waterers may be positioned at appropriate level so that the birds find comfortable to use. Make provisions to adjust the height of feeders/waterers so that their brim is hiked to the level of the back of the bird. The growth of broilers has to be monitored, weekly. For this, 10 birds, at random may be picked up, weighed and compared with standard chart as given below in Table 18.

Table 18: Growth performance and feed efficiency of broilers

Age (wk)	Average body weight (g)	Feed intake/1000 birds/day (kg)	Cumulative feed intake per bird (g)	Feed efficiency	Water intake 1000 birds/day (litre)
0	42	-	-	-	-
1	170	19	146	0.86	46
2	380	37	426	1.12	89
3	720	68	945	1.31	165
4	1170	102	1730	1.48	245
5	1680	134	2720	1.62	320
6	2220	168	3996	1.80	405

The table gives average weight of each bird, anticipated at the end of the week, and daily feed and water consumption by 1000 birds at the respective age even though water and feed consumption will vary depending on season. If the growth rate is lower, the farmer has to check the quality of feed, managemental flaws or possibility of presence of any subclinical infection. Also watch out for daily consumption of feed and water as any drastic change has to be investigated.

Litter Management for Broilers

Broilers are invariably reared on litter. The commonly used litter materials are, paddy husk, saw dust, chopped straw, ground nut husk, bagasse etc. To start with a litter the thickness of 5 cm is sufficient. The litter may be maintained practically dry (day matter of 75-80 %). If the moisture level exceeds 25%, excess ammonia will be produced. After 2 weeks, every day the litter has to be raked with the help of spade/spike so that caked material is broken up. Before raking the litter all feeders/waterers are to be removed from the floor.

The ammonia level inside brooder house, if exceeds 25ppm may cause stresses. The younger birds suffer the most. There will be irritation of eyes and nasal membrane leading to poor feed consumption, growth and lameness. The broiler will be predisposed to respiratory and coccidiosis problems. To assess moisture level in the litter, take a handful of it and squeeze. If the litter forms a cake then it can be assumed that the moisture level is high. If it crumbles into fine dust, moisture is very low which will make the environment more dusty. It has to remain as a loose mass, if the moisture level is less.

Lighting Management for Broilers

Normally 23 hours of continuous light (photoperiod is natural daylight + artificial lighting) is used in the building with one hour of darkness each day to prevent the birds from becoming frightened and resulting in piling ups and smothering, if a power failure should occur. A high intensity of light is usually given during first 14 days to help the chicks get started on feed and water.

Battery Cage Management

The Californian system of cages is the most commonly used in commercial egg production. In high humid regions like North-east India battery cage would be more appropriate. Just below the cages a shallow pit of 6-8 inches is dug to accommodate all the fecal materials to fall in. The accumulated materials must be regularly removed from this pit. The cages are fitted on 2-3 tiers on either side of the walk area. Of late, ***'elevated or high raised cage houses'*** are preferred in which cages are fitted at above 5-6' height from platform. This arrangement widens the gap between birds and their droppings, facilitates quicker drying and easy removal of droppings. In such houses the droppings are removed even after several years using lorry or JCB. In such houses smell, disease spreading or fly problem become minimal. Though cage system of rearing is gaining popularity over deep litter system, it has following advantages and disadvantages.

Advantages of cage system	Disadvantages of cage system
1. Increased production and feed efficiency.	1. More broken eggs are produced.
2. Less space per bird is required.	2. Few birds will exhibit the symptoms of cage layer fatigue.
3. Less labour requirement.	3. Fly problem.
4. Culling of unproductive birds become easier.	4. Problem of removal of litter.
5. Clean eggs are produced.	5. No chance of getting nutrients form litter.
6. No problem of wet litter.	6. Initial investment per bird is higher.
7. Higher stocking density.	
8. Layers are provided with better sanitary and hygienic environment.	
9. Broodiness is eliminated.	
10. Parasitic problems are lessened.	
11. Lesser incidences of cannibalism.	

Question Bank

I . Choose the Correct Answer

1. The floor space requirement per bird for commercial growers under deep litter system is: 1240/1260/ 1280 cm^2. (1260).
2. The feeder space requirement per bird for commercial growers under deep litter system is: 2-4/6-8/10-12 cm. (6-8).
3. The waterer space requirement per bird for commercial growers under deep litter system is: 2/4/6 cm/ (2).
4. The growers require only 7/9/11 hours of light per day. (9).
5. The growers may be dewormed at 14th /15th/16th week of age with appropriate dewormer. (16th).
6. Usually, one nest box for every 5/7/9 layers is sufficient. (5).
7. For proper intensity of light for layers one watt per 3/4/5 sq ft is recommended. (3).
8. For proper lighting the bulbs of 25 to 40 watt should be firmly attached 7/8/9 ft above the floor and 4-8/8-12/13-16 ft apart. (7, 8-12).
9. A floor space allowance of 410-419/420 – 450/451-479 cm^2 is allowed within cages for layers. (420 – 450).
10. The pullets start laying from 17th/19th/21st week. (21).

11. The ammonia level inside brooder house, if exceeds 15/20/25ppm may cause stresses. (25).

II. True / False.

1. Water requirement is increased during hot days. (true).
2. No artificial lighting is given to growers other than natural day light. (true)
3. It is advisable to provide *ad libitum* feeding during growing stage. (false).
4. A grower bird may take 120-130 g feed per day. (false).
5. The feed wastage is about 25 to 30% when feeder is filled full and about only 10% when filled two third.(true).
6. A light intensity of 0.5 to 1 foot candle is sufficient for egg production. (true).
7. The bottom floor is provided with 1/6 slope downwards to the front to facilitate rolling of the eggs to the cage front. (true).
8. The breadth of caged layer house is depending on the number of rows and tiers; whereas, the length can be adjusted as per the number of birds to be housed. (true).
9. When the egg production goes below 75%, it is uneconomical to retain. (false).
10. It is advisable to collect eggs in baskets rather than in filler flat.(false).
11. If the litter moisture level exceeds 15%, excess ammonia will be produced. (false).
12. In cage system of rearing of birds lesser space per bird is required as compared to deep litter system. (true)
13. Higher stocking density is achieved under deep litter system of rearing as compared to that of cage system. (false).

III. Fill in the blanks

1. Growers may be fed with mash containing .... % CP and .... Kcal/kg ME. (16 and 2600.).
2. Layer mash should contain .... % CP, ... Kcal/kg ME, ... % calcium and .... % available phosphorus. (18, 2700, 2.75 and 0.8, respectively).

3. The mortality rate during growing period must be lower than .... per cent.(3).
4. At the end of .... week growers are transferred to layer house to take special care (18th)
5. The commercial layers may be reared on good quality litter with floor space allowance of .... cm^2 (1800).
6. The feeders should be filled only to .... level to avoid wastage. (2/3).
7. The feeders should be distributed in a way that the birds do not have to walk more than .... meters for feed. (3).
8. The nest boxes may be adjusted to at about .... cm height.(45).
9. For layers the lighting program should commence from .... week or from the commencement of .... % egg production, whichever is earlier. (20th and 5)
10. Under step up lighting programme for every week the lighting period should be increased by .... minutes till a maximum of .... hours of photoperiod per day is reached. (15, 16).
11. The distance between 2 tube lights (florescent) should be .... ft.(15).
12. Normally .... hours of continuous light (daylight + artificial lighting) are used in broiler raising. (23).
13. For each broiler chick the floor space allowance is .... cm^2 up to 18 days and .... cm^2 afterwards till market age. (450, 1000).
14. Feeder and waterer space allowances are .... cm and .... cm for each broiler chick up to 18 days of age. (3 and 1.5, respectively).
15. Broiler chickens may be fed with mash containing .... % CP and .... Kcal/kg ME from 1st four weeks and .... % CP and .... Kcal/kg thereafter. (21, 2900, 21 2900-3000, respectively).
16. In case of '*elevated or high raised cage houses*' the cages are fitted at above .... ft. height from platform. (5-6)
17. A high intensity of light is usually given during first .... days to help the broiler chicks get started on feed and water. (14).

20

Poultry Judging

D. Sapcota

In India, poultry judging refers to selection of birds on the basis of their physical appearances, breed characteristics and production performances; however, in other countries, like USA judging is also used for eggs, carcasses and further processed products. The Directorate of Extension, Ministry of Agriculture, Govt. of India annually conducts livestock and poultry shows in various parts of the country in collaboration of state governments. Besides, state Agricultural/ Veterinary Universities or other institutions also conduct such shows. In these shows judging contests are carried out mostly for the undergraduate students by using a score card to grade birds either for production characters or breed characters. The winners are awarded trophies and cash prizes. The birds meant for judging are kept in individual cages and the participants are requested to score under various sub-headings and to finally rank the bird. Any deviation from "*ideal*" or "*perfection*" (as described by the American Standard of Perfection or the British Poultry Standards) but not serious enough to constitute a disqualifications in the show room is considered to be a defect. Serious defects are regarded as disqualifications and will bar a bird from winning any prize. Both layers and broilers can be physically evaluated for their performance rating.

For purpose of judging the bird may be divided into the following groups:

1. Exhibition or show class.
2. Utility or production class (layers or broilers).
3. Exhibition cum game group.

Objectives

1. To develop healthy competition among breeders/owners and encourage them to develop superior quality birds based on the present day need.
2. To exchange views and opinions among poultry farmers and extension workers.
3. To become aware of the birds available and breeding programmes carried out elsewhere.

Judging of Layer

Judging of a good layer is based on certain extrinsic characters and related measurements expected to indicate a laying bird. Accordingly, layers can be graded based on the following score card.

Scorecard

		Points
Health and vigour of bird	:	25
Body conformation and abdominal capacity	:	25
Moulting and plumage	:	15
Pigmentation	:	10
Condition of head, wattle, vent and others	:	25

Health and Vigour

Bird should be active and alert and respond immediately to external stimuli. It should be healthy and should not show any sign of disease. Eyes should be round, bright and prominent. Poor layer without the above signs, will have pale skin and shrunken eyes.

Body Conformation and Abdominal Capacity

Body conformation in a good layer is characterized by broad back, spacious body with less abdominal fat and large, full, soft and pliable abdomen. Abdomen will be shrunken or fatty in a poor producer. The abdominal capacity is measured by the distance between pubic bones, which should be more than two-finger space and the distance between pelvic bone and keel bone should be a minimum of four fingers distance. Skin should be thin and velvety, thick and coarse skin indicates poor laying.

Moulting and Plumage

Moulting is an annual physiological phenomenon of shedding of old feathers and replacing them with new feathers. In a good layer, moulting commences at the end of the first laying season and completes the moult early. In a poor layer, it will commence early and is prolonged. There is a definite pattern. It starts from the head, passes on to neck, back and tail and then the primary and secondary feathers. Moulting is also governed by physical conditions such as season, light, feed etc.

A good layer will have dirty, worn out feather, whereas a poor layer will have bright velvety feathers. A good layer converts feed into eggs, while the poor layer diverts the feed for feather making and maintenance.

Pigmentation

Pigmentation is also a good indication of reproductive status of a layer, but can be depended upon only in a bird with yellow skin and the feed also has adequate carotenoid pigments. The pigmentation is full and intense at the start of lay throughout the entire skin, shank, beak, earlobe and eye rings. As the bird starts laying, the above parts get bleached in the following order.

Vent 0-7 days,
Eye ring 7-14 days,
Ear lobe 2-3 weeks
Beak (back to tip) 4-6 weeks
Bottom of feet 2 months.

As the bird stops-laying, pigments reappear in the reverse order. Vent portion is lastly pigmented. A poor layer will have intense pigmentation of the above parts relative to the production level. Depending on the level of pigmentation, the bird can be described as well bleached, fairly well and bleached poorly.

Conditions of Head, Wattle, Comb and Vent

Head of the bird can be defined as refined head, crow head (more tapering), beefy head (meat type), masculine head, etc. Fully-grown and bright in a good layer, they are warm, soft and velvety without any discoloration or scale formation. Poor layer will have a less shrunken comb, dry, scaly and discoloured or bleached and would be cold and rough to touch. Large, oval, moist and warm to touch in a good layer. It will be small, round, dry and pluckered in a poor layer.

Table 19: Characteristics of birds to be accounted in judging

Sl. No.	Character	Distinguishing features for good birds	Features of poor or bad birds
1.	Head a. Nature	Strongly* feminine in females and masculine in males, square and broad at the top. All parts well proportionate	Tendency to be masculine in females; coarse, crow headed, narrow and tapering at the top
	b. Comb, wattles and beak	Full, red, waxy, warm, velvety stocky, well curved, broad and rather short	Dry, scaly, shriveled, cold, coarse. Narrow, very long, thin, sharp and pointed
	c. Eyes	Bright, alert and well set	Dull, sleepy, may have squint
	d. Earlobes	Full, waxy, velvety, colour as per breed specification	Shrunken, wrinkled, coarse, off-colour to the breed
2.	Neck	Stocky and rather short	Long and thin
3.	Body		
	a. Nature	Capacious	Limited capacity
	b. Back	Broad and straight	Narrow, pinches and crooked
	c. Sides	Deep and straight	Shallow, barrel shaped
	d. Keel bone	Long, properly curved, flexible	Short, crooked and hard
	e. *Pubic bone	Wide apart, thin, soft and pliable. Distance between two pubic bones is more than 2 to 3 fingers	Close together, thick and stiff. Distance between two pubic bones is less than 1 to 2 fingers
	f. *Distance between keel and pubic bones (for females)	More than 4 to 5 fingers	Less than 2 to 3 fingers
	g. Skin	Thin, soft, oily and silky	Thick, dry, rough and underlaid with fat.
	h. Abdomen	Large, soft and free from lumps of fat	Small, hard and with lumps of fat
	i. *Vent	Large, oval and moist	Small, dry and round
	j. Plumage and colour	Tight, compact, slightly dull coloured but colour specific for breed and variety	Loose, scattered, brightly coloured but may be off coloured for breed and variety
4.	Legs Shank Toe-nails	Thin, soft and flat at back. Stocky, well curved	Thick, hard and rounded at the back Long, thin and sharp pointed
5.	Temperament	Friendly and always happy	Shy, nervous, squakes when caught
6.	Appetite	Hearty eater and crop always nearly full	Mincing appetite and poor eater
7.	*Pigmentation	Pigment bleaches out from beak, skin, vent, shank and eye ring as laying advances and they will appear faint in colour	Due to non-bleaching beak, skin, vent, shank and eye-ring are brightly coloured because of poor or non-laying

*These characters are especially important for females, while others are of common importance.

Descriptive Score Card for Egg Laying Contests

			Points
a.	Vigour and Sex (General health indication & femininity or masculinity)	:	15
b.	Breed characteristic 1. (Type 6 points) trueness to type for variety. 2. Colour 6 points, trueness to colour for variety	:	12
c.	Head 1. Comb, wattles & earlobes (6 points) cut points for too coarse, too thick, too velvety or too thin. Poor shape, lopped comb in straight comb varieties, straight comb in lopped comb varieties, high rear blade, too many or too few points, etc., 2. Shape of head (8 points) cut points in case of head too long, too short, too narrow, round on top, shallow or lacking balance (face 3 points) cut for enamel white on face, feathered face, shrunken or fat and bloated face. 3. Eye (7 points) cut for lacking prominence or proper colour, dull expression or droopy eye lids.	:	24
d.	Body 1. Depth (8 points) Back to rear end of keel (3 points) shoulder to front end of keel (2 points); span of abdomen (3 points) cut if shallow or narrow 2. Width (8 points) heart girth (2 points) loin (small of back) (1 points) hip to rump (3 points) 3. Length (8 points) cut if short	:	24
e.	Pigmentation Deep in all section, normal for variety, shank, beak etc.,	:	5
f.	Shanks & toes Cut for incorrect number of toes for variety	:	5
g.	Handling quality 1. Size, shape and condition of vent; cut for small, dry, round vent 2. Softness and pliability of abdomen skin; cut for dry, tough skin and hard, tough abdomen	:	5
h.	Actions i) Female disposition & laying temperament ii) Male, disposition, friendly, active, alert, curious as contrasted with flighty & excitable	:	10
	Total	:	100

Judging Broilers for Meat Production

Broilers are young immature chicken of either sex usually below 5-6 weeks of age, tender meated with smooth textured skin and a soft pliable breast bone cartilage.

Scorecard for Judging of Broilers

		Marks
General appearance	:	10
Health and vigour	:	15
Breast	:	30
Back and rib	:	15
Leg and thigh	:	15
Feathering	:	15

General Appearance

Bird should have a compact body, broad and fleshy comb should be medium in size with bright and prominent eyes. Birds should be free from common defects such as breast blisters, crooked keel, split wing, coarse beak, injuries etc. skin should be smooth and pliable.

Health and Vigour

Birds should be apparently healthy and free from any signs of disease like unthriftness, pale or cyanotic comb etc. Excessive fat is undesirable.

Breast

Wide and heavily fleshed, keel bone should be straight, long and parallel to the back. May have very slight curve but should not be crooked. Breast can be measured in terms of breast angle and by measuring the girth.

Back and Rib

Back should be broad and long from front to tail, ribs wide enough.

Legs and Thigh

Bird should have normal legs of moderate length and well fleshed. Long and thin legs are undesirable, while thick plumpy legs are preferred.

Feathering

Should be closely feathered spreading uniformly on the body. It may have small area of scattered pin feather which when present should be long enough for easy removal upon processing. Bare back grades down the broilers.

Judging for Breed Characteristics
The Standard Scorecard

For meat type breed			For egg type breed		
Type	:	25	Type	:	30
Comb	:	10	Colour	:	30
Ear lobe	:	10	Head & eyes	:	10
Eyes	:	5	Legs & feet	:	10
Legs	:	10	Condition	:	10
Breast	:	5	Quality & texture	:	10
Size	:	5			
Colour	:	20			
Condition	:	10			
Total	:	100	Total	:	100

Preparation of Poultry for Show

A. Selection of birds

Select only healthy birds since only such birds will have good physical condition and bright appearance for which the chances of winning prize will be better.

B. Training of birds

It is very necessary that the bird shows its best worth to the judges and do not get excited in the pen when visited.

Select the bird at least one week before the show, place each show-bird in a cage similar to the one used during poultry show. Handle each bird two to three times a day in a manner similar to that used during judging so that the birds get trained and do not get excited during the show. Do not expose the solid red coloured breed to direct sunlight for several hours because it will fade the plumage colour.

C. Washing the birds

Washing may be necessary in white birds arranged for the show. The birds are washed with detergent solution (avoid the detergents which makes the feather brittle). If external parasites are present, birds may be dipped in certain mild pesticide like 0.25 to 0.50 per cent Sevin solution (active ingredient, Carbaryl). A bird can be washed in 15 to 20 minutes and the bird should be placed in a drying cage and it gets dried in 12 to 18 hours. The birds should be dried slowly for best results.

D. After washing

A small piece of cloth is moistened with baby oil or vitamin E and is rubbed over the comb, wattles, beak and shank of the bird. A mixture of equal parts of alcohol, glycerine and olive oil makes an excellent cleaning and polishing solution for shank, feet, comb and wattles. The nails and beak may be trimmed, if necessary.

E. Transporting the birds

Transport the birds in a clean cage with straw or wood shavings as bedding material. Do not provide water since it will spill and spoil the bedding material. If the birds are to be transported to a long distance, water should be provided at intervals during transport.

F. Care of birds during show

Make sure that the birds are provided with plenty of feed and water during the show.

G. Care of birds after the show

After the show, the birds should be quarantined and should not be mixed with other birds in the farm immediately because it may transmit some diseases which has been acquired during the show from other birds. After 14 days of quarantine, they can be mixed with other farm birds.

Culling among layers

Culling is an important managemental procedure to be practiced in case of layers and breeder females. It is a continuous operation once laying starts because all the layers/ breeders, despite of good start may not be persistent in laying for complete laying period. Therefore, usually monthly culling is followed to improve economy by removing unproductive birds.

Most of the characters in judging pertaining to productive features are evaluated during culling. If the productive characteristics are up to the standards, then general defects counted in judging are not given any weightage for culling. The characters that distinguish poor layers are given in Table 20.

Table 20: Body characteristics of birds for culling

Character/ body part	Good layer	Bad/ poor layer
Health	Healthy, vigorous, well fleshed but moderately fatty	Appearance sick, sluggish, thin or debilitated or extremely fatty
Feathering	Tight and close feathering, tail and wings well carried up	Loose and scattered feathering, tail and wings are droopy
Plumage	Initially bright and dark coloured but faint and dull in latter stage	Always bright and dark coloured
Comb and Wattles	Large, glossy, red and warm	Small, dry, scaly, pale and cold
Eyes and expression	Bright and alert	Sunken and dull
Abdomen	Well developed, soft and pliable	Contracted, hard, tight and fatty
Pubic bone	Soft and flexible, well spread, distance between two pubic bones 2 to 3 fingers	Hard, brittle, tightly placed distance between two pubic bones less than 2 fingers
Keel bone and distance	Soft, flexible, distance between keel and pubic bones is more than 4 to 5 fingers	Hard, brittle, distance between keel and pubic bones is less than 3 to 4 fingers
Skin	Soft, thin, loose, silky	Rough, thick, tight and under laid with fat
Vent	Large, oval, dilated and moist	Small, round, contracted and dry

Table 21: Some important defects and disqualifications for standard breeds

Parts of fowl	Defects	Disqualifications
Colour of plumage	Brassiness (White and barred varieties), Creaminess (White varieties), Irregular barring (Barred varieties), Slate undercolour (red varieties)	White feathers in black varieties, black feathers in white varieties
Comb	Frosted combs. Too many or too few points of comb on single comb Thumb mark (single comb)	Combs foreign to breed, split comb.
Head and adjuncts	Coarse texture of wattles. Positive enamel white in face of cocks and hens (Leghorns)	Positive enamel white in earlobes of red earlobes breed.
Deformities of shape and plumage	Pinched or 'gamy' traits (Leghorn)	Deformed beaks or backs, wrytail, split wing
Shanks and toes	Crooked toes	Bowlegs or knock-knees feathers on shank in breeds of unfeathered shanks.

Question Bank

Choose the correct answer.

1. The poultry judging is carried out to develop healthy competition among poultry corporate/poultry breeders /poultry processors. (poultry breeders).
2. In good layers the space between pelvic bones and keel bone should be a minimum of 2/3/4 fingers. (4).
3. The eyes of good layer must be sleepy/bright/pale. (bright).
4. The plumage and colour of good layer must be loose/tight/flabby. (tight).
5. The earlobes of good layer must be coarse/wrinkled/waxy. (waxy).
6. The keel bone of good layer must be short/long/medium.(long).
7. Bleaching/moulting/preening is an annual physiological phenomenon of shedding of old feathers and replacing them with new feathers.(moulting).
8. After the show the birds should be quarantined for 10/12/14 days to avoid transmitting the diseases which may have been acquired during the show from other birds. (14).

Fill in the blanks

1. The Directorate of .... Ministry of Agriculture, Govt. of India annually conducts livestock and poultry shows in various parts of the country. (Extension).
2. The judging contests are carried out mostly for the students by using a .... to grade the birds. (score card).
3. In India, poultry judging refers to selection of birds on the basis of their .... appearances, ... characteristics and .... performances. (physical, breed, production).
4. Any deviation from "*ideal*" or "*perfection*" but not serious enough to constitute a disqualifications in the show room is considered to be a .... (defect).
5. Once the bird starts laying it requires .... days to bleach the vent and .... months to bleach the bottom of feet. (0-7 and 2).
6. If the birds to be exhibited are infested with external parasites the same may be dipped in .... per cent Sevin solution. (0.25 to 0.50).
7. In good layer the distance between 2 pubic bones is .... fingers. (2 to 3).

True/False

1. The birds meant for judging are let loose in the field and the participants are requested to score.(False).
2. Serious defects are regarded as disqualifications and will bar a bird from wining a prize. (True).
3. Only layers and not the broilers can be physically evaluated for their performance rating. (False).
4. The objective of judging is to exchange views and opinions among poultry farmers. (True).
5. Judging of a good layer is based on certain intrinsic characters and not the extrinsic ones. (False).
6. Good layer will have pale skin and shrunken eyes. (False).
7. The body conformation in a good layer is characterized by narrow back with more abdominal fat and smaller abdomen. (False).

21

Poultry Litter Management

M.M. Kadam and P.L. Shinde

Management of the poultry house environment forms an essential aspect towards maximizing production performance. Generally, proper maintenance of poultry litter is seldom given emphasis. The condition of litter significantly influences bird's performance and ultimately affects the economy for rearing. The litter is defined as the bedding materials of around 5-6 cm height consisting of locally available materials like rice husk, peanut hull, wood shavings, paper shreds, sawdust or groundnut hulls. These materials can be used alone or in combination to rear the birds on floor under deep litter system of management. The excreta, feathers, spilled feed and water are mixed with bedding material, get further decomposed due to heat and bacterial action resulting in built-up-litter towards the end of rearing.

Important functions of bedding material

- Due to absorbing quality, litter material reduces the moisture from the droppings.
- Litter dilutes fecal material, thus reducing contact between birds and manure.
- Litter bedding helps in thermoregulation, provides protection and cushion for the birds.

Characteristics of good litter material

- Ideal litter materials should absorb water and subsequently release the same to the atmosphere and minimize litter caking
- Help to store/spread and clean out after rearing of birds
- It must be soft, light in weight and free from sharp objects
- It should be readily available in sufficient quantities and non-toxic in nature.
- Most importantly, it should be economical.
- In addition, a bedding material must be compatible as a fertilizer or soil amendment.

Table 22: Advantages and disadvantages of some of the commonly used bedding materials

Rice husk	A good litter material usually available at competitive price. Young chicks may be prone to litter-eating (not a serious problem).
Peanut hulls	An inexpensive litter material in peanut-producing areas. Tends to cake and crust but can be managed. Susceptible to mold growth and increased incidence of aspergillosis.
Sand	Field trials show comparable performance but more difficult to maintain suitable floor temperatures during extreme weather.
Sugar cane bagasse	Readily available in sugar cane production areas. Less moisture absorption capacity compared to other litter materials and prone to wet litter condition.
Crushed corn cobs	Limited availability. May be associated with increased breast blisters.
Processed papers	Various forms of processed papers have proven to be good litter material in research and commercial situations. Tendency to form cake with increased particle size. Top dressing paper base with shavings may minimize this problem. Careful management is essential.
Saw dust:	Preferred litter material but becoming limited in supply and expensive in certain areas.

Litter Quality and Performance

Litter quality mostly depends upon amount of excreta voided and litter moisture percentage, which indirectly affect bacterial proliferation and ammonia production. Excess moisture in the litter increases the incidence of breast blisters, skin burns, scabby areas, bruising, condemnations and downgrades. Wet litter condition promotes the proliferation of pathogenic bacteria, molds and cause increased ammonia emission which is serious environmental concern affecting broiler production. Many producers underestimate the detrimental effects of ammonia. The human nose is able to detect ammonia levels near 15 parts per million (ppm) but will lose even this level of sensitivity with long-term exposure. Ammonia concentration of 50 to 110 ppm can cause irritation of eyes which may induce possible health risks to farm workers. Prolonged ammonia exposure at high levels (50 to 100 ppm) can result in keratoconjunctivitis (blindness) in birds. However, ammonia levels of just 25 ppm for longer duration causes depressed growth, drop in egg production and immuno-suppression. In addition, a greater incidence of air sacculitis, viral infections and condemnations have been linked to ammonia levels at this concentration. Most of the time improper ventilation can lead to wet litter problem and ammonia fumes develop in wet litter at faster rate. Ammonia volatilization from poultry litter can also cause air pollution and lower fertilizer value of litter due to nitrogen loss.

Litter that is too dry and dusty can also lead to problems such as dehydration of new chicks, respiratory diseases and increased condemnations. Ideally, litter moisture should be maintained between 20 to 25%. Ammonia production starts when moisture exceeds 30% and increases further as surrounding temperature increases. As time passes, used litter can become seeded with pathogens. High humidity, warm temperatures and high pH favour the proliferation of pathogens in the litter. Bad litter acts as predisposing factor for several viral and bacterial diseases known to spread easily through contaminated litter. In addition, fungi that produce mycotoxicosis and aspergillosis (Brooder Pneumonia) have been isolated in broiler litter. In India, coccidiosis is a serious problem whereas; good hygiene can greatly reduce the number of oocysts. Wet litter further aggravates coccidiosis by providing the proper environment for oocysts to sporulate.

Management Practices to Improve Litter Quality

Initial thickness of litter should be 5 cm during summer and 7 cm during winter; whereas the final litter thickness will be ranging between 10 to 12 cm depending on season and growing period. The successful litter management mostly depends on skillful management of litter moisture during entire period of rearing. For instance, if new litter is not stored properly and becomes damp before it is spread as bedding material, wet litter problems may occur. It can be avoided by properly stirring of litter, which also called as raking. Sprinkle a mixture of wood ash and fertilizer grade superphosphate before raking litter, to prevent ammonia gas release from litter. Nutrition also influences litter quality as certain dietary ingredients (especially salt and potassium), when fed in excess, cause broilers to consume and excrete large amounts of water and result in wet litter conditions. Some drugs (diuretics) also stimulate excess water consumption and excretion.

Environmental conditions such as wet and humid weather, condensation or very cold temperature can cause wet litter if the ventilation system is not able to eliminate moisture, effectively. Drinker lines, foggers and evaporative cooling pads, if not managed and maintained carefully, can contribute greatly to wet litter problems.

Key points for better litter management

- Proper house preparation to release ammonia trapped in the litter is necessary to minimize ammonia accumulation during brooding. Heating and ventilating the house 24-48 hours prior to chick placement will help to accomplish this.
- Use exhaust fans to remove air from shed. The fans help to dry the litter by moving warm air (which can hold more moisture) off the ceiling and down to the floor. The relative humidity in deep litter house should be around 40%.
- Check watering systems to prevent leaks. Never fill the waterer to their full capacity. Keep the height of waterer at back-height of birds. Adjust drinker height and water pressure as birds grow to avoid excessive water wastage into the litter.
- Preferably use nipple drinkers at rate 1:10 birds and keep their height just above the chick head level.
- If leakage or spillage occurs then wet litter should be removed from the house promptly and replaced with clean, dry bedding.
- To avoid damp litter and to prevent release of ammonia gas from litter, a mixture of wood ash and fertilizer grade super phosphate in the ratio of 4:1 may be sprinkled over the litter at the rate of 5 kg per 10 m^2 area.
- Slaked lime powder should not be used on the litter, because this will increase the pH of the litter, which in turn release more ammonia from the litter and also favour growth of *E. coli*.
- In winter season depth of litter may be increased by 3-5 cm to manage heat production and *vice versa* in summer.
- Make sure no moisture is getting in from the outside. Check grading and drainage around the building to ensure that rainwater is being diverted away and not causing seepage.

Disposal of poultry manure

Oxidation ditches: Aerobic fermentation of manure occurs in open ditches. Bacteria decompose organic matter into simpler substances like CH_4 /NH_3 sludge and liquid manure, which can be used as NPK (fertilizer) elements in agricultural field. The solid sludge contains vitamin B_{12} and minerals, which is a good source of feed in the animals after proper processing.

Solid disposal: The stacked heap of manure on compression generates heat inside litter and kills microbes making the material sterile, which can be used as fertilizer. Some people prefer to spread the manure on ground in thin layer, which dries fast and can be applied to soil as good fertilizer

Lagoons: Shallow covered ponds in which manure is dumped along with liquid waste and covered are called as lagoons. Here, anaerobic fermentation decomposes manure and after 3-5 months enriched manure can be obtained.

Utility of poultry litter

It is natural organic manure, which prevents leaching of soil, a major problem with chemical fertilizers. Poultry manure is richer as fertilizer when compared with cow dung. It contains about 3, 2, and 2 percent nitrogen, phosphorus and potash (NPK), respectively which are major fertilizer constituents. A hen produces about 16 kg dried manure per annum in cage, whereas a broiler produces around 1.5 kg manure till marketable age. It can be used as a good fertilizer for wide variety of field crops. As it contains fair amount of protein and energy it can be used as cattle, pig, fish and poultry feed ingredient after proper processing and drying. Processing of poultry litter is necessary for destruction of potential pathogens, improvement of handling and storage characteristics, and maintenance or enhancement of palatability. Poultry litter can be used up to certain level (5 to 10%) as a feedstuff for cattle. The anaerobic digestion of organic wastes results in the generation of biogas. Poultry manure may be increased at 15-20% level along with cow dung. Non-contaminated and properly dried poultry manure can be recycled as poultry litter again.

Table 23: pH, organic carbon content and nutrient composition of poultry litter.

	Type of litter	
Parameter	Layer litter	Broiler litter
Organic C (%)	15.3	32.5
pH	8.1	6.4
Macronutrients		
Nitrogen, %	3.3	4.1
Phosphorus, %	2.9	2.1
Potassium, %	3.6	2.7
Sulfur, %	1.0	0.73
Calcium, %	17.9	4.0
Magnesium, %	0.8	0.7
Micronutrients		
Boron, ppm	42.7	33.5
Copper, ppm	163	163
Iron, ppm	2040	3254
Manganese, ppm	647	444
Molybdenum, ppm	10.7	6.2
Zinc, ppm	403	383

Recycling of old litter

The old litter can be recycled after treatment. The common treatment followed will be heaping and reheaping. During reheaping, the top layer of the previous heap will go to the bottom and the bottom layer will come to the top. During heaping and reheaping the litter get fermented, which will generate sufficient heat to kill all the harmful microbes and make it safe for the next batch of birds reared on it. While heaping, a disinfectant solution should be sprayed on the floor and heaped litter to reduce the microbial load. The heaping period may be up to 7-10 days after which the litter is sprayed again to rear the next batch of broilers. The used litter may be reused up to 2 times after treatment. If any serious outbreak has occurred in the previous batch the same litter must not be used again. Before, recycling the old litter (built-up litter) price and availability of fresh litter must be considered.

Question Bank

Q. 1. State true or false

i. Approximately a hen produces 16 kg dry litter per annum in cage (True)

ii. As management practice the height of waterer should be at back level of birds (True)

iii. Initially litter thickness should be 5 cm in height (True)

iv. A broiler produces around 1.5 kg manure till marketable age (True)

v. Relative humidity of poultry house should be maintained at 40 % (True)

Q. 2. Fill in the blanks

i. Built up litter contains about.............,.............,.............%NPK, respectively.

ii. The used litter may be reused up to .... times after treatment.

iii. In India, ..., an important litter-born disease causes heavy economic losses to industry

iv. Excess level of moisture in litter produces .... condition.

v. Ammonia level of poultry shed should not exceed .... ppm

Answers: i, 3, 2, 2; ii, 2; iii, coccidiosis; iv, wet litter; v, 20.

Q.3. Write short notes on:

i. Characteristics of good litter

ii. Key point to reduce litter-born issues

iii. Utility of poultry litter

iv. Thumb rule to detect litter quality

22

Special Management of Poultry

N. Panda and S.C. Mishra

Any deviation from optimum state could be referred as stress. Every living creature has to pass through one or the other type of stresses in life. Most of the farm animals including poultry suffer from various types of stresses. These include due to:

1. Adverse environment
2. Managemental practices
3. Diseases
4. Nutritional deficiency
5. Transportation *etc.*

Stresses affect welfare of poultry. Thermal stress is a major stress. Every animal has a thermo neutral zone where it performs optimum. For broiler, the ideal temperature is 10-22^{0}C whereas for layer it is 10-30^{0}C. Birds being endothermic regulate their body temperature close to a set point by controlling either heat production or heat loss independently of the ambient temperature. If the lower ambient temperature is lower than the zone of neutrality, it is also a stress to the birds but not as serious as the higher temperature. Body reacts to lower temperature in many ways like increased metabolism, huddling together to prevent loss of heat, involuntary movement of various parts of the body including peripheral muscles to generate heat. Birds need more energy for maintenance of temperature in addition to normal requirement. It is partly accomplished by increasing the feed intake.

Stress due to Adverse Weather Condition

When environmental temperature goes beyond the critical temperature in real term we call it as adverse condition, which is otherwise called as *heat stress*. Heat stress can result significant losses to production. When such temperature is coupled with high humid condition it becomes stressful and detrimental for poultry. More severe cases lead to heavy mortality. Losses in production efficiency will occur long before significant mortality rates are observed. These stresses can be minimized by adopting following special management and care:

a) Housing and building site

Orientation of poultry shed, amount of insulation and overhang have direct bearing on inside temperature of the shed. The orientation of the buildings should be such that the prevailing winds are used to an advantage and can move freely. In the Indian context the axis of house should be East-West with open space (wire netting) in North and South directions. There should be sufficient overhang a minimum of 3 ft, so that the sunshine does not fall directly to the house. Adequate ventilation should be provided above the ceiling. Insulation of the roof plays a vital role to reduce the temperature inside the shed. Roof surface should be kept free of dust and rust. Roof reflectivity can be increased by cleaning and painting with metallic zinc or by installing an aluminum roof or by white washing the asbestos roof. These practices are particularly effective for buildings those are insulated. Location of the poultry house also plays a major role to maximize air movement around the building. Grasses, shrubs and weeds should not be allowed to grow over 5-6 inches tall, low overhang tree limbs should be removed because these decrease the flow of air through the poultry shed. Tall trees can be planted near the building.

b) Housing light reflectors/insulators

The incandescent bulb produces 20 lumens per watt whereas the fluorescent gives 70 lumens per watt. During summer for brooding of chicks the fluorescent light is preferred during day time as it gives less temperature than incandescent ones. Similarly the reflectors also increase effective light by up to 50%. Depending upon the environmental temperature and birds' comfort the numbers of bulbs, height of the bulbs are also determined.

c) Sprinklers and foggers

To reduce radiant heat built up on the roof, water sprinkling can be practiced. Sprinkling can be accomplished by using sprinkler hose or by dripping water through holes. The sprinkling interval should be determined for each poultry shed but likely need to be at 20-30 minutes. The volume of water used should be just enough to wet the roof surface without wasting water at the eaves. Foggers reduce air temperature in the house where there is low humidity, especially during mid day. These foggers are accomplished by injecting fine water particles into warm environment. As the water vaporizes, heat in the environment is decreased.

d) Fan and pad systems

Another system of evaporative cooling is the fan and pad systems, in which all incoming air passes through a moist pad. If properly designed, the fan and pad system should reduce air temperatures to within five degrees. To get maximum benefit from the system, the material used to provide surface area from which the water evaporates should be properly wet at all times.

e) Ventilation

Using outside air is the principal method of removing heat from the poultry house. There are two parts to a ventilation system: a) Natural ventilation b) Forced ventilation; that must complement to each other. In naturally ventilated house the area of wire netting and the height of the house determine the amount of ventilation. In curtain sided houses with no mechanical ventilation, the curtains should always be adjusted to allow maximum air movement. The distribution of air to pickup heat and moisture before it leaves the house will improve the birds' comfort. Circulation fans in curtain houses are spaced to increase air movement and body heat loss from the birds. These circulation fans should be controlled by thermostats turning on at 85^0 F in hot summer and turning off when temperature drops below the set point of 85^0 F.

f) Forced ventilation

In forced ventilation system the air is moved entirely by fans in the building walls. It is also referred as "Controlled environment". The houses that are environmentally controlled depend entirely on fans in the sidewalls to exchange air. These power-ventilated houses can provide good, uniform airflow patterns under hot summer conditions by maintaining correct static pressure and avoiding airflow obstructions.

g) Tunnel ventilation

This method involves moving air along the building axis from inlets to exhaust fans, which provides high velocity air. This increases the convective heat loss reducing the effective temperature that the bird is feeling.

Dietary Modification to Ameliorate Heat Stress

Birds maintained in hot environment reduce their feed consumption naturally. The reduction in feed intake results in decrease daily intake of nutrients responsible for growth. Thus, the broiler can cope with the heat to certain period. But in prolonged hot weather and in extreme condition, the birds may not be able adopt the situation. So the following dietary modifications needs are practiced.

a) Time of Feeding and Withdrawing of Feed

The birds are to be fed at cooler, especially in morning part of the day. Metabolic heat production reaches its peak at about 3-5hrs after feeding and the increase of heat production is associated with 1-2°C rise in body temperature. Therefore management strategy for broilers is to withdraw feed 4-6 hours prior to peak warm temperature in the afternoon i.e. withdraw feed prior to the anticipated time of peak temperature so that it may take an unneeded heat load of the bird. In layers feeding during the later part of the day will ensure the availability of ionic calcium while the shell calcification is in active process. Feed can be reintroduced after peak temperatures have started to recede which allows feeding during night hours when cooling is expected.

b) Providing Adequate Cool Drinking Water

More water has to be consumed by the birds during hot weather in order to prevent dehydration occurred through panting. Provide cool drinking water round the clock stimulates feed intake. The waterer should not be empty in any time. Cool water absorbs body heat. Usually anything that results in increased water consumption during heat stress will benefit the survival rate.

c) Increasing Energy Density of Diet

Reduction in feed intake due to heat results in decrease in the daily intake of nutrients for growth and production. Therefore dietary nutrient, especially energy content of the diet should be increased by addition of fat at a level of 5% or more. The concentration of other nutrients especially minerals and vitamins are to be adjusted depending on the feed intake.

d) Balancing Amino Acids with Low Protein Diet

Higher protein level with imbalanced amino acids leads to produce more heat increment in birds than lower protein with balanced amino acids. Protein contributes more metabolic heat production than do carbohydrates and fats. The percentage of protein level should be lowered and the diets should be supplemented with lysine and methionine.

e) Providing Vitamins and Minerals

In high temperature there will be destruction of some vitamins like vitamin A, vitamin E and decrease synthesis of vitamin C. Therefore natural/synthetic antioxidants should be added. Vitamin C and vitamin E also help as antistress agent during heat stress. Some trace minerals like Zinc and Selenium help in increasing the immunity in birds.

f) Supplementing with Electrolytes

The electrolyte balance in the birds is altered during heat stress due to panting as it increases carbon dioxide loss. Heat stress also depletes potassium and other minerals like sodium, phosphorus and magnesium in the body. On the other hand Potassium chloride supplement appears to increase water intake at concentration range of 0.5 to 0.6%. The supplement should occur prior to heat stress period. Use of carbonated water or sodium bicarbonate in the feed is useful for layers during egg production.

Special Management During Rainy Season

- Litter must be changed at the start of rainy season and wet litter must be replaced from time to time with dry litter.
- Feed must be stored in dry places.
- Groundnut cake and maize have often been contaminated with fungi for which antifungal drugs may be added.
- Water reservoir and sources must be disinfected regularly.
- Preventive doses of medication against Colibacillosis, mycotoxicosis, coccidiosis may be given before commencement of rainy season.

Special Management During Winter Season

The adverse effect of cold weather seems to be more prominent when temperature drops below 10^0 C as mostly seen in the northern parts of India.

- The temperature of the poultry house should be increased by covering open sides with curtains.
- Avoid droughts of cold wind without obstructing ventilation.
- The roof may be insulated to conserve heat. A simple thatch can help to keep the shed warm.
- If required electric or coal heaters may be used to increase the temperature of the shed, particularly during brooding.
- The litter depth should be increased to a minimum of about 10-15 cm which help in warming.
- The stocking density may be increased to 10%.
- The energy contents of the feed be increased about 100-150 Kcal/kg.

Management During Debeaking, Transportation and Vaccination Stresses

- The vaccination, debeaking and transportation should be done at the cooler part of the day.
- Avoid unnecessary handling during the processes. Care should be taken to prevent huddling.
- The vaccination should be done at proper site with appropriate dosage.
- If vaccines are given through water, then withhold the water for 2 hours beforehand.

Question Bank

Q.1. Fill in the blanks

a) The ideal temperature for broiler raising is ....

b) In the Indian context the axis of poultry house should be ....

c) .... and .... vitamins are given during summer stress as antistressors.

d) The length of overhang should be minimum of ....

e) Heat stress depletes mostly .... mineral.

f) Reflectors increases the affectivity of light to the extent of ....%.

g) Forced ventilation is also called as ....

h) Ground nut cake should be avoided during rainy season due to ....

Q. 2. State True/False.

a) The feed intake of birds decrease during cold season.

b) Moist heat is more stressful than dry heat.

c) Metabolic heat production reaches its peak at about 3-5hrs after feeding.

d) To tackle heat stress the energy content of feed should be decreased.

e) During summer the incandescent bulb is better than fluorescent bulb.

f) During heat stress the energy density of the feed is to be increased to compensate the lower intake.

g) Population density inside the shed should be reduced during winter season.

h) The depth of litter should be increased during winter season.

Q. 3. Multiple Choice

a) The ideal temperature of poultry bird rearing is (i) 10-20 °C (ii) 10-30 °C (iii) 30-40 °C (iv) all of the above

b) Due to high temperature changes in the bird performance are i) Low FCR ii) Drop in egg production iii) Reduction of quality of eggs iv) All of the above

c) To combat heat stress the energy content of the diet should be increased by addition of fat at a level of i) 5 ii) 10 iii) 15 iv) 20 % or more

d) Roof reflectivity can be increased by i) cleaning ii) white washing iii) insulating iv) all of the above

e) Foggers are mostly useful for reducing the temperature in areas of (i) high humid (ii) Low humid (iii) both condition (iv) none of the condition

f) Fan and pad systems are a type of i) evaporative cooling ii) conductive cooling iii) convectional cooling iv) None of the above

g) During summer in layer birds feed should be provided at i) morning ii) noon iii) afternoon iv) any time

h) During summer stress the protein levels of the diet of poultry should be i) increased ii) decreased iii) remains same iv) none of the above

Q. 4. Define the following

a) What is stress and name different types of stresses that affect the poultry birds?

b) What is fan pad system of cooling?

c) What are antistress vitamins?

d) Which electrolyte is mostly required for during summer stress?

Answers

1. a) 10-22 ^{0} C
   b) East-West
   c) Vitamin E and C
   d) 3 ft.
   e) potassium/sodium
   f) 50
   g) controlled environment
   h) Fungal infestation (*aflatoxicosis*)

2. a) false
   b) True
   c) True
   d) false
   e) false
   f) True
   g) false
   h) True

3. a) ii
   b) iv
   c) i
   d) iv)
   e) ii
   f) i
   g) iii
   h) ii

23

Vices in Poultry and Their Remedial Measures

J.D. Mahanta

Vices of poultry are undesirable behavioural pattern manifested by the bird in the flock and spreads fast among the members resulting in financial losses.

Types of Vices

1.Pecking

2.Cannibalism

3.Egg eating

1. Pecking

It is a common vice particularly seen in light breeds of poultry. It is one of the means of social contact among birds mainly to establish social ranks. This kind of pecking takes as an extreme character in bad climate and environmental conditions. In natural conditions birds are seen plucking each other's feathers, eating small particles just for curiosity or to complete their diet. Pecking may be of various types, *viz*. toe pecking, vent pecking, head pecking and wing or tail pecking. Toe pecking is commonly seen in chicks. Hunger often initiates this practice. Due to mismanagement chicks may not find feed when feeders are placed too high or too far for eating. In such case he will peck at his own or his neighbour's toes. If the intensity of light in brooder house is very high, the blood vessels of toe start shinning. It is known that poultry has special affinity for coloured or bright objects. Red seems to attract maximum attention and is eagerly touched with beak. Once this toe pecking leads to bleeding, the smell and taste of blood leads to more aggressive pecking. Dead and injured birds should therefore be eliminated as early as possible.

Pecking of the vent or the region of the abdomen several inches below the vent is the severest form that leads to cannibalism. This type is generally seen in pullet flock during high production. Predisposing factors are prolapse or tearing of the tissue by passage of an abnormally large egg. Head pecking usually follows injuries to the comb and wattle caused by freezing or by fighting among males. It is observed in debeaked birds kept in separate cages; they will reach through the wire and peck at the neighbouring bird or grasp the ear lobes or wattle of the bird. Wing and tail pecking is most frequently seen in flocks kept in close confinement due to lack of sufficient exercise. External injuries and irritation caused by lice and mites may induce feather pecking.

2. Cannibalism

Cannibalism usually results from continued pecking by members of the flock at the exposed cloaca of the bird immediately after she has laid an egg. The cloaca and portion of the intestine may be eaten, so that the birds succumb to injury. Cannibalism in fowl is a costly and vicious habit that poultry producers cannot afford to ignore. Under the intensive management conditions used by today's industry, this condition can occur at any age among all breeds, strains and sexes of fowl. The lighter breeds or white varieties are more susceptible to cannibalism than heavier breeds. Such breeds are characterized by their flighty nature and are hypersensitive to environmental factors.

The important behavioural problems of cannibalism in the poultry industry can include the following activities:

i. Feather pulling in older birds from the body.

ii. Vent pecking in older birds.

iii. A dominant bird pecking at a more submissive member of the flock.

iv. Mutual pecking where birds in close proximity peck each other.

The birds that have been bred for high egg production usually have a more nervous temperament and thus often to start pecking. Due to cannibalism, the mortality rate in some places may even exceed 25%. This vice is more prevalent in some families of birds and can be eliminated through selective breeding.

Causes of vices

Different factors are responsible for development of vices in poultry ranging from inborn behaviour, managemental stress or nutritional deficiencies/ excesses.

Natural causes

a) **Inherent behaviour**: The problem may simply arise because of the normal pecking behaviour when searching for food or exploring an environment. Once one hen has picked up this technique other hens, observing the behaviour will learn from the initial pecker and a serious episode will develop.

b) **Slow feathering birds are most prone to cannibalism**: Most cannibalism occurs during feather growth in young fowl. Birds with slow feathering have immature tender feathers exposed for longer periods of time leaving them open to damage from pecking.

Managemental causes

a) **Overcrowding**: Keeping too many birds in one unit results in overcrowding. This is especially serious in brooding when the birds fill the available space as they grow older.

b) **Excessive light**: Extremely bright light or excessively long periods of light will cause birds to become hostile towards one another. Constant light can be stressful to birds.

c) **Excessive heat**: When the birds become uncomfortably hot they can become extremely cannibalistic.

d) **Absence of feed or water or a shortage of feeder and waterer space**: If the birds have to fight for food and water or if the birds are hungry they will increase pecking.

e) **Mixing different types and colours of fowl**: Mixing different ages of fowl or fowls with different traits promotes pecking.

f) **Abrupt changes in environmental or management practices**: If young birds are transferred to a new location, it is better to move some of their feeders and waterers with them in order to help them adapt.

g) **Brightly lit nests or shortage of nesting boxes**: During egg laying process the cloaca may become distended specially with the passage of large eggs and this protrusion of the vent may be an attractant to other birds due to its stark colour difference against white body.

h) **Condition of litter**: Accumulation of feed and filth around the toes of chicks are irritating. Their presence may give rise to toe picking and other forms of cannibalism.

i) **Allowing cripples, injured or dead birds to remain in a flock**: Fowl will peck on cripples or dead birds in their pens because of the social order and curiosity. Once pecking starts it can quickly develop into a vicious habit.

Nutritional causes

a) **High energy and low fibre**: Extremely high energy and low fibre diets cause the birds to be extra active and aggressive which in turn will make birds to peck others.

b) **Protein deficiency**: Feed, lacking protein and other nutrients, particularly methionine will also cause birds to peck feathers.

c) **Imbalance in the sodium level may lead to cannibalism**: High salt content in feed / water and lack of adequate drinking water increases pecking disorder.

d) **An abrupt change in the palatability** or form of a flock's ration may also be a contributing factor for the onset of cannibalism.

3. Egg eating

The incidence of floor laying in a deep litter house poses a major problem of egg breakage. Eggs laid on the floor are often trampled by the hens. Egg breakage favours *egg eating* vice to develop in a flock. The vice is also developed when the laying nests are not darkened.

Remedial measures

The best method of control is to prevent it from starting itself, since once it has begun it will be very difficult to stop. The vices can be prevented by adopting the following measures:

i. The recommendation for floor space, feeder space and drinker space should always be followed while rearing birds. Floor space may be increased during summer and rainy seasons. The feeders and waterers should be well designed and placed properly.

ii. Careful attention to light intensity should be given. White bulbs of more than 40 watts should not be used in poultry sheds. More than16 hours of light per day should not be used.

iii. The flock should constantly be supplied with balanced feed and water.

iv. Proper temperature and adequate ventilation must be made available. In hot weather, more ventilation should be provided to keep birds cool.

v. Adequate number of nest should be provided to avoid floor laying. One individual nest for every five birds should be given. Nests may be darkened to attract and protect layers.

vi. Birds should be offered balanced feed. Feeding oyster shell or limestone or grit will help to build strong shell. Changing of feed from chick to grower or layer should be gradual.

vii. Never brood different species of birds together.

viii. Debeaking is used as an immediate control and preventive measure. For replacement pullets, the debeaking at 4- 6 weeks of age has proven successful. If necessary, birds again can be debeaked at 12- 15 weeks of age. After 16 weeks debeaking should not be done until in exceptional condition.

Question Bank

I. Fill in the blanks

1. Keeping too many birds in one unit results in ....
2. The vice of egg eating is developed when the laying nests are not ....
3. The deficiency of the amino acid .... also cause birds to peck feathers.
4. White bulbs more than .... watts should not be used in poultry sheds.
5. .... is used as an immediate control and preventive measure.
6. Toe pecking is commonly seen in ....

II. Match the following

1. Pecking - a) Prevent cannibalism
2. Egg eating - b) Older birds
3. Debeaking - c) Floor laying
4. Prolapse - d) Light breed of poultry
5. Vent pecking - e) Abnormally large egg

III. What do you mean by vices in poultry?

IV. What are the different types of vices in poultry? Describe the causes of vices in poultry.

V. How will you control vices in a poultry farm?

Answers

I. (1) Overcrowding (2) darkened (3) Methionine (4) 40 (5) Debeaking (6) Chicks

II. (1) d (2) c (3) a (4) e (5) b

24

Water Quality in Poultry Rearing

R. Prabarkaran

Water is the most important and abundantly required nutrient for poultry. A continuous supply of clean, fresh and wholesome potable water is essential for poultry. Poultry rearing is becoming more and more intensive with which the chances of the infectious diseases being sustained in the different flocks also increase. Consequently, the need for effective disease control measures to be adopted also gains further importance.

Most often, poultry farmers get alarmed only when the mortality level or death rate in a farm is high. However, even the existence of disease at a sub-clinical level may hinder the performance of the birds, in terms of body weight or egg number; such economic losses, sometimes relatively less and unnoticed, may mean the difference between success or failure in the poultry business. Treatment of a sick flock after the onset of any disease becomes costlier and more frequently impracticable. The recovered birds may not regain their production to original levels and may also continue as source of infection to other healthy birds. Hence, the adage 'prevention is better than cure' applies more to poultry industry than any other field.

Water Contaminants

The drinking water for birds contain three major types of contaminants namely minerals, micro-organisms and organic matter including pesticide residue. The diseases caused by micro-organisms like bacteria, viruses or parasites which are difficult to treat and cause extensive economic losses can be controlled by effective disease prevention measures. Higher the number of organisms in the environment of the birds, more severe will be the disease. Some organisms quickly overcome the birds' resistance which is termed as virulence. When birds are suffering from some stress, even lesser number of organisms / less virulent organisms may also cause a disease. Hence, it is the duty of the farmer to provide appropriate environment (proper layout of houses, design of houses, potable water, ventilation, space allowance, quality feed, disinfection procedures, biosecurity measures, vaccinations and medications etc.) to make the bird have optimum body resistance and to minimize the load of the organisms in the bird's environment which are the two basic principles in disease prevention.

Disease producing organisms gain entry into poultry farm through various sources. Water remains as the major source of infections, especially the *E.coli* infection. Supply of potable water, free from pathogenic micro-organisms and substances which affect palatability is essential. Most often poultry farmers fail to provide good quality water to the birds. Both microbial and chemical quality of water needs to be tested before establishing a poultry farm in the area. Microbial contamination of water may happen at origin like in ponds, rivers, open wells and public water supply system; during transportation and storage and in the overhead tank/ bins also, it may be contaminated. Unhygienic practices in the farm results in disease spread. The microbial load shoots up during flood. Faecal contamination of water will exhibit the presence of coliform organisms. Mineral levels in water depend on soil conditions and show only minor fluctuations based on season and water table. They lead to hardness in water and affect the taste and palatability. The desirable quality guidelines for drinking water in poultry farms are given in Table 24.

Table 24: Desirable quality guidelines for drinking water in poultry farms

Water quality	Maximum permissible level	Desirable level
1. Total hardness (ppm)	350	60-180
2. pH	6.0-8.0	6.8-7.5
3. Nitrate	25 mg/litre	10 mg/litre
4. Nitrite	4 mg/litre	0.4 mg/litre
5. Total bacterial count	1000 ml	0/ml
6. Coliform count	50/ml	0/ml
7. Calcium chloride	250 mg/litre	60 mg/litre
8. Sodium	500 mg/litre	50 mg/litre
9. Sulphate	250 mg/litre	125 mg/litre

Removal of excess dissolved minerals by cheaper and simpler methods is not practicable and the farmers should change for other water sources in case of excess minerals in water. Chlorination is the best and cheapest method to get rid of micro-organisms. Five to eight grams of bleaching powder with about 35% available chlorine should be added to 1000 litres of drinking water to maintain a chlorine level of 1 to 2 ppm at delivery. A minimum contact time of one hour should be given before offering the water to birds.

Where storage facilities are not available, liquid chlorine preparations like chlorine dioxide, 5% sodium hypochlorite etc., may be used at a level of one ml per 10 litres of water. Iodophores containing 1.6% available Iodine is also used as water sanitizers at the same dosage level. Quaternary ammonium compounds like quat, quatovet, encivet, sokrena etc. may be used as water sanitizers as per manufacturers' specifications. By providing sanitized water to the birds, the chance of water borne infections is reduced and the cost of medication is saved. The life of pipelines and storage tanks is increased and overall growth / egg production efficiency will be improved.

Question Bank

I. Write True or False against the following statements.

1. Water is the most important and abundantly required nutrient for poultry. (T)
2. Chlorination is not a good method to get rid of micro-organisms. (F)
3. Water remains as the major source of infections, especially the *E.coli* infection. (T)
4. Mineral levels in water depend on soil conditions. (T)
5. Quaternary ammonium compounds are used as acidifiers. (F)
6. The maximum permissible level of pH of drinking water should be 6.0-8.0, (T)

II. Fill in the blanks with appropriate word (words).

1. Drinking water for birds contain three major types of contaminants namely ...., ... and .... including pesticide residue.(minerals, microorganisms, organic matter)
2. Quaternary ammonium compounds like ...., ..., ... and ....may be used as water sanitizers. (quat, quatovet, encivet, sokrena)

3. Iodophores containing .... % available Iodine is also used as water sanitizers. (1.6)
4. The desirable level of pH of drinking water should be .... (6.8-7.5)
5. By providing sanitized water to birds, the chance of .... borne infections is reduced. (water)

III . Write down the guidelines of quality drinking water for poultry.

25

Biosecurity

V. Ravinder Reddy and T. Srilatha

Biosecurity means protection against infectious biological agents. These agents include bacteria, viruses, protozoa, fungi, parasites, and any other agents capable of introducing infectious diseases into a poultry flock. Biosecurity therefore means maintaining a flock, poultry house or premises in such a way that infectious agents do not have a chance to enter to cause diseases. The biosecurity may be categorized into three: Conceptual biosecurity, Structural biosecurity and operational Biosecurity.

Importance of Biosecurity

In modern poultry production, birds are reared under intensive system where large numbers are concentrated in small area. As a result, when an infectious agent enters a poultry house, there is probability for widespread dissemination if it is not contained. Besides, the broiler and egg industry of today is under increasing consumer and regulatory pressures to guarantee food safety and meet export requirements. As a result, broiler and layer operations around the world require the supply of breeding stock free of salmonellas specific to avian species (such as *S. pullorum* and *S. gallinarum*) and those that could cause outbreaks of human food-borne illness. Inadequate biosecurity can contribute to wide epidemics of highly pathogenic or exotic diseases. An infection by a virulent organism within a facility can be devastating, reducing without overt signs of disease. Once contaminated with pathogens, poultry facilities are extremely difficult and expensive to clean, sanitize and disinfect. Prevention of disease is always less expensive than treatment. The cost of implementing biosecurity system is smaller when compared to financial profit that can be made from production. Good biosecurity is therefore vital requirement in the best possible control of disease.

Biosecurity Programme

An efficient biosecurity programme should be designed in such a way that it must be user friendly, flexible and cost effective and follow common sense of protocols. In developing a suitable biosecurity program it is necessary to analyze the various methods by which diseases can be transmitted. Infections such as lymphoid leucosis, Salmonellosis and mycoplamosis can be transmitted by the vertical route. Most avian pathogens are spread by more than one route. Viral respiratory infections, such as Newcastle, laryngotracheitis and infectious bronchitis can be transmitted over distances of up to 5 kilometers. Maintaining strong levels of immunity in flocks reduces the probability that a pathogen introduced into a population will multiply and exceed the outbreak threshold. There should be everyday implementation of good farming practices like providing adequate heating, cooling, and ventilation; offering good-quality feed and water using proper medication (when needed); vaccinating for specific diseases; early removing and efficiently disposing of dead birds; composting or deep stacking manure and litter; and providing an overall stress-free environment.

Sources or Reservoirs

Sources or reservoirs refer to animals, birds, feed or water that naturally carry the specific agent and are capable of passing it on to other living things like poultry. The common sources are:

1. Diseases may be introduced by people — employees, service representatives, truck drivers, vaccination crews, veterinarians, etc.
2. They may be transferred via new poultry — chicks, pullets, breeding males, semen, etc.
3. They may arise from previously contaminated and improperly cleaned premises or equipment.
4. They may be introduced by vectors — rodents, wild birds, insects, wind or water.

Vectors

The vectors may be animate (living), or inanimate (nonliving). It is capable of harbouring infectious biological agents that when moved or carried around is capable of disseminating and spreading the agents. It can be people, fomites (clothing, boots), pets, rodents, insects, birds, vehicles, equipment (crates, egg flats, inseminating tools), and so forth. By far the most important vector in spreading poultry diseases is the human being.

General considerations on biosecurity

- The house should be located at least 1-3 km away from other commercial or other private facilities.
- The farm should not be located adjacent to a public road.
- The houses should have natural drainage and contours.
- The farm area should be fenced and its houses should not be located closer than 150 ft from the fencing line.
- The design and construction of the broiler house should prevent wild birds and animals from entering it. It is preferable to have a concrete foundation of floor to prevent rodents from burrowing into the house.
- Clear and level an area 15 meters (50 ft) around all houses so that vegetation can be cut quickly and easily.
- The water supply should be free from pathogenic bacteria and preferably chlorinated at a level of 2ppm.
- There must be an approved method for timely treatment and disposal of wastes.
- Roads and walk ways on the premises should be constructed with all weather materials.
- Farm should be provided with an adequately equipped change room having shower facility for farm personnel and visitors.
- Designing a farm premise should include a one-way traffic route for personnel and vehicles, and poultry from younger birds to oldest birds, from cleaner areas to dirty areas, and from individual poultry houses to common use of employ areas.
- Aerosol transmission of disease should be considered while designing the poultry houses. The air intakes of one poultry house should be located away from the outflow vents of other houses.
- Visitors to the farm premises should be discouraged since they may pose great risk for the introduction of pathogens.
- Minimize the number of visitors to the poultry farm by locking the entry gates and posting no trespassing/no visitors signs.

- If supervisory personnel must visit more than one farm per day, they should make an effort to visit the youngest flocks first. Always visit flocks with disease problems last.
- All persons entering the farm should follow a biosecurity procedure. The requirement that all workers and visitors shower and use clean farm clothes is one of the best procedures to prevent cross contamination between facilities. If this is not possible, all workers and visitors should put on clean coveralls and boots upon arrival at the farm.
- Maintain a record of visitors, including name, company, purpose of visit, previous farm visited and next farm to be visited.
- When entering and leaving each poultry house, workers and visitors must wash and sanitize their hands and boots.

Decontamination of the Poultry House

All-in-all-out placement programms are recommended to prevent diseases. Complete depopulation of the entire farm at the end of each growing or laying cycle is necessary. Farms are effectively depopulated only when all flocks and their litter and biological materials are removed from houses. As a general rule the greater the value of the flock the longer will be downtime between flocks; minimum period of 4 weeks for pullet houses, 6 weeks for laying houses.

The following points may be considered to decontaminate a poultry house:

I. Bird removal

- Remove all dead birds from the building including the birds which run outside.
- Immediately begin vector control procedures during bird removal.

II. Cleaning of the farm

- Turn off power of electrical equipments prior to dry or wet cleaning.
- Clean fans and other air inlets from outside.
- On the inside, brush, sweep, vacuum and wipe dust and other dirt from ceilings, light fixtures, beams, ledges, walls, fans, air inlets and walkways. Move from top to bottom.
- Promptly open feeder lines and remove feed from troughs.
- Hard surface (concrete) floors can be cleaned faster and more easily than clay or earthen floors. Completely remove litter. Hand sweeping and

shoveling will be necessary around the perimeter, doorways, walkways, support poles, and corner. Manure should not be spread near poultry facilities.

- Wet cleaning includes soaking, washing and rinsing steps. Use of hot water is preferred. Detergents and other surfactants are often added to washing solution to loosen debris and films and allow better penetration of cleaning agents.

III. Repairs

- All repairs to the house should be made at this point.

IV. Disinfection

- Only clean potable water should be used for disinfection.
- All disinfectants work best at temperatures above 18.3^{0}C. Each disinfectant is the result of careful formulation. For economy, efficacy and human and flock safety, manufacturer's label instructions must be followed carefully.
- Use of pressure sprays or thermal devices is advisable to help force disinfectants into wood pores, cracks and crevices. Spray pressures of 500-1000 psi have been suggested.
- Dirt floors are virtually impossible to fully disinfect. Diluted disinfectant has been applied to the floor at 4 liters per 10 sq. ft.
- Decontaminate feed bins, boots, augers, hoppers and carts.
- Sanitize waterlines. Be careful – metallic and non-metallic components of watering systems can be damaged and lines plugged from improper use of sanitizing agents. Routine chlorination of poultry drinking water to a minimum 1 to 1.5 ppm free chlorine level has been reported to reduce the spread of salmonellas. Rodent bait should be placed in selected areas of house.

Daily sanitation practices

Attention should be paid for the proper management and disposal of dead birds, spilled feed, manure and refuse daily.

Disposal of poultry waste

Dead birds act as a source of disease that can be spread by rats, mice, dogs, cats, flies, beetles, mosquitoes, free flying birds and insects. Methods of disposal may vary from farm to farm and area to area. The two most acceptable methods are:

Incinerators

A good incinerator is probably the best means of disposal.

Disposal Pit

A less desirable but acceptable method of dead bird disposal is through the use of an adequately designed and tightly covered disposal pit.

- This saves labour.
- Birds cannot be dug up by dogs or rodents.
- It has no noticeable odour if tightly covered.
- No fire hazards.
- Pit can be used year round.
- Birds decompose fairly rapidly without the use of chemicals.

A pit of 6 ft (1.83 m) in diameter and 6 ft (1.83 m) depth is large enough to take care of one 10,000 capacity broiler unit.

Composting

The composting process is one that must be monitored and managed well.

Hatcheries

- The hatchery is the central hub of all integrated poultry operations. Since all of the chicks pass through here, it is the central place where transmission of pathogens can reach every chicken house in the farm.
- Infectious agents such as Chronic Respiratory Disease (CRD) and Salmonella can be transmitted vertically from infected breeder flocks.
- Hatchery biosecurity procedures should detect these infections early and either prevent their introduction or limit the horizontal spread.
- The hatchery should have a perimeter fence. Only egg-collection and chick delivery trucks be permitted to enter, after cleaning and disinfection.
- Workers and visitors should park outside the fence, and required to shower before changing into hatchery clothing.
- All egg-collection and chick delivery vehicles should be fumigated daily.

- The design of the hatchery should provide cleanable non-porous surfaces, slightly sloping floor to facilitate frequent washing and disinfection.
- Setters and hatchers should be cleaned and disinfected after each use.
- Periodic microbiological monitoring provides a quality assurance for the entire sanitation program.

Feed

- Feed is a well known source of *Salmonella*, as well as other bacteria and mycotoxins, and must be handled properly, treated to eliminate pathogens and not allowed to be reused after treatment.
- The design of the feed mill should provide for a separate ingredients-side and a finished feed-side.
- Rodents and wild birds need to be taken care of to prevent the introduction of pathogens.
- Animal by-products such as fishmeal and meat-cum-bone meal are higher risk ingredients. These should be moved and stored in separate bins by separate equipment.
- Recognizing the risk of contaminated ingredients, the practice of pre-conditioning and pelleting and conditioning and acidification of finished feed be widely practiced.
- Spilled feed should not be allowed to amass in and around poultry houses.

Question Bank

Q 1. Fill in the blanks

i) .... means protection against biological agents (Biosecurity)

ii) .... refers to the object that naturally carries the specific agent and is capable of passing it on to other living things that can then catch the disease (Reservoirs).

iii) The chlorine levels in water supply should be less than ....(2ppm)

iv) .... management systems favor the elimination of disease agents that do not survive well outside of the chicken (all-in-all-out).

v) Increasing the down time directly .... the persistence of disease causing organisms in poultry house (reduces).

vi) .... serves to carry a disease producing agent from one premise to another (Vector).

vii) The distance between the poultry houses and other commercial or other private facilities should be .... Km (1-3)

viii) All disinfectants work best temperatures above .... °C. (18.3)

ix) .... and .... are the major vertically transmitted disease in breeder flocks. (Chronic Respiratory Disease, Salmonellosis)

x) The distance between the poultry houses and other commercial or other private facilities should be .... Km. (1-3)

Q.2 State true or false against the following statements:

i) The agents for fowl cholera and coccidiosis are present in the litter (T)

ii) The vector that transmit pox virus is mosquito (T)

iii) Traffic should flow from oldest to youngest birds (F)

iv) All disinfectants work best at temperatures above 65 °F. (T)

v) The most important vector in spreading poultry diseases is people (T)

vi) Disinfectants are substitutes for cleanliness (F)

vii) Avian influenza transmitted by wild migrating water fowl (T)

viii) The greater the value of flock, the lesser the down time between the flocks (F)

ix) In all biosecurity programmes there should be balance between cost and risk (T)

x) Longevity of avian influenza virus away from the bird is years (F)

Q.3. Choose the appropriate answer of the following statements:

i) Which of the following disease spread by air borne transmission

a. Newcastle disease b. avian influenza

c. chronic respiratory disease d. all (a-c)

ii) Traffic flow in poultry hoses should be

a. Dirty to clean area b. sick birds to healthy birds

c. older to young d. none

iii) which one of the following is best method for disposal of birds in the areas where there is poor soil drainage

a. incinerators b. disposal pit

c. composting d. none of the above.

iv) The chlorine level in the water should be

a. 0.5ppm b. 2ppm

c. 6 ppm d. 5ppm

v) contaminated feed is source of

a. Mycotoxins b. Salmonella

c. both d. none of the above.

Answers Q3 (i) d, (ii) d, (iii) a (iv) b, (v) c

26

Poultry Behaviour and Welfare

Asma Khan

For maximization of productivity in any kind of poultry venture the knowledge on the behaviour of birds and its application play very significant role. *Behaviour is the reaction of the whole organism to certain stimuli, or the manner in which it interacts to its environment.* Behavioural patterns are not inherited as such, but develop through the process of growth and get differentiated under the influence of genetic and environmental factors. Primary function of behaviour is to enable the bird to adjust itself to some changes in condition, whether external or internal. Most animals have a behavioural pattern which can be tried out in a given situation and in this way they learn to apply one or the other according to that which produces the best adjustment.

Factors Governing Behavioural Responses

The number of factors those influence the behavioural responses of fowls are:

1. **Genetic**: The bird's genetic make-up has an important influence on its reaction to any stimuli. Some strains are more docile than others.
2. **Experience**: Chicks know instinctively how to eat because of their behaviour is innate, but they do not know what to eat or where to find it. In the natural situation, the hen teaches her brood what to eat and where to find it.

3. **Age**: Some of the behaviours like the development of the peck order and reproduction behaviour is expressed only when the chickens attain appropriate ages.
4. **Environment**: High light intensity tends to increase activity which is a beneficial response in very young chickens but, in older birds it can lead to harmful behaviour such as cannibalism.

Social behaviour

Factors influencing social behaviour:

a. Individual recognition
b. Communication
c. Pecking and the peck order

a) Individual recognition

Generally fowls recognize each other by appearance based on the shape of the comb, wattles and head. Colour changes in plumage are identifiable, with intense colours being more noticeable than the lighter. Members of flocks those are broken up forget each other within 3 to 4 weeks.

b) Communication

The fowl uses a variety of sounds in order to communicate with other fowls. The most commonly used are food calls, predator alarm calls, pre- and post-laying calls and rooster crowing. Chick-distress calls draw immediate attention from their broody mother. The clucking calls of the broody hen to her brood will result in all of the chicks gathering close to her. Fowls also communicate with others by displays and changes in posture such as head up or head down, tail up or tail down, or feathers spread or not spread. Displays play an important part in mating behaviour. Thus, communication plays an important part in the maintenance of individual personal space, flock organization and integrity in a group situation.

c) Pecking and the peck order

Pecking as a skill is recognized as being species for fowls. They peck to escape from the shell, to feed, to drink, to obtain and keep personal space and to establish relationships as well as for other reasons. Submission is usually demonstrated by escape or crouching. The pecking habit is used to establish a hierarchical organization or ranking structure in the flock of dominant and progressively subordinate members. This organization is established separately for males and females in the same flock is called the peck order, the organization commences at an early age and, depending on flock size and complexity, is established by 10 to 16 weeks.

Non-adaptive or displacement behaviour

While poultry are known for their adaptability, they do possess innate behaviour needs that, if they are not given an opportunity to carry out may lead to non-adaptive or displacement behaviour. Examples of this behaviour include escape behaviour, preening, redirected pecking and various other types of movements. The situations that lead to these types of activity are believed to produce a level of frustration in the birds. This in turn may develop to where production efficiency is adversely affected.

Nesting behaviour in free range

In the free-living state hens select a nesting site with great care, often accompanied by a male if there is one present. Nesting is characterized by secrecy and careful nest concealment. Nesting behaviour has four stages:

i) Seeking a place to lay is a quite protracted activity as she becomes restless, and paces about giving pre-laying calls and showing characteristic body postures. In litter houses she will often examine the walls and corners.

ii) Inspecting a number of nest sites before selecting one and entering it.

iii) Settling, squatting and forming the nest by rotating her body several times, she usually stands to expel the egg.

iv) After laying she examines the egg and leaves the nest, cackles and joins the rest of the flock.

Nesting behaviour in cages

In cages the hen tries to adopt the same procedure, but because of the restrictions applied by cages, she cannot feel free and consequently is believed to suffer a degree of frustration as demonstrated by the display of non-adaptive behaviour. She searches the cage, pushing other hens away till she settles.

Welfare

Welfare is defined as organized efforts designed to promote the basic well-being, happiness, health and interests of individuals in need.

Welfare of bird and code of practice

Several developed countries have planned the code of recommendations for the welfare of poultry to encourage all those responsible for looking after birds to adopt the highest standards of husbandry. The United Kingdom Farm Animal Welfare Council stated that husbandry systems should provide freedom from: 1) hunger and thirst, 2) thermal and physical discomfort, 3) pain, injury and disease, 4) fear and distress and 5) insufficient space or facilities in which to exercise most normal patterns of behaviour.

Implementation of welfare code

Although the five freedoms mentioned under animal welfare are desirable, they are not likely to be entirely achievable. The level of compromising the bird's welfare with higher productivity may be ascribed to a number of factors like culture, economics, religious and philosophical beliefs, scientific knowledge and aesthetics. When balancing the socio-economic condition of any country and the welfare of birds it mainly concentrate on suitable poultry house design, sufficient floor space in cages and cage design and optimal environmental conditions around the bird.

Poultry housing for bird welfare and higher productivity

The modern housing systems are aimed to reduce labour and housing cost per hen by making higher density environments in the multiple tier cages. After the publication of the book *Animal Machines* (Harrison, 1964) started criticisms over intensive housing systems and such criticisms gaining momentum in the recent past. While considering the bird's welfare, the productivity of the birds over investment also to be kept in mind. Hence poultry housing should satisfy both the bird's welfare and economics of the poultry farm.

Poultry house design (Open sided)

Poultry house should have elevated ceiling to keep heat radiation away from birds. The height of roof should be 2.5 to 3.0 m (8 to 10 feet) at eaves and 4 to 5 m (13.5 to 16 feet) at ridge is preferable in tropical areas. To protect birds from exposure to direct sunlight and splashing of rainwater into the poultry house, the roof at both eaves will be extended as overhangs for about 3 to 5 feet on either side. As a thumb rule, the ideal width of the overhang will be half the height of open space at eaves. The effect of different roofing materials on microclimatic elements on birds housed is different. Asbestos roofed cage houses exerted significantly lower mortality rate and better feed efficiency than those housed in asbestos roofed deep litter; tile roofed cage; and tile roofed deep litter houses.

Cage floor space and cage design

The floor space of cage birds should provide adequate freedom to stand normally, turn around and stretch their wings. European Union welfare directives imply a minimum of at least 600 cm^2 per bird against the floor space of 450 cm^2 per bird adopted in India. For improving the welfare of the cage birds several manufacturers in western countries introduced different cage designs as enriched cages or welfare cages allowing sufficient floor space per bird (600 cm^2 per bird) plus extra room for a nesting box (156 cm^2 per bird) and a dust bath (120 to 156 cm^2 per bird). These additional provisions will necessarily increase the cost of cages and labour. By considering the fact of welfare of the birds and cost of investment per bird in India, the floor space may be increased by 10 per cent to that of present cage floor space allowance i.e. to 500 cm^2 per bird (Leghorn type layers).

Environmental conditions around the birds

Under intensive systems of rearing of birds to compensate the loss of freedom, comfortable living environment is necessary. Any variation in environmental temperature below 18^{0}C and beyond 24^{0}C range will affect the productivity of the birds. Hence special heating / cooling systems should be installed in the poultry houses to protect the birds during cold or hot periods. Adequate air movement in the house, effective ventilation and dry litter are to be maintained. To achieve proper oxygen level inside the poultry house, the speed of entry of fresh air and expulsion of exhaled foul air from the house should not be less than 0.5 cubic foot per bird per minute. Since carbon dioxide is relatively heavier than other gases, it remains at bird-level if ventilation is inadequate. Ammonia is another gas produced in warm and humid houses. Since it is lighter in nature, it rises and if easy exits are not available, accumulates near the ceiling room where it can be pushed down again by fans. When ammonia reaches a level of 15 to 20 ppm it will affect the growth and production performance of the birds.

Management practices and welfare issues

Debeaking

To reduce problems with feather pecking and cannibalism, most commercial laying chicken have their part of beak cut off. The practice has come under scrutiny because of associated pain, both immediate and chronic.

Stocking density

Stocking density is the number of birds placed into a given area. Production per bird tends to remain constant until flock size reaches a certain number. As this number is increased above what could be called the maximum stocking density, mortality will increase and production will probably decrease. Stocking of more number of birds in limited area than the recommended floor space required by those birds, is against bird's welfare.

Forced moulting

Conventional forced moulting based on long term feed removal is life-threatening, causing physiological stress in the commercial layers and is considered as inhumane method of rejuvenating birds.

Question Bank

Q. I. Fill in the blanks

a. .... and .... are the two most popular systems of housing birds.

b. Nesting is characterized by .... and careful nest ....

c. Captivity of birds in commercial production introduced new ....

Q.II. Justify the following statements.

a. Forced moulting is inhumane practice in birds..

b. Enriched cages are recommended over the California cage.

c. While constructing poultry houses roof hang extended 1 meter beyond walls.

d. Width of poultry house should not be more than 35 feet.

Q. III. Answer the following in brief.

a. Enlist various factors that governed behavioural responses of the birds.

b. Define the term welfare. Discuss in detail about the poultry housing for birds welfare and higher productivity.

Q. IV. Define the following

a. Peck order

b. Stocking density

c. Preening

d. Displacement behaviour

Q. V. Write short notes on the following

a. Ideal environmental condition for birds

b. Enriched cages for commercial layers

c. Welfare code

Answers

i. Deep litter, cage (b) secrecy, concealment (c) stresses-boredom

27

Feeding of Poultry

D. Sapcota

Digestive System and Digestion in Chicken

Studies on structure and functions of digestive system of chicken play important role for their nutrition and feeding. Functions of each part are given below (Fig 35):

Mouth: Birds feed through the beak. The horny upper and lower mandibles form the beak. Lips, teeth, cheek and soft palate are absent. The dagger-like tongue helps to force the feed into the esophagus. Chicken has 24 taste buds with high sense of taste. Absence of teeth makes the particle size of the feed important.

Esophagus (Gullet): It is made of loose fibrous tissue and serves as a tube to pass the food from mouth to crop. This is relatively long because of the long neck of the fowl.

Crop: (Ingluvius): It is a pouch like structure of esophagus to store, moisten and soften the food. It gives information about the feeding habits of the fowl.

Proventriculus (Glandular stomach or True stomach): It is an enlarged glandular ovoid structure of the esophagus connected to gizzard. It secretes pepsin and Hydrochloric acid.

Gizzard (Muscular stomach): Disc shaped muscular organ with two pairs of strong thick muscles and lined internally with a thick horny epithelial covering called the *Koilin* layer. Coarse materials are ground well by its powerful contractions with the support of the grit that birds consume.

Small Intestine: It comprises of duodenum, jejunum and ileum. It is the site of digestion and absorption. The duodenal loop supports the pancreas that secretes pancreatic juice. In chicken, the absorptive regions of the small intestine have a capillary bed instead of central lacteals of the villi.

Caeca (double caecum): Two blind ended pouch-like structure that demarcates the small and large intestines. Here microbial digestion of the undigested food material takes place.

Large intestine: This part of gut is very small and the size is double the diameter of small intestine with a short rectum. This is the site of water absorption.

Cloaca: This is a bulb like structure at the end of the digestive tract that serves as the common exit for digestive, reproductive and urinary tracts. Faeces and urine pass out simultaneously as a brownish black mass with white uric acid cap on its top.

Vent: This is the external opening of the cloaca.

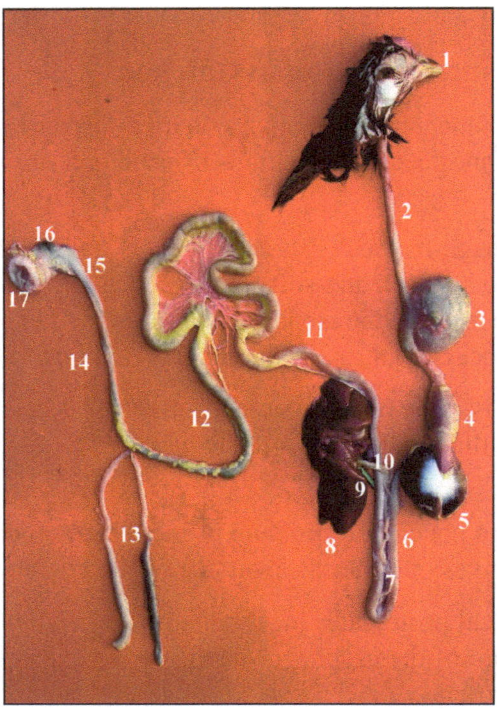

1. Beak
2. Esophagus
3. Crop
4. Proventriculus
5. Gizzard
6. Duodenum
7. Pancreas
8. Liver
9. Gal bladder
10. Hepatic duct
11. Jejunum
12. Ileum
13. Caecum
14. Colon
15. Rectum
16. Cloaca
17. Vent

Fig. 35. Digestive system of chicken.

Digestive System of Poultry

Supplementary digestive organs

The supplementary digestive organs to assist the digestive process are the pancreas and the liver.

Pancreas: It secretes the pancreatic juice that is conveyed into the duodenum through the pancreatic duct. The pancreatic enzymes digest the carbohydrates, proteins and fats.

Liver: It secretes greenish yellow sticky bile that helps to emulsify the fat for digestion and to neutralize the acid condition of the digestive tract.

Table 25: Enzymes of the digestive tract of chicken their substrates and products

Location	pH	Enzyme/Secretion	Substrate	Product
Mouth	7.0-7.5	Saliva	Lubricates and softens the feed	
		Amylase	Starch Dextrin	Dextrin Glucose
Crop	4.5	Mucous	Lubricates and soften the feed	
Proventriculus and Gizzard	2.5	Hydrochloric acid	Lowers digesta pH and initiates protein cleavage	
		Pepsin	Protein	Polypeptide
Duodenum	6.0-6.8	Amylase	Starch Dextrin	Maltose Glucose
		Trypsin, Chymotrypsin	Proteins Peptides	Peptides Amino acids
		Carboxypeptidase	Peptides	Amino acids
		Bile	Emulsification of fats	
		Lipase	Fat	Fatty acids Mono-glycerides Di-glycerides
		Cholesterol esterase	Cholesterol esters Cholesterol	Fatty acids
Jejunum	5.8-6.8	Maltase Isomaltase	Maltose Isomaltose	Glucose
		Sucrase	Sucrose	Glucose and fructose
		Peptidases	Peptides	Dipeptides, Amino acids
Caeca	5.7-5.9	Microbial activity	Cellulose, polysaccharides, starch and sugars	Volatile fatty acids, Vit K and B-Vitamins

Classification of Common Feed Ingredients and Their Nutrient Compositions

Conventionally, poultry feed ingredients can be widely participated as: energy source, proteinaceous source and mineral supplement. The nutrient compositions of common feed ingredients are given in Table 26.

1. **Energy source:** Maize, rice polish, wheat bran, de-oiled rice bran, molasses, sorghums, fats and oils.
2. **A) Proteinaceous (animal origin):** Fish meal, meat meal, slaughter house by product meal, hydrolyzed poultry feather meal, hatchery by-product meal and silk worm pupae meal.

2 **B) Proteinaceous (plant origin):** Soybean meal, ground nut/pea nut cake, cottonseed cake, sesame cake and canola meal.

3 **Mineral supplement:** Dicalcium phosphate, Limestone and oyster shell

Table 26: Nutrient composition and level of inclusion of common poultry feed ingredients

Ingredient	Crude protein %	M.E. (Kcal/kg)	Lysine %	Methionine %	Inclusion level %
Yellow maize	8.8	3300	0.24	0.20	0-60
White jowar	9.0	3100	0.22	0.18	0-40
Bajra	12.0	2650	0.45	0.25	0-40
Ragi	10.0	2550	0.24	0.20	0-15
Broken rice	8.7	2900	0.24	0.15	0-30
Wheat broken	10.0	3100	0.34	0.18	0-25
Rice polishing	12.2	3000	0.57	0.22	0-30
Deoiled sunflower cake	28.0	1900	1.17	0.60	0-15
Deoiled Groundnut cake	45.9	2200	1.76	0.45	0-30
Expeller groundnut cake	42.0	2500	1.64	0.42	0-30
Rotarary groundnut cake	38.0	2800	1.49	0.38	0-20
Deoiled soybean cake	46.0	2300	2.93	0.65	0-20
Dry fish	45.0	2580	3.28	1.32	5-10
Meat meal	55.0	2100	2.80	0.70	0-4
Molasses	3.2	2000	—	—	0-4

Nutrient Requirements of Different Age Groups

As birds are fed in groups, the nutrient requirements are not expressed on individual basis; but are expressed on unit weight of feed and hence feed intake by the bird influences the nutrient requirements. Nutrient requirements of birds are influenced by the age, sex, size of the bird, production level, energy content of the ration, physical form of diet, nutritional adequacy of the diet and environmental temperature. Hence, prescribing a common list of quantities of nutrients required for birds at all seasons, for different ages and under all conditions is an extremely difficult task.

To allow for variations in composition of feed ingredients, to avoid loss during storage, to allow for nutrients destroyed in the digestive tract and to allow for stability of the nutrients, an increase in the supply of the nutrient over the minimum requirement is made as a safety margin which is termed as *nutrient allowance*. Minerals and vitamins are more prone for destruction. For majority of the vitamins, usually twice the requirements are added as safety margin. Likewise, for major minerals, 20 to 30 per cent of the minimum requirement is used as allowance. The nutrient requirement of different age group of chickens is given in Table 27.

Poultry Feed Formulation

Feed is the largest component of expenditure which accounts for more than 75% of the total cost of poultry production. Moreover, the cost per kilogram of feed is ever increasing. A major portion of poultry feed is prepared on farm or by custom-mixing. Hardly, around 20% of the requirement is met by the organized sector.

Nutrients

Nutrients are essential substances that are present in feeds. These are required for growth, maintenance and reproductive process of a living body. Poultry require more than 40 such nutrients which are classified into six major groups based on their chemical nature, their functions and the method of determination. These are: 1. Proteins, 2. Carbohydrates, 3. Fats, 4. Minerals, 5. Vitamins and 6. Water and are present in the feed but get split up upon digestion within the birds' body, absorbed and rebuilt in tissues. These nutrients are briefly described as under:

1. Protein

Proteins constitute about 20% of chicken meat and 12% of egg. They are considered as the building blocks of the body. They are essential for proper growth and health buildup. Grains generally contain lower level (8-9 per cent) of crude protein, whereas, animal or vegetable protein source contribute higher levels (30-50 per cent). The demand for protein during early age is very high. Further, energy level of the ration also decides the protein requirement; higher the energy level, greater the percentage of protein required.

Table 27: Nutrient requirements for different age groups of chicken (BIS)

Age (wk)	Category	Type of feed	ME Kcal/kg	Protein (min) %	Crude fibre (max) %	AIA max. (%)	Ca (%)	P (Available %)	Salt (%)	Aprox qnty. reqrd. (kg)
0-8	Chick	Starter mash	2800	20	4	3	1.0	0.5	0.6	2.0
9-20	Grower	Grower mash	2600	16	7	4	1.0	0.5	0.6	5.5
21 and above	Layer	Layer mash	2650	18	6	4	3-3.5	0.5	0.6	40
21 and above	Breeder	Breeder mash	2700	18	6	4	3-3.5	0.5	0.6	-
0-4	Broiler	Broiler starter	2900	22	3.5	3	1.0	0.5	0.6	1-1.25
5-6	Broiler	Broiler finisher	3000	19-22	4	3	1.0	0.5	0.6	1.7-1.9

Note: AIA is acid insoluble ash. Feed should not contain >11% moisture.

Protein is made up of several amino acids and it is necessary to know the composition of any protein rich feedstuffs in terms of its constituent amino acids. Among amino acids ten are considered to be *essential* for poultry since the birds cannot synthesize these. They are Arginine, Histidine, Isoleucine, Leucine, Lysine, Methionine, Phenylalanine, Threonine, Tryptophan and Valine. Among these, lysine and methionine are considered as *'critical amino acids'*, since poultry feed is likely to be deficient in these two amino acids. Amino acids synthesized in the body are called *non essential amino acids*.

The amino acids composition of proteins from different protein sources vary widely. Deficiency of essential amino acids in poultry diets result in poor growth, poor egg production or poor feed efficiency. Hence, amino acid inputs to the required levels is one of the most important factors in formulating poultry feed.

2. Carbohydrates

Carbohydrates occur in feed as a soluble form which is mostly starch, sugars and crude fibre. The crude fibre in chicken is digestible not beyond 7%. Every one per cent increase in the crude fibre lessens the digestibility of food by 2% and useful energy by 3-6%. Birds require energy to maintain their body heat and to keep the body systems running. They derive their supplies of energy from two major groups of nutrients, known as carbohydrates and fats/oils. The most frequently used to describe the energy value of ingredients is the metabolisable energy (ME). It is calculated as gross energy minus energy voided through droppings (faeces + urates) and gases and is expressed as kilocalorie per kg of feed. 1 Kcal = 4.18 KJ.

Energy content of the feed determines the quantum of feed intake. Lower the energy level, higher is the feed consumed per day and *vice versa.* Hence, absolute intake of other nutrients in the feed is also influenced by the energy content of the feed. It is then necessary to adjust the density of different nutrients present in poultry feed not only to the requirements of the birds; but also to the expected feed intake per day determined by the energy content of the feed. Since most of the vitamins and minerals are normally provided in poultry feed well in excess of the daily requirement, it is customary to adjust only its protein content to the energy content. This relationship is referred as *calorie: protein ratio* or C: P ratio which is more important than absolute requirement of energy or protein. It is the number of energy units for every per cent of crude protein in the compound poultry feed. Wider the ratio, the relative proportion of energy content is high and narrower the ratio, that of crude protein is high in the feed.

In summer, feed intake goes down. It is then necessary to reduce the energy content of the diet and increase nutrient density, especially of critical amino acids and trace minerals. In winter, the energy requirement to maintain body heat is high and hence feed intake increases; it is then necessary to widen the standard C: P ratio. During disease conditions, the appetite and in turn, the feed intake is poor. Hence, net intake of all the nutrients becomes less. The bird then suffers from nutrient deficiencies also, their disease resistance goes down and the effect of disease on production becomes more intense.

3. Fats

Fats are concentrated source of energy and yield 2.25 times more energy than carbohydrates. In feed it reduces dustiness, increases palatability, gives high energy, supplies essential fatty acids and to some extent fat soluble vitamins. However, excess of fat in the feed may lead to rancidity and spoilage. All edible oils and animal fats included up to 5 per cent in poultry rations.

4. Vitamins

Vitamins are essential, but trace organic substances required in small amounts for overall health, growth and reproduction. Good growth, prevention of leg weakness, egg shell thickness all need precise vitamin supplement. Vitamins occur in many naturally available feed ingredients. They cannot be synthesized by the body, therefore should be added as supplements to meet the birds' requirements. Vitamins are classified into two groups, viz. fat soluble vitamins (A,D,E and K) and water-soluble vitamins (B complex group of vitamins and vitamin C). Vitamins in B complex group are thiamin (B_1), riboflavin (B_2), niacin(B_3), pantothenic acid, pyridoxine (B_6), biotin (Vit-H), choline, folic acid (Vit-B_9) and cobalamine (B_{12}). Vitamins, A, B_2 and D_3 are called *'critical vitamins'* for poultry as any deficiency in their availability severely impairs growth rate and egg production.

Vitamin supplements need storage in light-proof conditions at temperatures below 72°F. Especially, vitamins A, D and E may be readily oxidized and destroyed by adverse conditions of heat, light, moisture and also by mixture with certain minerals. Contrarily, water soluble vitamins like biotin, riboflavin, folic acid, pyridoxine, choline etc. are more stable and losses normally do not arise during the process of milling and mixing. Thiamine (B_1) is sensitive to heat and light.

5. Minerals

These are essential for bone, blood and egg shell formation. They aid in digestion, absorption and utilization of other nutrients. About one per cent of the broiler meat and 11% of the egg are made up of minerals while bones contain about 40 per cent. Feed ingredients of animal origin contain more minerals than the vegetable counterpart. Minerals found in common feedstuffs may not supply the birds' requirements for which they are added to the ration to overcome the possibility of deficiency. The minerals required for poultry are classified as *'Macro'* minerals, *'Micro'* minerals and *'Trace'* minerals depending on their level of requirement. These are described in Table 28.

Table 28: Minerals and their functions

Minerals	Important functions	Deficiency symptoms
Macro Minerals		
Calcium	Formation of bone, blood clotting, heart function, egg production	Poor growth, soft bones, thin shelled/shell-less eggs, poor egg production
Phosphorous	Bone development, egg production, utilization of carbohydrates	Poor growth, soft bones
Magnesium	Several vital metabolic functions	Slow growth, lethargy, loss of appetite, spasms
Sodium and potassium	Constituents of blood, bile and body fluids, for growth, digestion, acid-base balance	Poor growth of muscles (excess: loose droppings, reduced production)
Micro Minerals		
Manganese	Bone formation and utilization of phosphorous	Staggering gait, enlargement of joints
Zinc	Activation of several body enzyme	Poor growth and feathering, shortening of leg bones
Iron &Copper	Blood pigment formation	Anaemia
Iodine	Body activity, constituent of thyroid	Impaired body response, lowered activity
Trace Minerals		
Selenium	Muscular functions, immunity development	Muscular dystrophy, poor immune response
Cobalt	Constituent of Vitamin B_{12}	Poor growth

Excessive levels of some minerals may also be harmful. In practice, however, the levels of calcium, phosphorous and salt (sodium chloride) are calculated and specific ingredients/ mineral mixtures are added to meet their requirements. Limestone, di-calcium phosphate, shell grit, common salt etc., serve the purpose. The trace minerals are supplied by adding commercial supplement and there is no necessity to consider each of them separately.

6. Water

Half of the chicken's body is water. It is essential for life and has to be supplied throughout, separately. Birds can survive for a long time (2-3 days) without taking feed but suffer even beyond 12 hours, if there is shortage of water. Feed ingredients also supply water, but it should not exceed 7-12%. The quality of feed depends on the moisture content, since excess of moisture leads to mould growth. Usually birds drink water double the quantity of feed.

How to formulate a poultry ration

Before formulating any ration one should remember that no feed ingredient is essential but all nutrients are essential.

The feed formulated shall be able to meet all the recommended nutrients, with the least possible cost. For this purpose one shall be aware of the followings;

- Type of feed to be formulated.
- Nutrient requirements of the birds at different ages.
- Local availability of different feed ingredients and their cost.
- Level of inclusion of particular feedstuff
- The nutrient composition of the feed ingredients.

During manual feed formulation, it is sufficient to check the critical nutrient levels like protein, energy, lysine and methionine. If these levels are met, as recommended, good quality mineral and vitamin mixtures are added at the recommended levels. Invariably, the feed will be a balanced one meeting all the nutrients. If computer is used in feed formulation, the level of all the nutrients can be checked.

First, formulate a tentative feed formula and calculate the critical nutrient levels with the help of the data and compare these values with the recommended levels. If the calculated nutrient levels are on par with the recommended levels, the feed formula can be adopted as such. If the tentative feed formula is not able to meet the recommended critical nutrient levels, make slight alterations in the feed formula, to satisfy the nutrient levels. Again check the composition and alter the formula if necessary until the recommended nutrient levels are met. Now add the feed additives/ supplements recommended. The formula is complete and proceed for mixing the feed.

Quality-wise own feed should be equally good as compared to the company feed and shall be cheaper. Based on the formula, calculate the exact quantities of different feed ingredients per batch. First, weigh all the ingredients to be ground like grains, oil cakes, fish etc. grind them together. Then add the weighed quantities of mineral mixture, meat meal, rice polishings etc. which do not need grinding. Prepare a premix of all the medicines/ supplements/ additives; mix them with small quantity of some ground ingredients like rice polish, oil meal or maize meal and then add to the rest of the feed ingredients and mix thoroughly. Avoid dustiness during grinding and mixing, to prevent loss of nutrients. Ensure thorough mixing in a horizontal/ vertical mixer. It is always safe to sun dry all grains, fish and oil cakes, before storing. Sun drying not only reduces the moisture level, but also kills the germs as well as checks the aflatoxin level. If needed, change the feed formulae based on the local availability, cost and quality of the feed ingredients. Never make drastic changes in the formulae, but bring only gradual changes, since drastic change may affect the feed intake and thereby the growth rate/ egg production.

Economics of Feed Formulation Cost/Unit Nutrient

Layer ration (Requirement: CP= 18%; ME =2650 Kcal/kg ; Ca= 3-3.5 %; P (Available)= 0.5 %; Lysine= 0.7% ; Methionine= 0.4%).

Ingredient	Quantity (kg)	Cost per ingredient (Rs)	Parameters	Level
Maize	40	640	Crude Protein	18.24
Rice Polish	24	340	ME Kcal/kg	2629.7
Wheat bran	5	85	Ca%	3.08
DOGNC	5	190	P% (available)	0.40
MOC	2	47	Lysine	0.49
Soya DO	5	205	Methionine	0.32
FM	8	235		
Meat meal	4	48		
Shell grit	2.5	34		
Bone meal	2	26		
Min. Mix	2	89		
Salt	0.5	2		
Total ingredient	100	1941		

Additive: Vitablend, dose @ 10 g/qntl, cost: Rs. 1200/Kg.
Cost of feed without Vitablend: 19.41
Cost of feed with Vitablend: 19.53
NB: The cost of compounded feed varies as per the geographical location, season, tax levied on ingredients by the state government etc.

Feeding Systems

Some of the popular methods or systems of feeding poultry are as follows:

1. Whole grain feeding

In this system birds are supplied with whole grains as a free choice feeding with a belief that they could balance their ration according to their individual needs. Certain advantages like simplicity and saving of labour were claimed for this method. However, differences were found in the response to different grains and the reaction of certain individuals and breeds. This is an old and abandoned system of feeding.

2. Mash and grain feeding

This system involves feeding of both mash and grain and is regarded as a slightly better method than the previous system. Along with the mash some grains or grain mixtures are also fed either in feed hoppers or as scratch grain. The advantage of this system is that it is flexible as one can increase or decrease the level of protein at will.

3. Complete mash feeding

This involves grinding of coarse materials and mixing together of all the feed ingredients in required proportions. It is a good system for feeding all types of poultry. The main advantage with this method is that it enables one to formulate a ration according to the nutritional requirements of the fowls. This system also prevents selective eating and thereby produces more uniform quality products (eggs or meat).

4. Pellet feeding

In this system complete mash is first prepared and then rolled into small cylindrical masses called pellets, in a pelleting mill. It allows less wastage of feed and does not permit the birds to pick some of the ingredients of their choice and leave others. Though pellet feeding is costly, improvement in growth rate and feed utilization have been found better under this system.

5. Crumble feeding

Large sized pellets are passed through blur mills, granulators or rolling mills to break them in varying sizes of crumbles. They are quite palatable and useful, when pellets are more hard and oversize for younger birds.

Feeding of broilers

The growth rate of broiler is very fast therefore, they are feed with high energy, high proteinous diet *ad libitum*. Broilers are fed with 'broiler-starter' diet up to 4 weeks and then shifted to 'broiler-finisher' diet thereafter. However, now-a-days in many commercial farms feeding of broilers with 'pre-starter' diet for the first 2 weeks is practiced with appreciable results.

Feeding of layers (Egg-type birds)

Egg type birds are fed with different diets depending upon their age such as from day-old to 8 weeks, chick mash; from 8 to 20 weeks, grower mash and from 20 weeks onwards layer mash.

The chicks should be fed with finely grounded maize or other cereal grains for the first day and from second day onwards with chick mash containing CP 20%, ME 2800 Kcal/kg, lysine 1%, Methionine 0.35%, calcium 1% and phosphorus 0.5%.

The grower mash contains CP 16%, ME 2600 Kcal/kg, Lysine 0.7%, Methionine 0.25%, calcium 1% and Phosphorus (available) 0.5 %. Shell grit should be provided from 18th week onwards. Change over from grower mash to layer mash may be done gradually when the pullets are at 18 weeks.

A layer mash contains CP 18%, ME 2650 Kcal/Kg calcium 3-3.5% and phosphorus (avl.) 0.5%.

Economization of poultry feeding

- Fill up the feeder only one-third at a time, increase frequency of feeding to 3-4 times a day.
- Feed in the poultry shed should not be stocked more than a day's requirement to avoid spoilage by rats.
- Storage should be organized to facilitate the first-in, first-out usage. Compounded feed should not be stocked for more than 1 – 1 ½ months to avoid rancidity or fungus.
- Feed in feeders should be stirred at 4-5 times a day to avoid formation of cake or fungal growth.
- Feed and feed ingredient bags should be stored on pallets and not directly on the floor and away from the walls to avoid dampness.

Restricted or Controlled feeding method

Several types of feed restriction programmes can be followed during the growing period of breeder pullets, usually from 6 – 20 weeks of age. Some of the common methods are:

- Restriction on quantity i.e. feed intake.
- Restriction of feeding time.
- Restriction of a nutrient, like protein or energy.
- Skip-a-day programme.
- Alternate day feeding programme.

Each method has certain advantages and disadvantages and none can be regarded as best suited under all conditions. The choice of a feeding system would depend upon the age of the birds, relative cost of mash and grains, the amount of time and labour available. Several advantages like reduced cost of feeding, delayed sexual maturity, better egg production curve, reduction in the number of small eggs laid, have been claimed for this method.

Separate male feeding

Males are reared separately for breeding purpose. For them specific ration is provided which will be beneficial for their maintenance of physiological conditions and fertility. This is also important because underfed males lose libido; whereas, excess feeding leads to overweight affecting fertility. The broiler breeder males are fed a ration containing CP 12-14 % and ME 2630 - 2800 Kcal/kg; whereas, broiler breeder females are fed a ration containing CP 17-18 % and ME 2760-2800 Kcal/kg.

Feed additives including herbal bio-enhancers

A feed additive or supplement is a substance or mixture of substances, other than the bulk and basic feedstuffs, used in small quantities, usually at less than one per cent level in the compounded feeds, in order to supplement and complement certain nutrients or non-nutrients to improve the quality of the feed and performance of the birds fed.

Functions of feed additives

Feed additives have one or more of the following functions:

- Prevent various deficiency diseases, other diseases of nutritional origin and certain bacterial or parasitic diseases.
- Improve the nutritive value of the feed and feed efficiency.
- Improve the growth rate and egg production.
- Protect the birds from stress and improve the immune status.

- Prevent the spoilage of feed due to microbes, rancidity and other physical conditions.
- Enhance the colour, flavour, palatability and general appearance of the feed.
- Help to prevent caking, dustiness and loss of feed during storage, handling and feeding.
- Improve the quality of the egg, yolk colour, shell thickness and meat quality.
- Have sparing action on certain nutrients and prevent nutritional imbalance.
- Certain non-nutrient feed additives cause thinning of gut wall and thereby facilitate better absorption of nutrients.

Based on their functions, the feed additives are broadly classified into two categories, namely,

- Nutrient feed additives and
- Non-nutrient feed additives.

Nutrient feed additives

The nutrient feed additives contain certain essential nutrients necessary for normal growth and production of the birds. Deficiency of these in poultry will lead to various anatomical and physiological abnormalities, deficiency diseases, poor growth rate, low egg production and low disease resistance. They need to be added if the formulated feed is not expected to contain such nutrients in required levels.

The nutrient feed additives can be further classified into the following categories:

1. **Vitamin Supplements**
   - *Fat soluble vitamins:* Such as Vitamins A, $D_{3,}$ E and K
   - *Water soluble vitamins:* Such as B-Complex group of vitamins and Vitamin C.
2. **Mineral Supplements**
   - *Macro minerals:* Such as calcium, phosphorous, magnesium, sodium, potassium and sulphur.
   - *Micro minerals:* Such as manganese, zinc, iron, copper and iodine.
   - *Trace elements:* Like selenium, cobalt, molybdenum and chromium.

3. *Essential Amino Acids:* Like lysine, methionine and tryptophan.
4. *Protein hydrolysates:* A predigested protein such as hydrolysed feather meal, hair meal etc. supplying essential amino acids and other nutrients.
5. *Liver extract:* Supplies essential nutrients in the most assimilable form.
6. *Live yeast and yeast extract:* Supplies essential nutrients, digestive enzymes and unidentified growth factors (U.G.F.).
7. *Fermentation by-products:* Supply various essential nutrients and U.G.F.

II. Non-Nutrient feed additives

This group of feed additives do not have any direct nutritional role, but are added to the feed in order to reduce the mortality and morbidity due to various diseases and stress factors; improve the feed efficiency by better digestion, absorption and utilization of nutrients; enhance the colour, flavour, consistency and quality of the feed and improve the shelf life of the feed by preventing caking, moulds, mustiness, oxidation and other physical, chemical and micro-biological degradations.

Classification, Uses and Examples

Based on their nature and functions the non-nutrient feed additives may be classified as follows,:

- ***Antibiotic feed supplements*:** Used to control sub-clinical bacterial infections and thereby boost the performance. Ex: Tetracyclines, lincomycin, bacitracin, flavomycin, avilamycin, zinc bacitracin, virginiamycin etc. However, several antibiotics have been banned in certain developed countries for their residual effects and development of resistant strains.
- ***Non-antibiotic antimicrobial feed supplements*:** Check bacterial infections and promote the performance. Ex: Furazolidone, chlorhydroxy-quinoline.
- ***Mould inhibitors/Antimycotic agents*:** Prevent mould growth and production of toxins. Ex: Gentian violet, copper sulphate, propionic acid, calcium propionate, sodium benzoate.
- ***Coccidiostats*:** Prevent outbreaks of coccidiosis especially under deep litter system. Ex: Dinitro-ortho-toluamide, salinomycin, robenidine, nicarbazine, monensin, maduramycin, ionophores etc.
- ***Anti-parasitic additives*:** Check various parasitic infestations. Ex: Dichlorophan, Niclosamide, Praziquantel etc.

- ***Anti-oxidants*:** These are used to prevent oxidative rancidity of fats present in ingredients like rice polish, fish meal etc. Ex. B.H.T., B.H.A., Ethoxyquin,vitamin E, selenium etc.
- ***Enzymes*:** The inherent enzyme of birds may not be adequate to digest their feeds properly for which extraneous enzymes are added to help in better digestion of the feed. Ex: protease, lipase, cellulase, amylase, pectinase etc.
- ***Arsenicals*:** Arsenicals (0.01% or less) promote growth rate, feed efficiency and carcass finish. Eg: 3-Nitro-4-hydroxy phenyl arsanilic acid.
- ***Adsorbents*:** Adsorb (bind) toxins and prevent their absorption from the intestine. Eg: Zeolites, activated charcoal, hydrated sodium calcium aluminosilicate (HSCAS).
- ***Pellet binders*:** Used for pelleting the feed in preparation of crumbled feed for broilers Eg-bentonite, sodium alginate, lignin sulphate, gelatine, lignosulphonate, carragenan, guargum etc.
- ***Emulsifiers*:** Emulsifiers increase the surface area of fat for digestion and absorption. These are fed especially in first week to improve fat digestion. Lecithin is a good emulsifier.
- ***Deodorizing agents*:** On feeding these agents ammonia production in the litter will be reduced. Eg: Yucca extract.
- ***Aromatics/ Flavouring agents*:** Added to improve the feed flavour or mask original unpleasant flavour or to impart new flavour. Eg: Essential oils, fish oils etc.
- ***Pigments*:** Impart attractive colour to the feed as well as to the products like egg yolk and skin. Eg: Canthaxanthin, Leutin, Zeaxanthin etc.
- ***Herbal preparations*:** Tone up the liver, protection against nephro-toxicity, stimulate immune response, improve the appetite and increase the disease and toxin resistance power of the birds. Eg: Extracts of herbs.
- ***Performance boosters*:** Improve the overall performance of the birds, by various means. Eg-nitrovin, avoparcin etc.
- ***Immunostimulants*:** Stimulate antibody production, cell mediated immunity and general resistance to diseases. Eg: Tetrahydropheny + limidazole, immogen, levamisole etc.
- ***Other miscellaneous feed additives*:** Perform certain specific functions in the body or feed and thereby improve the performance. Eg: electrolytes, egg-up, egtonner etc.

- ***Probiotic or Direct Fed Microbials (DFM)*:** Probiotic is a live microbial feed supplement which beneficially affects the host animal by improving its intestinal microbial balance and the host animal responds with a better performance in terms of growth/feed efficiency. Probiotic preparations are made from bacteria, yeast and fungi. Among bacteria, strains of *Lactobacillus, Leuconostoc, Bifidobacterium, Pediococcus* and *Streptococcus* and among fungi, strains of *Aspergillus* and among yeast, strains of *Saccharomyces* are commonly included in probiotic preparations in various combinations. In general, probiotic preparation increases the growth rate in broilers, egg production in layers and reproductive performance in breeders. However, the effect of probiotic is profound in stressed birds than healthy ones.
- ***Prebiotics*:** These are non digestible feed ingredients that beneficially affect the host by selectively stimulating the growth of gut bacteria. Ex: DOS, MOS, Inulin etc. It is observed that the effect of probiotics is always better if exposed to proper prebiotics.

Herbal bioenhancers are phytomolecules that at low doses promote and augment the bioavailability or bioactivity of drugs. Their development is based on ancient knowledge of *Ayurveda*. They may reduce the dose, shorten the treatment period and thus reduce drug resistance problems. Due to dose economy, they make treatment cost-effective, minimize drug toxicity and adverse reactions. They are effective when used in combination with a number of drug classes such as antibiotics, antiviral and antifungal drugs. They may improve oral absorption of a wide range of nutrients such as vitamins, minerals, herbal extracts and amino acids. They act through several mechanisms of action affecting mainly the absorption process, drug metabolism or action on the drug target.

Anti-Nutritional Factors and Toxins

Anti-nutritional factors or antinutrients are the substances found in the animal feed that have the potential to adversely affect health, growth and productive performance of the bird. These may include compounds of both plant (endogenous) and microbial origin (exogenous). The plant origin may affect the digestion, absorption and metabolism of nutrients, some important are given below:

Table 29: Some antinutrients of plant origin

S No	Antinutrients	Occurance
1.	Trypsin inhibitors,Antigenic proteins, Protease inhibitors.	Soybean
2.	Haemagglutinins (lectins)	Legume seeds (Castor bean, kidney bean, soybean).
3.	Cyanogens	Cassava root
4.	Glucosinolates	Rapeseed
5.	Gossypol	Cottonseed
6.	Phyto-oestrogens	Clover; lucerne; soybean

However, these antinutrients may be removed, though partially, by using various methods like heat treatment, soaking in water, ammoniation, solvent extraction etc.

Mycotoxins

Mycotoxins are those secondary metabolites of fungi that have the capacity to impair poultry health, productivity or sometimes death. No region escapes this silent killer. According to the FAO, approximately 25% of world's grain supply is contaminated this mycotoxins. Common mycotoxins occurring in feeds are given in Table 30. Contamination may occur during harvesting, processing and storage of feedstuffs or whenever environmental conditions are appropriate for the spoilage fungi. Moisture content and ambient temperature are key determinants of fungal colonization and mycotoxin production.

Table 30: Certain common mycotoxins occurring in poultry feeds.

Mycotoxins	Fungal species
Aflatoxins	*Aspergillus flavus; A. parasiticus*
Ochratoxin A	*A. ochraceus; Penicillium viridicatum; P. cyclopium*
Zearalenone	*F. culmorum; F. graminearum; F. sporotrichioides*
T-2 toxin	*F. sporotrichioides; F. poae*
Fumonisins; moniliformin; fusaric acid	*F. moniliforme*
Diacetoxyscirpenol	*F. sporotrichioides; F. graminearum; F. poae*
Deoxynivalenol	*Fusarium culmorum; F. graminearum*
Cyclopiazonic acid	*A. flavus*
Citrinin	*P. citrinum; P. expansum*
Patulin	*P. expansum*
Citreoviridin	*P. citreo-viride*

Aflatoxins

This group includes aflatoxin B_1, B_2, G_1 and G_2 (AFB_1, AFB_2, AFG_1 and AFG_2, respectively). The aflatoxigenic *Aspergilli* are generally regarded as storage fungi, proliferating under conditions of relatively high moisture/humidity and temperature. Aflatoxin contamination is, therefore, almost exclusively confined to tropical feeds such as oilseed by-products derived from groundnuts, cottonseed and palm kernel. Aflatoxin contamination of maize is also an important problem in warm humid regions where *A. flavus* may infect the crop prior to harvest and remain viable during storage.

Ochratoxins

The *Aspergillus* genus includes a species (*A. ochraceus*) that produces ochratoxins, a property it shares with at least two *Penicillium* species. Ochratoxin A (OA) and ochratoxin B are two forms that occur naturally as contaminants, with OA being more ubiquitous, occurring predominantly in cereal grains and in the tissues of animals reared on contaminated feed. Another mycotoxin, citrinin, often co-occurs with ochratoxin. The ochratoxins and citrinin are nephrotoxic to a wide range of animal species.

Fusarium mycotoxins

Fusarium mycotoxins are the trichothecenes, zearalenone (ZEN) and the fumonisins. The trichothecenes are subdivided into four basic groups, with types A and B being the most important. Type A trichothecenes include T-2 toxin, HT-2 toxin, neosolaniol and diacetoxyscirpenol (DAS). Type B trichothecenes include deoxynivalenol (DON, also known as vomitoxin), nivalenol and fusarenon-X.

Question Bank

I. Choose the Correct Answer.

1. The pH in proventriculus of adult chicken is found to be 2.5/5.5/7.5. (2.5).
2. Chicken require more than 40 nutrients which are classified into 2/4/6 major groups based on their nature and functions. (6).
3. The crude fibre in chicken is digestible not beyond 7/9/11 percent. (7).
4. The crude protein content in chick diet should be 18/20/22 % and ME content 2600/2800/3000 kcal/kg. (20 and 2800).
5. The antimycotic agents commonly used in poultry ration is ionophores/ copper sulphate/flavomycin. (copper sulphate).

6. Aflatoxin is produced by the fungus *Penicillium viridicatum* /*Aspergillus flavus*/ *F. sporotrichioides*. (*Aspergillus flavus*).
7. The edible oils and animal fats included up to 5/7/9 % in poultry ration. (5).
8. The ME content in maize is 2300/3300/4300 kcal/kg. (3300).
9. The crude protein and ME contents of grower mash should be 14/15/16 % and 2600/2700/2800 kcal/kg. (16 and 2600).
10. An adult layer hen consumes on an average 80/110/130 G. of feed per day. (110).
11. A broiler chicken eats around 2.50/3.50/4.50 kgs of feed till it reaches its market age. (3.50).

II. Fill in the blanks

1. Chicken has .... Nos of taste buds with high sense of taste. (24 N0s).
2. Proventriculus is also known as .... stomach; whereas, the gizzard is known as............. stomach. (Glandular or True and muscular).
3. The thick horny epithelial covering inside gizzard is also called as .... layer. (Koilin).
4. In .... (part of intestine) microbial digestion of the undigested food materials takes place. (caeca).
5. Bile helps to .... fat for proper digestion. (emulsify).
6. The additives are usually used less than .... per cent in compounded poultry feed. (1).
7. Fats are concentrated source of energy and yield .... times more energy than carbohydrates. (2.25).
8. Feed is the largest single item of expenditure which accounts for more than .... % of the total cost of poultry production. (75).

III. True/False.

1. While preparing poultry ration the fish meal can be incorporated up to a safe level of 25%. (False).
2. The oyster shell is used to provide phosphorous in poultry diet. (false).
3. The dietary requirement of calcium for the layers is more than 3.0%. (True).

4. Vitamins A, B_2 and D_3 are called as ‘critical vitamins’ for poultry. (True).
5. Restricted feeding is ideal for commercial broiler raising. (False).
6. In poultry ration the adsorbents are used to bind the dietary mycotoxins. (True).
7. All feed ingredients should contain more than 11% moisture level. (False).
8. Usually, broiler starter ration contains more level of energy than that of broiler finisher ration. (False).

28

Health Care

B. Mohan

Common Poultry Diseases

Infectious diseases

Bacteria

Commonly known as "germs", bacteria are very small living microorganisms. Only a few bacteria cause diseases. In birds these include Salmonella, Clostridia, Pasteurella, Vibrio, Staphylococci, Streptococci, Mycoplasma, Hemophilus, and Mycobacterium etc.

Viruses

Viruses are the smallest microorganisms known, and can multiply only within living cells. Viruses are not responsive to drug treatments. Important viral diseases include Ranikhet disease, Infectious bronchitis, Laryngotracheitis, Fowl pox, Infectious Bursal Disease, Avian Encephalomyelitis, Avian Influenza, Marek's Disease and Lymphoid leucosis.

Mycoplasma

These are very small organisms. Many mycoplasma serotypes are infectious for birds. The disease producing organisms are *Mycoplasma gallisepticum, M. synoviae, M. meleagridis and M. gallinarum*

Protozoa

Similar to bacteria, but usually much larger include coccidia, histomonads (black head), hexamita, trichomonads, toxoplasma.

Parasites

Ectoparasites include mites, lice, fleas and others. Endoparasites are mainly worms and consist largely of ascarids, cecal worms, tape worms and capillaria.

Fungi

This group contains the molds. There are two important diseases in this group, Aspergillosis (brooder pneumonia) and Moniliasis (candida). There are others as Thrush and Favus.

Non-Infectious Diseases

Nutritional Deficiencies

The ration of the modern, fast growing bird must be nutritionally balanced. There is continued need, however, for refinements in the nutritional quality of feeds in order to parallel continued advances in the genetic improvement of birds. As birds grow faster on less feed, greater attention must be given to the refined nutritional requirements of the particular genetic makeup of a given bird. The nutritional requirements of these birds will vary markedly.

Poisons and Toxins

The major intoxication of birds is mycotoxicosis. Others include botulism, excess dosage of medicaments, excess intake of salt, ingestion of insecticides or fungicides, and occasionally heavy metal poisoning with special reference to arsenic.

Nutritional Deficiency Diseases

Vitamin A

Vitamin A is essential for normal vision, growth, egg production and reproduction.

Deficiency Symptoms: Retarded growth, weakness, ruffled feathers, absence of liquid from the tear glands, Xerophthalmia and blindness may result. There are cheesy exudates of the eyes in adult birds. Egg production and hatchability are impaired. The incidence of blood spots in eggs increased. The resistance of the bird to some poultry diseases are lowered.

Vitamin D (Cholecalciferol)

Vitamin D in poultry aids in absorption of calcium and phosphorus from the intestinal tract, thus increasing the amounts of these two minerals available for bone development and the amount of calcium for egg shell deposition.

Deficiency Symptoms : Rickets – Calcium and Phosphorus are not deposited in the bones in normal amounts. The hock joints are enlarged. General unthriftiness, soft shelled eggs, lowered egg production and reduced hatchability.

Vitamin E (Alpha-tocopherol)

Vitamin E (tocopherol) is necessary for adequate productivity of the cells and for blood formation.

Deficiency Symptoms: (a) Nutritional encephalomalacia - evidenced by a twisted neck, prostration, curled toes and 'crazy chick' disease. (b) Exudative diathesis – there is some indication that selenium is involved, as addition of this mineral have been shown to reduce the deficiency. (c) Muscular dystrophy- the signs are usually unapparent, but locomotor problems could occur.

Vitamin K

This vitamin is necessary for the synthesis of prothrombin, a chemical necessary for blood clotting.

Deficiency Symptoms: There is a hemorrhagic syndrome. Hemorrhages that are pin point in size at first and large later occurs on the flesh. If skin of the chicken pulled off, bleeding may be seen on the breast, thighs and ribs.

Thiamin (B_1)

Thiamin is necessary to stimulate the appetite, to form certain enzymes necessary for digestion and to prevent nervous disorders that culminate in polyneuritis.

Deficiency Symptoms : Deficiency of this vitamin causes polyneuritis, which is characterized by loss of appetite, convulsions, retraction of head, paralysis of wings and neck and emaciation.

Riboflavin

Riboflavin is a part of an enzyme probably needed by all living cells.

Deficiency Symptoms : 1. Curled-toe paralysis – The toes curl and sometimes the legs are affected to produce paralysis. 2. Poor hatchability – Embryos not hatching are dwarfed and have abnormal down termed 'clubbed down'.

Pantothenic acid

This vitamin is associated with many protein molecules and is involved with protein, carbohydrate and fat metabolism. It is relatively unstable.

Deficiency Symptoms: Retarded growth in young chicks, ruffled feathers, granulated and stuck eyelids in young chicks, scabs at the corner of the mouth, dermatitis of the feet, lowered egg production and lowered hatchability.

Niacin (Nicotinic acid)

This vitamin is an important component of 2 co-enzymes: NAD and NADP. The chick requirement for niacin is relatively high, but it is low for laying birds. Growing embryos have a high requirement.

Deficiency Symptoms: Swollen hocks similar to perosis, but the tendon seldom slips from the condyle, retarded growth, inflamed tongue and mouth (black tongue), scaly skin and feet and ruffled feathers, reduced feed consumption and increased deposits of liver- and body fat in layers.

Pyridoxine (Vitamin B_6)

This vitamin is a growth stimulator in chicks and is abundant in most feedstuffs. It forms a part of several enzymes and is a muscular conditioner.

Deficiency Symptoms: Most practical diets do not produce symptoms, but laboratory diets low in pyridoxine show reduced growth of chicks,

Choline

The chick's demand for choline is great. Choline forms a part of the phospholipids, lecithin, rather than an enzyme. Therefore, choline is seldom considered a true vitamin.

Deficiency Symptoms: Perosis, fatty liver syndrome and retarded growth.

Biotin

Biotin seems adequate in the diet when the composition of normal feedstuffs is concerned, but only about half is available to the chicken.

Deficiency Symptoms: Scaly dermatitis, mild perosis, retarded growth and reduced hatchability.

Folic acid

Folic acid is a complicated chemical compound necessary for many physiological functions like growth, muscle formation, blood formation and feather growth. Diets are seldom low in this vitamin.

Deficiency Symptoms: Depressed growth, poor feathering with feathers lacking pigment, anemia and increased embryonic mortality.

Vitamin B_{12} (Cobalamin)

This vitamin is associated almost entirely with feeds of animal and fish origin. Plant products contain little or no vitamin B_{12}. Microorganisms of the intestinal tract as a cobalt-containing compound synthesize it. The birds own dropping is a source of vitamin B_{12}. Therefore birds raised on cages are more likely to show a deficiency than those kept on a litter floor.

Deficiency Symptoms: Anemia, reduced chicken growth, poor hatchability and fatty liver.

Ascorbic acid (Vitamin C)

In all probability vitamin C is not required in the feed of chickens, for they synthesize an adequate amount. In extreme weather, the birds need excessive amount of vitamin C to alleviate stress. Ascorbic acid helps embryo growth, aids bone development in young chicks and stabilizes body fat.

Other Important Nutritional Deficiency Diseases

Nutritional anemia

Cause of the disease : Iron and copper deficiency

Deficiency Symptoms : Reduced hemoglobin content, reduction in RBC and WBC counts, loss in weight, ruffled feathers, emaciation, reduced egg production and hatchability.

Goose stooping

Cause of the disease : Zinc and magnesium deficiency

Deficiency Symptoms : With zinc deficiency there is abnormal bone formation, short and thickened tibiotarsus, reduced bone ash, thin shelled eggs, low hatchability, dermatitis, parakeratosis, poor

		feathering. With magnesium deficiency there is cerebellar ataxia, poor feathering and mortality.

Perosis (slipped tendon)

Cause of the disease	:	Manganese deficiency.
Deficiency Symptoms	:	Deformity of one or both the hocks with enlargement, twisting and slipping of gastrocnemius tendon from condyles.

Vaccination in a Poultry Farm

Vaccination is one of the most effective ways of preventing specific diseases by building up immunity in the birds. Not all vaccines however impart lifelong immunity. So it is important to know the period of immunity, the age at which the bird must be vaccinated, the dosage and route of administration and the storage condition for stocking vaccines. Success of vaccination programme depends on potency and purity of the vaccine and its application under the condition for which it is specifically intended. Vaccination essentially produces a mild form of disease.

Types of vaccines available in the market

Live vaccines with mild strain and killed or inactivated vaccines adjuvanated with oil emulsion to produce sustained higher antibody production are available in the market

Methods of vaccination

Intranasal or Intraocular method

It is a common method of vaccination in young chicks to give primary vaccine response in early stages. The freeze dried, live attenuated vaccines are reconstituted with diluents and instill one or more drops either in nostrils or in eyes or in both is a common practice.

Intramuscular or Subcutaneous

In modern cage managemental practices, the live vaccines such as RDVK and Fowl Pox intended for subcutaneous or wing web method respectively, are to be administered through intramuscular route. This facilitates easy to administer, less handling and induce minimal stress to birds. However, the farmers maintaining their birds in deep litter system adopt the subcutaneous route of administration of those vaccines.

Wing web method

To prevent the Fowl Pox disease in a flock, vaccines intended for this disease is given through wing web puncture method. 7 to 10 days after the vaccination the vaccinated flock should be examined for the evidence of "takes". 'Take' consists of swelling of skin or a scab at the site where vaccine was applied and is the evidence of successful vaccination. Immunity will develop normally in 10 to 14 days post vaccination.

Vaccination through drinking water

Because of labor saving, easy to administer and avoid handling of birds, most of the poultry farmers adopt such type of vaccine administration. However, the drinking water in which the vaccine is mixed should be free from disinfectant and water sanitizers. Dried skim milk powder if added to water will protect the vaccine. Water vaccination should be preceded by an adequate water withdrawal time.

Aerosol spraying method

To ease the vaccination procedure and induce less stress, this method of vaccination is preferred. The spraying should be evenly distributed like mist on the birds.

Compatibility of vaccines and with medicines

Sometimes antibiotics are mixed with vaccines during vaccination; however, it is not advisable. The antibiotics may severely alter the pH of vaccines and may affect its potency. Likewise, some of the vaccines may not be compatible with other. Combination of vaccines must be tested before they are used indiscriminately.

Vaccination programme in a poultry farm

Vaccination in a poultry farm is not a substitute for good management. Disease is multifactorial involving the pathogenic agents, the host and the environment. There are three general philosophies regarding timing of vaccination.

1. High levels of antibodies are produced in breeder hens.
2. These maternal antibodies are transferred from the hen to the chicks through the yolk (passive immunity), so as to make chick vaccination programme to minimal.
3. Chick must be vaccinated, if breeder hen antibody levels are low.
4. *In ovo* vaccination (active acquired immunity prior to hatching).

Table 31: Vaccination Schedule

Sl. No.	Age of the bird	Type of vaccine	Route of administration	Remarks
For Commercial Layers				
1.	Day old	Marek's	Subcutaneous	At hatchery
2.	5 -7 days	RDVF/B1/LaSota	Intra nasal/ocular	
3.	14 – 16 days	IBD intermediate	Intra ocular	
4.	20th day	IB	Intra ocular/Drinking water	
5.	24 -26 days	IBD intermediate	Intra ocular	
6.	30th day	RD LaSota	Intra ocular	
7.	35 – 40 days	IBD intermediate	Intra ocular	
8.	8th week	RDVK/R2B	S/C or I/M	
9.	10th week	Fowl Pox	W/W or I/M	
10.	13th week	IB	Intra ocular/Drinking water	
11.	18th week	RDVK/R2B	S/C or I/M	
12.	After 30th week	RDVK/R2B	S/C or I/M	
Check immunity titre for RD and IB every two months and administer vaccines accordingly				
For Commercial Broilers				
1.	Day old	Marek's	Subcutaneous	At hatchery
2.	5 -7 days	RDVF/B1/LaSota	Intra nasal/ocular	
3.	14 – 16 days	IBD intermediate	Intra ocular	
4.	24 -26 days	IBD intermediate	Intra ocular	Optional
5.	30th day	RD LaSota	Intra ocular	
For Breeders				
1.	Day old	Marek's	Subcutaneous	At hatchery
2.	1st day	IBH	Intra ocular	
3.	4th day	Leechi-Inactivated	Subcutaneous	
4.	5 -7 days	RDVF/B1/LaSota	Intra nasal/ocular	
5.	14 – 16 days	IBD intermediate	Intra ocular	
6.	20th day	IB	Intra ocular/Drinking water	
7.	24 -26 days	IBD intermediate	Intra ocular	
8.	30th day	RD LaSota	Intra ocular	
9.	35 – 40 days	IBD intermediate	Intra ocular	
10.	8th week	RDVK/R2B	S/C or I/M	
11.	9th week	Fowl cholera and AE	S/C	
12.	10th week	Fowl Pox	W/W or I/M	
13.	10th week	I. Coryza	I/M	
14.	11th week	Reo	S/C	
15.	12th week	Fowl Pox	W/W or I/M	
16.	13th week	IB	Intra ocular/Drinking water	
17.	14th week	FC + IC	I/M	
18.	18th week	RD+IBD+IB+Reo	S/C	
19.	19th week	Leechi-Inactivated	Subcutaneous	

Pre and post vaccination care

1. Before charting out vaccination schedule, it is advisable to monitor maternal antibody level of the day-old chicks. This will allow one to make good judgment as to when the progeny become susceptible.
2. Use proper methods of shipping, storage, mixing, and administering vaccines.
3. Perform vaccination in healthy flocks only.
4. All birds within a house should be vaccinated on the same day.
5. During any outbreak of diseases, the vaccination programme should be postponed.
6. Vaccines should not be used in a flock affected with other diseases.
7. Keep stress factors at a minimum.
8. Until ready to use, keep all vaccines under refrigeration. At the time of vaccination the reconstituted vaccines particularly live viral vaccines should be kept in ice. Follow the manufacturer's instructions strictly.
9. Use speed but don't sacrifice accuracy and thoroughness.
10. Destroy all empty vials, bottles and unused vaccines. Cleanup and disinfect all equipment and clothing after the job is over.
11. Vaccination does lead some reaction and stress among birds. Such stress or limited reaction is a sign of proper 'take' of the vaccine.
12. For minimizing stress in summer, vaccinations should be performed at night or in the early hours of the day.
13. During vaccination, often the needles should be changed. Preferably use one needle for every 500 birds. Correct gauze-size needle should be used to avoid injury to the muscle.
14. A stabilizer such as skim milk powder should be used in the drinking water when vaccine is administered through drinking water.
15. The vaccination should be performed by trained personnel under the guidance of qualified veterinarians.
16. Keep a record of the brand, kind, and batch number of vaccines and date of vaccination.

General considerations on administering medication through water and feed

Medication is formulated to be delivered in the feed or the water, although water medication is preferred because often sick birds will not eat but will continue to drink. Proper administration of drugs and parasiticides when required is essential to minimize disease and restored health of the bird.

When chickens are sick, veterinarians must diagnose the disease quickly and correctly respond with the appropriate treatment, at the recommended level.

Sick birds eat less. One unfortunate scenario is of lower consumption of feed containing a coccidiostat leading to an outbreak of coccidiosis in addition to the primary disease. Conversely, an increase in medicated food or water consumption (such as increased water consumption during hot weather) can result in drug toxicity.

The following relationships should be understood in the medication of birds:

- In general, about 5 days medication is required for the successful treatment of a disease.
- Following single injections, drug activity is rarely prolonged more than 8 – 12 hours. The problem could be overcome by repeating the injections at 8-hour intervals.
- For continuous medication, drugs must be administered orally in the feed or water. Many drugs, however, do not absorb, and most or the entire drug ingested passes in the droppings.

Disinfection of poultry farms

Definition

Disinfection refers to inactivation of disease-producing microorganisms. It does not destroy bacterial spores. Disinfectants are used on inanimate objects in contrast to antiseptics, which are used on living tissue. Disinfection usually involves chemicals, heat or ultraviolet light.

Disinfectants

Usually disinfectants are "cidal" in that they kill the susceptible potential pathogenic agents. A powerful tool of poultry farm biosecurity should have the following qualities to be a good disinfectant,

- Broad spectrum of activities – Effective against wide range of disease causing organisms including bacteria, virus, fungi, bacterial spores, protozoa etc.

- Safe and non-toxic to both birds and personnel working in the sheds
- Effective in the presence of organic matter
- Should have longer residual activity
- Should not taint the surfaces, equipment etc.
- Should be cost-effective
- Non-corrosive to the equipment
- Should have minimum contact time

Disinfectant effectiveness depends on many factors. These includes,

- Type of contaminating microorganisms – Each disinfectant has unique antimicrobial attributes
- Degree of contamination – This determines the quality of disinfectant required and time of exposure
- Amount of proteinaceous material present – High protein based materials absorb and neutralize some chemical disinfectants
- Presence of organic matter and other compounds such as soaps may neutralize some disinfectants
- Chemical nature of disinfectant – It is important to understand the mode of action in order to select the appropriate disinfectant
- Concentration and quantity of disinfectant – It is important to choose the proper concentration and quantity of disinfectant that is best suited to each situation
- Contact time and temperature – Sufficient time and appropriate temperature must be allowed for action of the disinfectant and may depend on the degree of contamination and organic matter load
- Residual activity and effects on fabric and metal should be considered for specific situations
- Application temperature, pH and interactions with other compounds must be considered.

Surfactant –An important component of disinfectant

Surfactant is one that reduces the surface tension and increases the surface area available for disinfectant to act. Surfactant hastens dirt and manure removal by increasing the wetting speed and breaking organic matter into very small particles so the disinfectants can act effectively. For deep penetration into the organic matter and kill the microbes the disinfectant need the support of a surfactant.

Type of Disinfectants

There are three types of disinfectants available in the market

Low level disinfectants

Phenolic disinfectants

Phenolic disinfectants are effective against bacteria, especially gram positive bacteria and enveloped viruses. Phenols maintain their activities in the presence of organic materials. Phenolic disinfectants are usually safe, but prolonged exposure to skin may cause irritation. Phenol liquid at 0.4 % giving advantage of continued suppression of bacterial and viral population in poultry sheds.

Quaternary Ammonium Compounds (QAC)

The quaternaries are odourless, non corrosive and good cleaning agents but high water hardness make them less microbial because it absorb the active ingredients. They act even in the presence of organic matter and are effective against Gram positive and Gram negative bacteria and enveloped viruses, but not effective against non enveloped viruses, fungi and bacterial spores. They are generally low in toxicity, but prolonged contact can be irritating.

Intermediate level disinfectants

Alcohols

These chemicals (Ethyl alcohol and Isopropyl alcohol) are rapidly bactericidal rather than bacteriostatic against Gram positive and Gram negative bacteria; they are also tuberculocidal, fungicidal and virucidal against enveloped viruses. Alcohols are not effective against bacterial spores and have limited effectiveness against non enveloped viruses. Their cidal activity drops sharply when diluted below 50% concentration. Alcohols require time to work and they may not penetrate organic material. They are generally too expensive for general use as a surface disinfectant.

Hypo chlorites

Hypo chlorites are the most widely used chlorine disinfectants and are available in a liquid (e.g. sodium hypochlorite) or solid (e.g. calcium hypochlorite, sodium dichloroisocyanurate) forms. They are unaffected by water hardness, are inexpensive and fast acting, and have a low incidence of serious toxicity. Hypo chlorites can eliminate both enveloped and nonenveloped viruses. They are also effective against fungi, bacteria and algae but not spores. Organic material such as faeces or blood inactivate chlorine based disinfectants, therefore surfaces must be cleaned before their use. In order to obtain maximum effectiveness with chlorine based disinfectants they must remain in contact with surfaces for several minutes. Chlorine based disinfectants diluted in tap water have a limited shelf life. Ideally solutions used for surface disinfection should be mixed fresh to ensure adequate levels of chlorine for antimicrobial activity. Chlorinated drinking water should not exceed 6 – 10ppm of free chlorine.

Iodine and Iodophor

These compounds are bactericidal, sporicidal, virucidal and fungicidal but require a prolonged contact time. The disinfective ability of iodine, like chlorine, is neutralized in the presence of organic material and hence frequent applications are needed for thorough disinfection.

High level disinfectants

Hydrogen Peroxide

The activity of peroxide is greatest against anaerobic bacteria. Stabilized hydrogen peroxides are effective against a broad range of pathogens including both enveloped and nonenveloped viruses, vegetative bacteria, fungi and bacterial spores. This solution sterilizes in 30 minutes and provides high-level disinfection in 5 minutes.

Gluteraldehyde

Gluteraldehydes are bactericidal, virucidal, fungicidal, sporucidal and parasiticidal. They are used as a disinfectant or sterilant in both liquid and gaseous forms. They have moderate residual activity and are effective in the presence of limited amounts of organic material. Gluteraldehydes are very potent disinfectants, which can be highly toxic warranting it to be handled by appropriate personal.

Formaldehyde

Formaldehyde is sold and used principally as a water-based solution called formalin, which is 37% formaldehyde by weight. The aqueous solution is bactericidal, fungicidal, virucidal and sporicidal. Formaldehydes should be handled in the work place as a potential carcinogen with an employee exposure standard that limits an 8 hours time-weighted average exposure to a concentration of 0.75 ppm.

Disinfection Procedure in a Poultry Farm

There is no substitute for cleanliness and neatness of a poultry farms for an effective disease controlling programme. Disinfectants, sanitizers and sterilizing compounds can be a valuable part of a sound biosecurity programme that limits the growing bird's exposure to pathogenic organisms. For more efficacious disinfection procedures thorough cleaning before disinfection is essential.

It is absolutely essential to read and follow the manufacturer's directions for use, whichever disinfectant is chosen. Usually, disinfectants are applied by spraying or foaming with a medium pressure sprayer. After disinfection, allow the house and equipment to dry completely. In a poultry farm, periodical use of different disinfectants is an important part of the overall strategy of biosecurity. To prevent microorganisms from building up resistance to any one particular disinfectant, the use of several disinfectants on a rotational basis is essential.

Question Bank

I. Choose the correct answers.

1. Avian Influenza is caused by

    a) Bacteria b) Parasite

    c) Virus d) Fungi

2. Coccidiosis is caused by

    a) Mycoplasma b) Protozoa

    c) Nutritional deficiency d) Toxins

3. The major intoxication in birds is

    a) Excess intake of salt b) Botulism

    c) ingestion of fungicide d) Mycotoxicosis

4. Xerophthalmia in birds caused by the deficiency of

    a) Folic acid b) Vit. B12

    c) Ascorbic acid d) Vit. A

5. Reboflavin deficiency leads to

    a) Perosis b) Curled-toe-paralysis

    c) Scaly leg d) Blindness

6. Vaccination to be done to prevent
   a) Parasitic diseases b) Viral diseases
   c) Nutritional deficiency diseases d) Mite infestation
7. Inactivation of microorganisms refers to
   a) Sanitation b) Disinfection
   c) Fumigation d) Prevention of disease
8. Farmaldehyde is used in the process of
   a) Fumigation b) Sanitation
   c) Treatment d) Vaccination
9. Hypochlorites are corrosive to metals at
   a) <200ppm b) 300-350ppm
   c) >500ppm d) 400ppm
10. Quarternary ammonium compounds are not effective against
    a) Gram +ve bacteria b) Non enveloped viruses
    c) Enveloped viruses d) Gram -ve bacteria.

Answers: 1. c, 2. b, 3. d, 4. d, 5. b, 6. b, 7. b, 8. a, 9, c, 10. c.

II. Tick the following statements are True or False

1. Clostridia are classified as protozoa ( )
2. Endoparasites are mainly worms ( )
3. Brooder Pneumonia is caused by Aspergillus ( )
4. Sulphur ointment is effective against red mite ( )
5. Vitamin D3 is measured in the unit of I U ( )
6. Vitamin B12 deficiency caused anemia in chicken ( )
7. Fowl pox vaccination is done by intra ocular method ( )
8. Low level disinfectants kills most vegetative bacteria and some fungi and enveloped viruses ( )
9. Disinfectants should have maximum contact time ( )
10. Iodine and Iodophors are well established disinfectants ( )

Answers: 1. F, 2. T, 3. T, 4. F, 5. T, 6. T, 7. F, 8. T, 9. F, 10. T.

III. Fill in the blanks with suitable words

1. Viruses are not responsive to ....
2. Exudative diathesis is a disease caused by the deficiency of ....
3. ....Vitamin is not required as feed supplement in chicken.
4. Zinc and magnesium deficiency leads to ....
5. Aerosol spraying should be evenly distributed like .... on the birds.
6. Vaccines are .... with some antibiotics.
7. Perform vaccination in .... flocks.
8. Coccidiostats have .... potential.
9. 7-10 days after the fowl pox vaccination the vaccinated flocks should be examined for the evidence of ....
10. .... is one that enhances the potential of the disinfectant.

Answers 1. Drug treatments, 2. Vitamin E, 3. Vitamin C, 4. Goose stooping, 5. Mist, 6. Incompatible, 7. healthy, 8. good absorption, 9. “takes”, 10. Non-ionic surfactant.

Short Questions

1. What is Bio-security ?
2. What is deworming ?
3. Write short notes on nutritional anemia.
4. What is “takes” ?
5. Give short answer on perosis.
6. What is vaccination ?
7. Define disinfection.
8. What is method of vaccination.
9. Describe compatibility of vaccines with medicines.
10. Describe disinfection and disinfectants
11. Describe high level disinfectants
12. Write on vaccination schedule for broilers.

29

Designer Egg and Chicken Meat

J.D. Mahanta and Rahul M. Warhadpande

"Let the kitchen be an apothecary, the foods be the medicines"
– **Hippocrates**

Chicken's eggs have been used as a food item by human beings since antiquity. The egg is composed largely of the proteins out of the three most important dietary essentials (proteins, fats and carbohydrates). The egg proteins are highly digestible and remarkably complete, containing the most important essential amino acids. The amino acid profile of egg is similar to the ideal balance of amino acids needed by humans. It also supplies various minerals, some in significant amounts, and contains a range of vitamins. The nutritive excellence of the egg enhances the value of any food in which it is incorporated. Meeting consumer demands is a constant challenge for the poultry industry. Present day consumers desire somewhat distinct products with respect to safety, healthfulness, freshness, taste, color, etc. To remain competent, various companies have developed several designer and specialty eggs which have appeared in supermarkets.

What is designer egg ?

The contents of the chicken egg can be changed in such ways as to be more healthful and appealing to a segment of our consumers who are willing to pay more for those improvements in the egg. '*Designer eggs*' are those in which the content has been modified from the standard egg. Designer eggs contain 600 mg of Omega-3 (n-3) fatty acids, equivalent to a 100 g serving of fish. The benefits of Omega-3 fatty acids include reduction in plasma triglycerides, blood pressure, clot formation, tumour growth and skin diseases. Vitamin E, a fat soluble vitamin as well as an effective antioxidant, is enhanced to 100 per cent in these eggs. Studies have shown that when 2-3 designer eggs are consumed every day, HDL levels are raised while LDL levels are decreased, blood fats are reduced and more than 60 per cent of the daily vitamin E requirement is fulfilled.

The Poly Unsaturated Fatty Acids (PUFA) are of 2 major types; namely Omega-3(n-3) and Omega-6 (n-6) fatty acids. The n-3 fatty acids are essential fatty acids, which cannot be synthesized by the human body. The n-6 PUFA is mainly linoleic acid which decrease both good (HDL) and bad (LDL) cholesterol. Hence, it is not having any net beneficial effect. On the other hand, n-3 PUFAs consist of linolenic, eicosapentaenoic, decosahexaenoic acids (DHA); which will selectively decrease the bad (LDL and VLDL) cholesterol. Hence these are really good for health. These acids in their natural form are highly instable and have off odour and hence consumers do not like to consume these products. Under these circumstances, egg is the best vehicle to incorporate the n-3 PUFAs, because it can be easily incorporated in the egg and is most acceptable food by all. Canadian scientist Professor Sim introduced this technology and therefore it was originally known as Professor Sim's designed egg and subsequently referred as Designer egg. Ordinary eggs will have about 0.3% n-3 PUFA and about 18% n-6 PUFA with a n-3/n-6 ratio of 1: 60, whereas a designer egg will have about 12% n-3 and 17% n6 PUFA with a n-3/n-6 ratio of 1: 1.5, which is a healthy ratio. Recently a range of bioactive peptides in eggs have been characterized with antihypertensive, phagocytosis-stimulating and opioid properties which may be beneficial for humans. It has been recorded that a designer egg, enriched in vitamin E, lutein, DHA and selenium can be not only a good nutritional product but also a good vector for the delivery of these 4 essential nutrients vital for human health. A crucial feature of these designer eggs is the synergistic combination of n-3 fatty acids with major antioxidants and said 4 nutrients, as an important approach to the improvement of the human diet

Vitamin Content

Two vitamins, A and E, are receiving the most interest as components of designer eggs. The vitamin content of the egg is variable and is somewhat dependent on the dietary concentration of any specific vitamin. In addition, the hen does not transfer different vitamins into the egg with equal efficiency. Because of this, the vitamin transfer efficiency and cost of the vitamin must be taken into consideration when determining the economic feasibility of marketing such eggs. Eggs higher in Vitamin E are currently available in stores.

Fat and fatty acid contents

The fatty acid profile (or the ratios of the different types of fatty acids) of egg yolk lipid can easily be changed, simply by changing the type of fat used in the ration. Consumption of polyunsaturated fatty acids has been reported to promote infant growth and reduce the risk of atherosclerosis and stroke in adults. Different feeds, such as flaxseed (linseed), sunflower oil, marine algae, fish, fish oil, and vegetable oil have been added to chicken feeds to increase the omega-3 fatty acid content in the egg yolk. Omega-3 fatty acid rich eggs may provide an alternative food source for enhancing consumer intake of these *'healthy'* fatty acids. There are designer eggs on the market those contain a lowered saturated to unsaturated fatty acid ratio. Canola oil is commonly used to alter the ratio of saturated to unsaturated fatty acids. Some producers produce eggs said to contain 25% less saturated fat than the regular eggs.

Diet composition and levels of Omega 3 fatty acids in the egg

The simplest way to produce n-3 designer eggs is by enriching hen egg with linolenic acid which is a precursor of DHA. For this purpose the hen's diet is usually enriched with flax seeds or its oil. As a result of such changes in the hen's diet egg yolk is enriched with linolenic acid and the level of DHA is also enhanced. Grasses have relatively high proportion of alpha-linolenic acid (53.4%) in total fatty acids and eggs from hens fed under free-range conditions had a higher concentrations of total n-3 fatty acids than eggs from hens fed commercial diet. The conversion of linolenic acid into DHA in human body is not always effective, especially in elderly and children, and most health promoting properties of n-3 fatty acids are associated with DHA. Therefore inclusion in the hen's diet of preformed DHA, usually in the form of fish (menhaden, herring or tuna) oil, is a more promising route however this may be associated with a pronounced fishy taste in the egg yolk. Enrichment of the chicken diet with n-9, n-3 or n-6 fatty acids was associated with different proportions of PUFAs in the egg yolk as shown in Table 32.

Table 32: Polyunsaturated fatty acids in the egg yolk depending on the diet composition

Fatty acid	n-9 rich diet	n-3 rich diet	n-6 rich diet	Control
18:2n-6	11.1	12.1	28.5	11.6
18:3n-3	0.2	5.8	0.3	0.9
20:4n-6	2.2	1.3	2.7	2.0
20:5n-3	0	0.3	0	0.02
22:5n-3	0	0.3	0.1	0.05
22:6n-3	0.8	2.7	0.5	1.5
Total n-3 PUFA	1.1	9.1	0.9	2.6
Total n-6 PUFA	13.4	13.4	31.2	13.6
n-6/n-3	12.7	1.5	34.3	5.3

In general, there are numerous n-3 fatty acid supplements used in poultry rations and the fatty acid profile of the egg is dependent on which supplement was fed with.

Mineral content

It has been possible to increase the selenium, iodine and chromium contents of the albumen and yolk through dietary supplementation of the hen. These three minerals are important in human health. However, success could not be achieved for calcium and phosphorus contents of the albumen and yolk.

Pharmaceuticals

Newer biotechnology is being used to develop genetically modified chickens to produce compounds which could be harvested from the eggs. The hen, like all animals, produces antibodies to neutralize the antigens (viruses, bacteria, etc.) to which she has been exposed to. These antibodies circulate throughout her body and are transferred to eggs as protection to the developing chick. Immunologists are taking advantage of the fact that the hen can develop antibodies against a large array of antigens and concentrate them in eggs. Specific antigens are now being selected and injected into the hen that develops antibodies against them. As new biotechnology knowledge is gained in this area, designer eggs in the future may be produced those contain a range of antibodies from treatment against snake venoms to the countering of microorganisms which cause tooth decay.

It has also been shown that there is no alteration in fatty acid profile of eggs enriched with n-3 PUFAs during cooking or during storage for seven weeks at 25^{0}C. On the other hand, n-3 enriched eggs are characterized by increased susceptibility to oxidation which can cause problems during egg storage and cooking. Enrichment of egg yolk in vitamin E is thought to be an effective means to resolve this problem significantly decreasing thiobarbituric acid values in the n-3 eggs. Likewise, the fishy taint of eggs due to rancidity of n-3 fatty acid could be tackled by using stabilized or microencapsulated oils in the diet of chickens.

Commercial production of enriched eggs

There are various enriched eggs available in supermarket shelves in different countries. In the UK there are free range eggs, organic eggs, free range organically produced eggs available. In some other countries eggs enriched with iodine (Japan) or DHA (Canada) are produced. The DHA enriched eggs are marketed by *OmegaTech* in the USA, Germany, Spain, Portugal, Belgium and Norway. In India n-3 enriched eggs are produced by M/S Suguna Poultry Farm and Panjab University.

Designer Meat

There has been growing interest of chicken consumers towards lean meat or carcass with lesser fat. Today's health conscious consumers are in need of safe poultry products, which are free from drug / pesticide residues and other harmful components. Moreover, they are ready to pay a premium price for such products, which are not only safe but also promote their health; due to the presence of special health promoting components like n-3 fatty acids, anti-oxidants, extra vitamins, minerals etc. These types of value addition are done mostly by combination of managemental and nutritional manipulations of birds. There are two types of value addition: Pre-slaughter and post-slaughter value addition.

Pre-slaughter value addition

Dietary manipulation is the major step in producing the pre-slaughter value added poultry products. Selenium enriched meat can be produced by feeding organic Se to birds which will increase the antioxidant properties of meat. Dietary incorporation of n-3 PUFAs at 5% level has been reported to decrease body fat while increasing lean meat of chickens. The designer meat, not only contain high levels of natural anti-oxidants like vitamin-E, selenium, carotenoid pigments and flavonoid compounds, but also contain synthetic anti-oxidants like Ethoxyquin and anti-oxidants of herbal origin such as Lycopene, Curcumin, Sulforaphene, Carnosine, Quercetin, depending upon the herbs used in the diet of the birds. Supplementation of these anti-oxidants in birds' diet will increase their levels in the meat.

The advantages of enrichment meat with anti oxidants include:

- Decreased susceptibility to lipid peroxidation
- Prevention of fishy odour to the product
- Retarding destruction of fat-soluble vitamins
- Preventing denaturation of natural fat-soluble pigments

The regulation for production of organic chicken varies from country to country. EC regulation, EC-2092/91 and its subsequent amendments, place restrictions on the ingredients that a manufacturer of organic food can use. There are nodel agencies in each country, to certify the product as organic. In India the APEDA (Agricultural Products Export Development Agency), in UK the UKROFS & OFF, in Europe the ECOCERT, Naturland & Skal and in USA the OCIA, OGBA, QAI and FVO are the prominent certifying agencies for organic foods.

Question Bank

I. Fill in the blanks

1. Designer eggs contain............ mg of Omega-3 fatty acids.
2. Poly Unsaturated Fatty Acids (PUFA) are of 2 major types; namely ...... PUFA and........ PUFAs
3. The n-6 PUFA is mainly................acid.
4. The n-3 PUFAs consist of..............., ... and.......................acids.
5. Ordinary eggs contain about.........n-3 PUFA and about......... n-6 PUFA with a n-3/ n-6 ratio of 1: 60.
6. A designer egg contains about..........n-3 and........... n-6 PUFA with a n-3/ n-6 ratio of 1: 1.5.
7. A large egg contains approximately................ mg of cholesterol.
8. Organic chicken is the earliest................................ value added product.
9. Chicken meat contains about ....mg of cholesterol per 100 g.

II. Match the following

1. linolenic acid	-	a) Yolk colour
2. Spirulina	-	b) Canadian scientist
3. Roche Color Fan	-	c) Blue-green algae
4. linoleic acid	-	d) Precursor of DHA
5. Professor Sim	-	e) n-6 PUFA

III. What is a designer egg?

IV. What are the benefits of Omega-3 fatty acids in human health?

V. Describe the importance of designer eggs in human health.

VI. Write short notes on the following

a. Vitamin and pigment contents of designer egg
b. Fat and fatty acid contents in designer egg
c. Commercial production of modified eggs

d. Safe poultry products

e. Advantages of enrichment of the egg and meat with anti oxidants

Answers

I.

(1) 600

(2) n-3 , n-6

(3) linoleic

(4) linolenic, eicosapentaenoic, decosa hexaenoic

(5) 0.3%, 18%

(6) 12%, 17%

(7) 200 – 220

(8) Pre-processing

(9) 60

II. (1) d (2) c (3) a (4) e (5) b

30

Breeder Flock Management

H.N. Narasimha Murthy

Breeder management includes pure line management, parent stock management, and grandparent stock management depending on the context. Except for small variations in management among these stocks basics are common within layer breeder stocks and broiler breeder stocks. The main objective of the breeder management is to produce more fertile eggs per pullet and increasing the hatchability by hygienic handling of these fertile eggs.

Location of the breeder farm

Location of the breeder farm should be away from commercial poultry farms in order to prevent the spread of diseases between the flocks. However, they must be in close vicinity of the city/town to have a good transport facility and other amenities such as water, electricity and availability of labour.

Three types of breeders with sex ratio are

Type of bird	Male	:	Female
i. Egg Type (White egg layers)	10-12	:	100
ii. Medium Type (Brown egg layers)	10-12	:	100
iii. Meat type (Broiler breeder)	12-15	:	100

Chick management

- **Sexing:** This is done by cloacal (vent sexing), machine or colour sexing methods.
- **Brooding:** Brooding of breeder chicks is done as for commercial chicks, described elsewhere in this book (Chapter N0. 10).
- **Vaccination:** Vaccination programme is different for broilers, breeders and layers, as detailed elsewhere in this book (Chapter N0. 28).
- **Dubbing** : Removal of a part of the comb in the early age is called as Dubbing. It prevents injury to the comb due to contact with equipment, cages or during fighting, provides better vision and lowers damage due to frost bite in the cold climate. It is not recommended for birds reared under tropical climate as combs have important role in thermoregulation. It should be done at day- old or at least within the first few weeks to minimize hemorrhage.
- **Clipping of toes:** It is recommended for breeding males. The inside and back toes of all breeding males are toe clipped to prevent tearing the back of females during mating. It should be done at day-old age. Obviously, female breeders or commercial pullets are not subjected to the toe clipping.

Grower management

i) **Debeaking (Beak Trimming):** Beak of cockerels is cut at equal size to help in holding females while mating whereas in pullets, lower beak is cut at 1/3rd and upper at 2/3rd level to help scooping of feed.

ii) **Dewatteling:** Dewatteling is trimming of wattles in cockerels of 12-14 weeks of age. It is not advisable to dewattle just prior to mating as it reduces fertility.

iii) **Selection at 5 weeks of age:** In meat type breeders it is essential to remove smaller males to attain uniformity and genetic vigour. Usually selection is done at 5 weeks of age for males whereas, there is no such selection for egg type lines at this age. Body weight should meet standard weight. Select birds with strong and straight legs apart from good toes. Keel should be straight with good conformation and feather cover all over the body. Select for masculine and refined head type with strong beak. Remove all runts, anaemic and diseased males at this point. About 18 to 20 males per 100 females should be sufficient.

iv) **Sex-wise rearing:** The male and female chicks are reared separately until 12 weeks of age for layer breeders and until 5 weeks for broiler breeders. It helps in better weight control, selection accuracy, early transfer to the laying house, enhanced flock fertility as results of improved semen quality, mating ability and livability.

Sexes intermingled: In this method chicks are separated only until they are reared in brooding guard after that they intermingled as per specified ratio. Sexing errors should be removed as early as possible to reduce expenditure. The males should be added in the breeding pen when pullets are at 5 per cent egg production. The males should be placed in the pullet pens late in the afternoon to reduce fighting.

Housing system

Breeders are housed in three systems of housing viz., (i) All deep litter or floor system, (ii). Slat and litter floor (or plastic floor) system and (iii) Cage system. Out of these systems, deep litter and cage systems are more common in India. Broiler breeders generally prefer deep litter system because of heavy body weight and layer breeders are more suited for cage system.

1. Deep litter or floor system

Under this system of housing eggs are layed over litter and are likely to be contaminated. Such eggs are ideal culture medium for bacterial growth, may explode in the incubator causing contamination of all other eggs. These eggs are also known as '*exploders*'. Providing adequate number of nest boxes with clean cushioning materials would reduce this problem.

2. Slat and litter floor (or plastic floor) system

Under this system 2/3 of the floor is slat and 1/3 is litter floor. The advantage of this system is more number of eggs per pullet can be obtained and floor eggs are reduced to the extent of 3 times as compared to all litter floor system. However, Layer house mortality is slightly higher in this system than all litter floor system.

3. Cage system

Under this system of rearing, eggs obtained are clean but percentage of broken eggs will be little higher Best suited for pedigree record keeping since artificial insemination can be practiced which also confirms higher fertility.

Rearing systems

Brood-grow system of growing: In this system, particularly the egg type strains are reared in a single house during the brooding and growing period by restricting the floor space during the initial 5 wk period and then allowing full space after that.

Brood-grow- lay system: In this system once the chick enters the house it is reared in the same shed for its life time. The shed has all provisions right from brooding to laying.

Grow- lay system: It is a popular system with brooding facilities capable of keeping the birds to 10 weeks of age. The birds are then moved to the permanent laying house.

Floor space requirements

The recommended floor space, water space, and feeder space requirements per breeder pullet are detailed in Table 33, Table 34 and Table 35, respectively.

Table 33: Floor space requirements per breeder pullet (males included)

Type of Breeder	Type of floor			
	Litter (sq.ft.)	Slat (wire and Litter) (sq.ft.)	Slat	Wire
Mini Leghorns	1.5	1.25	1.00	1.0
Leghorns(conventional)	2.0	1.75	1.25	1.25
Medium-size, egg type	2.25	2.0	1.5	1.5
Mini-meat-type	2.25	2.0	1.5	1.5
Meat-type (conventional)	3.0	2.5	1.5	2.0

Source: Commercial chicken production manual, (Mack O North, 2006)

Table 34: Water space requirements for breeder birds

	Space per bird (in)
Mini Leghorns	0.60
Leghorns(conventional)	0.75
Medium-size, egg type	0.85
Mini-meat-type	0.85
Meat-type (conventional)	1.00

Source: Commercial chicken production manual, (Mack O North, 2006)

Table 35: Feeder space requirements for breeder birds

	Space per bird (in)
Mini Leghorns	2.0
Leghorns(conventional)	2.5
Medium-size, egg type	2.5
Mini-meat-type	2.5
Meat-type (conventional)	2.5

Source: Commercial chicken production manual, (Mack O North, 2006)

Selection of Breeder Flocks : A breeder needs fewer males than females. Therefore, rigorous selection of cocks is an important component to a sound breeding program. It is better to hatch more chicks from selected hens.

Basic qualities for selection

1. **Rate of Growth:** The rapid weight gain influences profitability and also indicates strength of the immune system as well as suitability for system of production. Excessively fast growing birds can be more prone to diseases because of thinner gastrointestinal tracts which allow both faster nutrient uptake as well as easier penetration by microbes. Extremely slow growing poultry have less robust immune systems.

2. **Mature size:** In order to reach ideal mature size, the bird should attain desired weight and have ample flesh in the sections important for that breed.

3. **Egg-laying ability:** Selection for egg laying ability is a trait of primary importance in egg laying breeds. Significant importance to dual-purpose breeds and of some importance even in meat producing breeds for high egg production is to be girer Selecting for earlier production reduces adult egg size.

4. **Breed type:** Type is comprised of body shape and conformation. It affects the size and shape of the internal organs and the distribution of flesh. Breeds like the Wyandotte, New Hampshire etc. have rather compact but deep and wide bodies which ideally suited to retaining heat. Thus, these breed do well in cold regions. The Leghorns, Minorca etc. tend to be rather longer and narrower proportionally and are well suited to hot climate. So breed type is an important consideration for the purpose of regional adaptation.
5. **Plumage colour:** Color can and does impact a breed's suitability for different systems of production. For example, white plumaged chickens are healthy but will not do well on pasture and are slightly more prone to predation.
6. **Fertility and vigor:** High levels of vigor and fertility are the foundation upon which economic value is built. Both of these traits are of the utmost importance and together they give the breed the ability to withstand challenges including inbreeding or disease.

Lighting management

Effect of light: Light rays when passes through eyes stimulate the hypothalamus to release certain factors which in turn cause the release of FSH and LH from anterior pituitary. These hormones control the maturation of follicles and ovulation, respectively. Ovipositon is induced by oxytocin is also influenced by light.

Threshold of photoperiod: A threshold exists for the photoperiod below which it does not influence the growing pullets and layers. This threshold is about 9 hrs photoperiod. During growing period, photoperiod must be below 9 hrs and preferably not more than 8 hrs. On the other hand, during laying period, photoperiod must exceed the threshold of 9 hrs. In practice 16-17 hrs photoperiod is allowed for layers. Growers may be placed on reduced photoperiod soon after the brooding period.

Available lumen: All the light given by the bulb is not available to the chicken. About 30 per cent is absorbed by walls, ceiling equipments. Reflectors increase the light intensity by 50 per cent at bird level. Bulbs have to be cleaned at least once in a fortnight or more often.

Light intensity threshold: The threshold for the light intensity is 0.04 foot candle at bird level above which pituitary gland is stimulated to influence sexual maturity and egg production. In practice one foot candle of light intensity at bird level is provided. Natural day light provides much higher light intensity than one foot candle. The higher intensity of light is not a problem for egg production but may be associated with certain vices like pecking, prolapse and nervousness. The minimum distance from the floor to the bulbs kept is about 7-8 feet. To provide one foot candle, usually one watt for each 4 sq ft of floor space is used. The distance between the bulbs within a row or between different rows is 2 times the distance from the bulb to the bird. i.e., 12 feet.

Lighting schedule for Layers

Brooding period (0-8 weeks of age): - 24 hrs lighting

Growing period (9- 20 weeks of age): No artificial lighting is provided and only natural day light is available.

Step up lighting programme - 21st week onwards

Starting with 13 hrs lighting per day, the photoperiod is increased by 30 min per every week until 16 or 17 hr photoperiod is attained. (Supplementing artificial light to natural day light).

Increasing the photoperiod: Artificial light is the only source of light for the photoperiod in environment controlled houses. In open sided houses, artificial light is used to supplement natural day light. The supplementation of artificial light may be effected in one of the following ways: Providing artificial light in the morning, evening or both.

Light for broiler breeders: A 14 hr photoperiod is sufficient. The light intensity may be about 0.5 foot candle at bird level. In environmentally controlled houses, red light may be used to control cannibalism. Red or blue light may be used to catch birds during the night.

Breeder nutrition: The nutrient supply to the broiler breeder is a sum of two parts, namely nutrient content of the diet and quantity of feed supplied to the breeder birds. Both parts need to be balanced to ensure correct daily nutrient supply. Maintaining uniformity and keeping close to bodyweight targets are essential factors in feeding parent stock. Over-feeding early in the laying cycle will induce over-development of the ovaries. If egg production falls below target, additional feed should not be given unless it seems likely that energy is the limiting factor. Giving excess energy at any stage will damage production. If a nutrient other than energy is limiting, and causing poor performance, then the feed should be re-formulated. In general, a high quality nutrient provision for the breeder is economically justified.

Restricted feeding: Growth and uniformity are influenced by feeding program and to a lesser extent, by feed formulation. Therefore, feed delivery time becomes critical management factor. Broiler breeders are subjected to restricted feeding to optimize the body weight at 20 weeks of age by checking the growth of chicks and without affecting the normal development of various body systems. It helps to attain optimum body weight of 2.2 kg at the age of 20 weeks in females and 2.6-2.8 kg in males. This can be achieved either through skip-a -day programme, alternate day feeding or restricting amount but feeding depending on the convenience of a particular farm. The traditional system of feed restriction has been skip-a-day, where birds are fed only on alternate days. Feed restriction can start as early as 2 weeks or as late as 4 weeks depending on the strain. The daily allowance of feed is reduced to the extent of 30 percent of the normal consumption. The quality of feed is also altered so as to meet the optimal requirements of all nutrients even when quantity is restricted. Whatever system of feed restriction is used, the goals are to obtain a uniform and consistent growth rate through to maturity. Ideally, the pullets and roosters will be close to target weight by 16-18 weeks of age, since attempts at major manipulation in growth after this time often compromises body composition (birds get fatter), maturity and subsequent reproductive performance.

Provide shell grit at the rate of 4 kg per 1000 pullets in separate feeder for one day in each week from 8th week onwards to stimulate the gizzard for grinding the feed. Roosters can be grown with the hens or grown separately, but in both situations, they will almost exclusively be fed starter and grower diets designed for the female birds. When males and females are grown together, the onset of restriction programs and feed allocation are usually dictated by progress in hen weight and condition. Growing roosters separately provides the best opportunity to dictate and control their development. Water restriction is also important for juvenile breeders. With feed restriction, birds can consume their feed in 30 minutes to 2 hr and so given the opportunity, these birds will consume excessive quantities of water simply out of boredom or to satisfy physical hunger. Pullets given free access to water seem to have wetter litter. Water restriction becomes more challenging in hot weather.

Pre-breeder feed: The purpose of a pre-breeder feed is to increase the calcium levels in the diet above the levels fed in the grower period to provide a calcium reserve for the initiation of eggshell formation. It is also used to stimulate the nutrient intake of protein and energy for pullets that are lower in body weight than standard body weight. The use of pre-breeder feed from 105 days (15 weeks) of age is strongly recommended. This will provide sufficient amino acids and other nutrients for satisfactory development of reproductive tissues. Additional calcium may also be provided to ensure maximum development of medullary bone. Provision of extra vitamins will maximize levels in body tissues before egg production commences. Energy level in the pre-breeder feed should be similar to that of the breeder feed.

Separate male feeding: High protein diet will affect the sperm quality and semen volume. Therefore, broiler and layer breeder *males* must be fed with a low protein diet having 15 and 16% protein, respectively; whereas the *female* broiler and layer breeders to be fed with 16 and 17% protein, respectively as per BIS. Therefore, separate feeding of breeder hens and cocks should be followed. BIS recommends 3.5% calcium for females. It is advisable to provide 40mg/kg of vitamin E to male breeders. The feeds for male and female breeders are offered in separate feed hoppers in slat and deep liter systems. The feeders for male are placed at a higher level to which the females cannot reach, while the feeders for female are kept at a lower level but the males cannot eat from it as the partitions in the feeders are small and only the female head can go through as the males' head is bigger. In cage system, the sex separate feeding can be followed with 100% accuracy, since they are reared in different cages.

Nutrient (Energy) requirements of breeders: Breeder nutrition must be tailored to produce the greatest number of fertile eggs, and as such, judicious rationing of energy and protein is the usual criteria. The breeder hens utilize nutrients to meet her requirement for maintenance prior to partitioning nutrients for production.

Protein requirements: An average protein level for a broiler breeder diet should be 16%. When breeders are fed diets containing 16% protein and provided 165 g feed/day, they are consuming approximately 26.4 g of protein. In breeder feeds it is important not to exceed an upper limit of crude protein because of the adverse effects of excess protein in egg and hatchability.

Mineral requirements: The major minerals, especially calcium, phosphorous, sodium, potassium, magnesium and chloride are involved in shell formation; improvements in shell quality generally lead to better egg and chick quality. The recommended strategy is to feed a constant and modest level of calcium in the feed and to use variable quantities of calcium grit (i.e. limestone or oyster shell) to provide additional requirement.

Vitamin requirements: Vitamins are involved in most of the metabolic processes and are integral part of foetal development. Their requirements are higher for hatchability than for egg production. Therefore, breeder birds should be provided with a higher level of vitamin supplementation than are birds used for commercial egg production. Vitamins account for about 4 per cent of the cost of a breeder feed, so economizing their inclusion is rarely a sensible option. The nutrient specifications for broiler breeder and layer parents are detailed in Table 36 and Table 37, respectively.

Table 36: Nutrient Specifications for broiler breeder parent stock

Nutrient	Chick starter (0-21 days)	Grower (22-119 days)	Pre-breeder (120-154 days)	Breeder 1, (155-314 days)	Breeder 2, (315 days and above)
Crude Protein %	17.50	15.00	15.50	16.00	15.50
ME Kcal/lb	1300	1300	1300	1300	1300
Fat %	3-4	3-4	3-4	3-4	3-4
Fibre %	3-4	3-4	3-4	3-4	3-4
Amino acids %					
Lysine	0.90	0.75	0.80	0.80	0.75
Methionine	0.40	0.35	0.34	0.34	0.31
Methionine+ Cystine	0.72	0.60	0.58	0.58	0.55
Minerals %					
Calcium	1.00	1.00	1.50	3.00	3.20
Available Phosphorus	0.45	0.40	0.40	0.40	0.40
Sodium	0.16	0.15	0.15	0.15	0.15
Chloride	0.18	0.16	0.16	0.16	0.16
Potassium	0.40	0.40	0.60	0.60	0.60
Trace Minerals ppm					
Copper	4.00	4.00	16.00	16.00	16.00
Iodine	0.50	0.50	4.00	4.00	4.00
Iron	5.00	5.00	20.00	20.00	20.00
Manganese	70.00	60.00	100.00	100.00	100.00
Magnesium	250.00	250.00	250.00	250.00	250.00
Zinc	50.00	40.00	100.00	100.00	100.00
Selenium	0.15	0.15	0.20	0.20	0.20
Vitamins					
Vit A IU	4550.00	4450.00	7300.00	7300.00	7300.00
Vit D IU	1600.00	1600.00	1600.00	1600.00	1600.00
Vit E IU	15.00	15.00	25.00	25.00	25.00
Thiamin mg	0.25	0.25	2.50	2.50	2.50
Riboflavin mg	2.25	2.25	7.00	7.00	7.00
Niacin mg	9.00	9.00	23.00	23.00	23.00
Pantothenic acid mg	3.70	3.70	9.00	9.00	9.00
Biotin mg	0.12	0.03	0.20	0.20	0.20

Table 37: Nutrient requirement of layer breeder parent stock

Nutrient	Chicks(0-8 weeks)	Growers (8-20 weeks)	Breeders
ME Kcal/kg (min)	2600	2500	2600
CP %	20	16	18
Crude fibre, %	7	8	8
Salt %	0.6	0.6	0.6
Moisture, %	11	11	11
Lysine, %	0.9	0.6	0.65
Methionine, %	0.3	0.25	0.3
Calcium, %	1	1	3
Available phosphorus, %	0.5	0.5	0.5
Manganese, ppm	90	50	90
Zinc, ppm	50	60	100
Iodine, ppm	1	1	1
Iron, ppm	120	90	90
Copper, ppm	12	9	12
Vitamin A, IU/kg	6000	6000	8000
Vitamin D3, IU/kg	600	600	1200
Vitamin E, ppm	15	10	15
Vitamin K, ppm	1	1	1
Thiamin, ppm	5	3	3
Riboflavin, ppm	6	5	8
Pyridoxine, ppm	5	5	8
Pantothenic acid,ppm	15	15	15
Nicotinic acid, ppm	40	15	15
Biotin, ppm	0.2	2.15	0.2
Folic acid, ppm	1	0.5	0.5
Cyanocobalamin, µg/kg	15	10	10
Choline chloride, ppm	1300	90	800
Linoleic acid, %	1	1	1

Health care

Vaccination of breeder flock: This program is similar to the vaccination program for commercial laying strains. Because of the desire for high levels of maternal antibodies in the chicks, killed vaccines for ND, IB and IBD are usually given. Breeders may be revaccinated during lay to keep maternal antibody levels high. Commercial broilers are marketed at early age (about 5 weeks) and are not subjected to many diseases those affect breeder birds. Hence different vaccination schedule is followed for commercial broilers and breeders. The breeder flock vaccination programme is detailed in Table 38.

Table 38: Breeder flock vaccination programme

Age	Vaccine	Strain	Route
1 d	Marek's disease	HVT	S/C
7-10 d	Newcastle Disease	F1/Lasota	Water
10-12d.	Infectious Bronchitis	Massachusetts-Connecticut	Water
	Infectious Bursal Disease	Intermediate	Water
28 d	Newcastle Disease	Lasota	Water
	Infectious Bronchitis	Massachusetts-Connecticut	Water
	Infectious Bursal Disease	Intermediate	Water
7 wks	Newcastle Disease	Lasota	Coarse spray
	Infectious Bronchitis	Massachusetts-Connecticut	Coarse spray
	Infectious Bursal Disease	Intermediate	Coarse spray
10 wks	Pox	Fowl	Wing-web
	Avian encephalomyelitis	Calnek	Wing-web
12 wks	Newcastle Disease	Lasota	Fine spray
	Infectious Bronchitis	Massachusetts-Connecticut	Fine spray
	Infectious Bursal Disease	Intermediate	Fine spray
16 weeks	Newcastle Disease	Killed oil emulsion	S/C
	Infectious Bronchitis	Killed oil emulsion	S/C
	Infectious Bursal Disease	Killed oil emulsion	S/C

Common diseases of breeders

The common infectious (Sl N0 1- 4) and metabolic (Sl N0 5) diseases of breeder flocks are as follows

1. Viral diseases

- Ranikhet disease/ Newcastle disease(RD/ ND)
- Avian influenza(fowl plague) or bird flu
- Fowl pox
- Marek's Disease(MD)
- Infectious laryngotracheitis (I.L.T.)
- Infectious bronchitis (I.B.)
- Avian leucosis/ Big liver disease
- Infectious Bursal Disease (IBD)/ Gumboro disease
- Egg Drop Syndrome (EDS)
- Avian encephalomyelitis/ Epidemic fever
- Inclusion body hepatitis (IBH)

2. Bacterial diseases

- Infectious coryza
- Fowl typhoid
- Pullorum Disease/ Bacillary White Diarrhoea (BWD)
- Chronic Respiratory Disease (CRD)
- Fowl cholera/ Avian pasteurellosis
- Colibacillosis

3. Fungal diseases

- Aspergillosis / Brooder pneumonia
- Favus (white comb)
- Aflatoxicosis

4. Protozoan diseases

- Coccidiosis

5. Metabolic disorders

Deficiency of minerals	Symptoms
Calcium and Phosphorus	Rickets: Rubbery bones, bowing of legs in young ones, reduced growth, osteoporosis, internal hemorrhage. Osteomalacia in adults: Bowing of legs, thin shelled eggs, reduced egg production and feed intake.
Selenium	Exudative diathesis, reduced growth, muscular dystrophy and encephalomalacia, in embryo absence of upper beak, eyes and limbs
Zinc	Cartilage become shortened and thickened, bones of embryo deformed, depletion of vertebral column, eyes underdeveloped, and missing limbs, post hatch mortality in hatched weaklings, "scaly limb" disease in adults.
Nickel	Enlarged hock joints.
Copper	Death at early blood stage with no malformation.
Iodine	Prolongation of hatching time, reduced thyroid size and incomplete abdominal closure.
Iron	Low blood haemoglobin, poor extra- embryonic circulation in candled egg.
Deficiency of vitamins	
Vitamin- A	Failure to develop blood system, Embryonic malposition.

(*Contd.*)

Deficiency of minerals	Symptoms
Hypovitaminosis and hypervitaminosis D	Stunted growth and rickets, soft extremities of bones, and junction of ribs. Cartilage swollen.
Vitamin-E	Avian encephalomalacia/ crazy chick disease- diseased chick appears to push head beneath breast, paralysis and death. In chicks bulging eyes and in mature birds drop in egg production. Haemorrhages in cerebellum and medulla oblongata. exudative diathesis, muscular dystrophy, enlarged hocks.
Riboflavin (B_2)	Atrophied leg muscle, curled toe paralysis, drooping of wings and head, dermatitis of eyelid, feet and mouth. Decline in egg production, embryonic mortality at 2nd or 4th week.
Vitamin-K	Prolonged embryonic blood clotting time, blood clot in embryo, haemorrhage, blood tinged faeces and mortality could reach up to 50%.
Niacin	Enlarged hock joints and legs bend outwards, diarrhoea, stomatitis, oesophagitis.
Pantothenic acid	Formation of scabs at commisure of mouth, eyelid and toes. Hyperplasia or cracks in the skin of foot pad, stunted growth abnormal feathering, subcutaneous haemorrhage.
Thiamine (B_1)	Bird sit on hock, Star gazing appearance-pulling head towards back.
Pyridoxine	Stunted growth, staggering gait, incoordination, jurking movement of legs and wings.
Biotin	Micromelia, shortening of long bones, parrot beak, twisted bones of feet.
Choline	Perosis, fatty liver syndrome, reduced egg production.
Vitamin (B_{12}).	Embryonic malposition, stunted growth, reduced capacity of feed intake.
Vitamin (B_6).	Reduced hatchability

The above diseases may be prevented by adopting proper vaccination programme and feeding standard balanced diets.

Economic parameters on returns from breeders

The economic parameters may be calculated on the following major components:

1. Sale of day-old commercial chicks.
2. Sale of unset table eggs.
3. Sale of spent hens and cocks.
4. Manure.
5. Gunny bags.

To calculate the costs of producing a dozen hatching eggs from egg type-, medium type- or meat type-breeder replacement females will include: pullet growing cost, feed cost, number of eggs produced, mortality, labour etc.

Selection and Culling of Breeder Flocks

- **Selection**: Any bird that is selected for breeding purpose must meet the established historic standards for the breed. A producer needs to retain far fewer males than females for breeding stock. For this, rigorous selection of the males is an important component to a sound breeding program. It should also be remembered that the adult female stock is selected on the basis of their body weight; undersized or otherwise poor quality females should not be retained. Usually males are selected based on their vigour and spermatozoa concentration. In case of natural mating, the mating ability of the males is important, in addition to its semen quality. Six basic qualities for selection of breeder stock are: (i) Rate of growth, (ii) Matured body weight, (iii) Egg-laying ability, (iv) Breed type, (v) Colour and (vi) Fertility and vigour.
- **Culling** : Culling refers to the identification and removal of the non-laying or low producing hens and poor or infertile males from a breeder flock. It is an important managemental tool to be practiced in case of breeder females. The most accurate method of measuring a bird's productive ability is by trapnesting method under deep litter system. However, only a small fraction of the total population can be culled by this method. Therefore, out of a practical necessity, birds have to be culled by external appearance. Usually monthly culling is practised. Hens eat feed whether or not they are laying. Thus, culling reduces the cost of egg production, reduces the incidence of diseases, and saves more feed and space for better productive birds.

Two types of culling are usually adopted:

- sight- culling at the time of housing and
- culling by individual inspection, which evaluates the bird's ability to lay or her past productive performance.

Question Bank

Q. 1. Fill in the blanks

a) There are three types of breeders viz., ..., ... and ....

b) Common methods of sexing chick are ...., ..., ... and ....

c) Brooding temperature recommended is ....^{0}C during first week with a gradual reduction at the rate of ....^{0}C per week.

d) Removal of comb is called as ....

e) The .... and .... toes of all breeding males are clipped to prevent tearing the back of females during mating.

f) Dewatteling should be done when the cockerels are .... weeks of age.

g) Quantitative feed restriction is carried out by ...., ... and daily restricted feeding.

h) Photoperiod availability for broilers, growers and layers is ...., ... and ....hours, respectively.

i) The light rays passes through the eyes and stimulate the .... to release .... and .... from anterior pituitary.

j) Ratio of male: female for White egg layers, Brown egg layers, Broiler breeders is ...., ... and .... respectively.

k) Vitamin-E deficiency causes ....

l) Caecal coccidiosis is caused by ....

m) Ranikhet disease is caused by ....

n) Marek's disease (MD) is caused by DNA Herpes virus.

o) ME requirement of layer breeder parent stock for chick, grower and layer is ...., ... and .... κcal.

p) CP requirement of layer breeder parent stock for chick, grower and layer is ...., ... and ....per cent.

q) Exudative diathesis is caused by deficiency of ....

r) Curled toe paralysis is caused by deficiency of ....

s) Vaccination to be made at day-old / hatch-day is .... and strain used is ....

Q. 2. State whether the following statements are **True or False**

a) Feed restriction starts at 12 week of age in broiler breeders. ( )

b) Vent sexing of chicks is usually carried out at 10 days of age. ( )

c) Removal of feather is known as Dubbing. ( )

d) Breeder pullets are subjected to the toe clipping. ( )

e) Debeaking increases cannibalism and feed wastage. ( )

f) The threshold photoperiod for growers is about 8- 9 hrs. ( )

g) In the layer house, minimum distance from the floor to the bulbs is about 7-8 feet. ( )

h) Red or blue light may be used to catch birds during the night. ( )

i) Floor space required for meat type birds under deep litter system is 2 feet. ( )

j) Feeder space requirement for Leghorn type chicks is 2.5 in. ( )

k) Skip-a-day programme is more efficient than everyday feed restriction. ( )

l) The use of pre-breeder feed from 77 days (11 weeks) of age is strongly recommended. ( )

m) Calcium requirement for broiler breeder male is 1-1.2 per cent. ( )

n) Egg drop syndrome affects 12- 14 week old birds. ( )

o) Infectious bursal disease (IBD) affects birds of 8-10 week age. ( )

p) Exudative diathesis is caused by deficiency of vitamin-D. ( )

q) Perosis is caused by biotin deficiency. ( )

r) Salmonellosis is vertically transmitted disease. ( )

s) Vitamins account for about 4 per cent of the cost of a breeder feed. ( )

Q.1. Answers

a) Egg Type (White egg layers), Medium Type (Brown egg layers), Meat type (Broiler breeder)

b) Vent, feather, colour, machine sexing
c) 35, 2.5
d) Dubbing
e) Inside, back
f) 12-14
g) Skip a day, alternate day
h) 24, 8-9, 17
i) Hypothalamus, FSH, LH
j) 10-12: 100, 10-12:100, 12/15:100
k) Crazy chick disease
l) *Eimeria tenella*
m) Paramyxovirus
n) DNA Herpes virus.
o) 2600, 2500, 2600
p) 20, 16, 18
q) Vitamin-E
r) Riboflavin
s) MD, HVT

Q. 2. Answers

a) F
b) F
c) F
d) F
e) F
f) T
g) T
h) T
i) F
j) T
k) F
l) F
m) F
n) F
o) F
p) F
q) T
r) T
s) T

31

Artificial Insemination in Poultry

J.D. Mahanta

Artificial insemination (AI) is the deposition of the semen or male germ cells (spermatozoa) in the female genital tract by artificial means (instruments). Artificial insemination includes collection of semen from the male, preservation, handling and deposition into the female reproductive tract hygienically replacing natural mating by a male. In India this technique is gaining momentum in chickens due to improved animal husbandry practices and economic considerations, initiated by IVRI, Izatnagar and JNKVV, Jabalpur. In many parts of the world, turkey, ducks, goose and guinea fowl are bred solely by AI. Chicken species are endowed with the behaviour and capacity of each male to mate several females and also 25 to 40 times a day. Further, the process of ovulation in birds is almost daily and stimulated by intensity and duration of light.

In modern poultry managemental practices of using cages, environmentally controlled houses and breeding and hybridization techniques employed for developing highly economical chickens, selection for faster growth and heavy body weight in broilers, which has led to loss of fertility and hatchability and use of dwarf female parents in broiler industry have demanded the use of AI in poultry.

Economic advantages of AI over natural mating

1. Fertility through AI is 5 to 10 per cent higher and consequently number of chicks produced per breeder is higher (6 chicks) compared to those from floor (93- 95% fertility with AI).
2. Fertility is ensured irrespective of the age of the bird and climate.
3. Fewer males are required than the natural mating (5% *vs.* 10- 20%) and thus reduce the feeding cost on males.
4. Production of inter-species hybrids (species hybridization) where natural mating is not possible. For example Mule ducks production between domestic duck (*Anas platyrhynchos* var. *domesticus*) and Muscovy duck (*Cairina moschata*).
5. Possibility of using large (7 to 8 Kg) males on dwarf females and *vice versa*.
6. Use of single ejaculate of semen to large number of females.
7. Infertility due to agonistic behaviour or preferential mating in both males and females is avoided facilitating every male and female to contribute genetically to next generation.

Semen collection

Semen collection from the cock is done with the help of manual massage technique. Both '*one-man*' and '*two-man*' collection methods are involved in chicken. *Two-man* method is fast, easy and efficient to operate. In this method males are trained for semen donation by lumber- reflex method which involves gently passing palm of the hand from back towards tail feathers, encircling root of tail between thumb and forefinger. The reflex action helps the cock to evert copulatory papilla, which can be gently pressed by forefinger and thumb of the operator waiting for evertion. Excessive pressure may cause bleeding. The birds should be picked up gently from cage and manipulated quickly avoiding struggling and excitement. This procedure, once cocks are trained for donation, does not take more than 10-15 seconds. The pre-requisite for obtaining good quality and quantity of semen is that cocks should be kept in wire cages individually for 5-7 days. Otherwise picking cock from floor pens might give disappointing response. It is advisable that feathers from cloacal region are removed during training period to avoid contamination. A glass or plastic funnel (5 cm) sealed with wax can be used as collection funnel. Semen is generally milked every alternate day for getting better quality semen. Average semen characteristics of different poultry species are given in Table 39.

Spermatozoa of chicken

Spermatozoa of avian exhibit a great deal of variation in size and shape depending upon the species. A fowl spermatozoon has 3 parts as shown in Fig. 36.

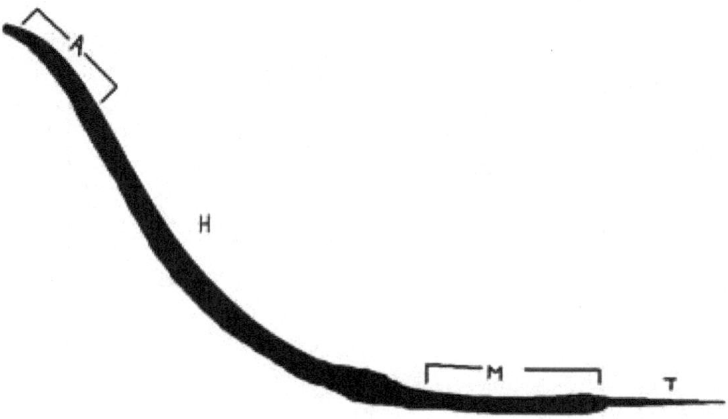

Fig. 36: Diagram of a fowl spermatozoon showing different parts. A= acrosome (2 ηm long)-part of the cell containing mechanism for penetrating the egg at fertilization; H= head (12.5 ηm long)-contains hereditary material; M= middle-piece (4 ηm long)- contains mechanism for creating energy for motility; T= tail (about 8 ηm long)- contains mechanism for propelling spermatozoon.

Semen dilution

The fertilizing capacity of avian semen is quickly lessened on storage. Therefore many poultry breeders use neat (undiluted) semen for insemination. It is very difficult to provide exact *in vitro* environment for prolonging the survivality of spermatozoa. In general, if semen has to be stored beyond one hour after collection, dilution with ideal extenders and careful handling throughout is essential. They can protect the semen up to 6 hours of storage under 4-5 °C. Extenders are used to dilute (increase volume) the semen rather than storage. Semen dilution ratio is 1:2 or 1:3 and insemination dose from such diluted semen is 0.03 to 0.05 ml given at every 5-7 days interval. The insemination dose of 20-25 million sperm is recommended for optimum fertility. The diluted semen should be inseminated within 20 minutes after dilution and 30 minutes after collection. All extenders may lower fertility by 2-3 per cent. The Table 40 below shows the composition of commonly used semen extenders for diluting semen.

Table 39: Average semen characteristics of different types of domestic poultry

Characteristics	Fowl		Turkey		Guinea fowl	Duck	Goose	Remarks
	Light breed	Heavy breed	Light weight	Heavy weight				
Volume (ml)	0.25-0.50	0.5-1.0	0.08-0.3	0.10-0.33	0.05-0.15	0.1-1.0	0.2-1.5	Volume varies
Sperm concentration (X 1000 million per ml)	4.0	5.0	9.0	9.5	6.0	4.0	0.25	Very highly concentrated
pH	7.0-7.6	7.0-7.6	7.0-7.2	7.0-7.2	-	-	-	Alkaline
Age at which semen can be collected (weeks)	20-22	22-24	-	-	-	-	-	-
Appearance	Pearly white	Pearly white	-	-	-	-	-	-
Doses required for insemination	20-25 million per dose	20-25 million per dose	-	-	-	-	-	Spermatozoa should be normal, active and progressively motile

Table 40: Composition of commonly used semen extenders

Ingredient	g per 1000 ml		
	Ringer's solution	Lock's solution	Tyrode's solution
NaCl	9.00	9.00	9.00
KCl	0.30	0.24	0.20
$CaCl_2$	0.25	0.42	0.20
$MgCl_2$	-	-	0.10
$NaHCO_3$	0.20	0.20	1.00
Dextrose	-	1.00	1.00
pH	7.00	7.00	7.00

Insemination technique

This phase consist of eversion of vagina and introduction of semen into the oviduct. The female placed on open door cage is caught by one assistant holding the shank and the palm of other hand and pressing abdomen forward and upward gently. The left side opening of the cloaca can be seen as vaginal portion of the oviduct and right side one being the large intestine. Then with the help of tuberculin syringe or inseminating cannula required quantity of semen is introduced at about 3 cm depth into the everted oviduct. The semen is not released from the syringe before the oviduct is allowed to regain its normal position. Insemination cannula should be rinsed with 1 per cent NaCl solution.

Dose: An undiluted semen dose of 0.03-0.05 ml.

Interval: Insemination in chicken is recommended at 5 to 7 days interval.

Time: AI is practiced during afternoon hours, usually after 1.00 pm because presence of egg in uterus may lower fertility.

AI equipments:

Collection cup: 5 cm diameter glass or plastic funnel with sealed stem serves as good collection cup.

Insemination cannula or tuberculin syringe: A plastic or glass cannula inserted into a piece of rubber tube mounted to the end of syringe or glass mouthpiece is commonly used for insemination. For mass insemination automatic insemination cannula fitted with graduated syringe and store cup is recommended.

Wash bottle: A wash bottle to keep 1% NaCl.

Cryopreservation of poultry semen

In order to meet the increasing demand of chicks stud farming in poultry has become very essential. To make the breeding programme successful cryopreservation of avian semen has become crucial. The main use of semen cryopreservation in birds is the management of genetic diversity. This diversity is rapidly decreasing due to the progressive disappearance of many small populations and the high specificity of selected commercial lines. In addition, the increasing risk of epidemic avian influenza in the past few years have emphasized the need for acceleration of *ex situ* conservation of genetic resources. In Europe, there are two main national germplasm cryobanks: one in the Netherlands managed by The Netherlands centre of Genetic Resources and one in France managed by the French National Cryobank of Domestic Animals.

Question Bank

I. Fill in the blanks

1. .... is the deposition of semen in the female genital tract by artificial means.
2. .... is the site of fertilization of ovum.
3. .... is the largest portion of fowl oviduct.
4. The spermatozoa can live in oviduct for at least.........to .... Days.
5. Insemination in chicken is recommended at .... to .... days interval.
6. An insemination dose of .... million sperm is recommended for optimum fertility.

II. Match the following

1. Sperm nest	-	a)	semen extender
2. Cock semen	-	b)	Uterus
3. Ringer's solution	-	c)	Alkaline
4. Left oviduct	-	d)	Infundibulum
5. Shell gland	-	e)	Functional

III. Write down the semen characteristics of different types of poultry?

IV. What are the economic advantages of AI over natural mating?

V. Describe the insemination technique in poultry.

VI. Describe the method of semen collection in chicken.

VII. Draw the structure of an avian spermatozoon.

VIII. Write short note on cryopreservation of poultry semen.

Answers

I. (1) AI (2) Infundibulum (3) Magnum (4) 5, 11 (5) 5, 7 (6) 20-25

II. (1) d (2) c (3) a (4) e (5) b

32

Hatchery Practices

S.J. Manwar

Principles of Incubation

Incubation is a process by which the embryo within egg develops into a fully formed chick capable of breaking free from the shell. Basically, when a hen incubates an egg, it means she is on the egg in order to keep it warm for a certain period of time, 21 days for chicken, until the chick embryo has fully formed and is ready to hatch. The incubation period in other species is given in Table 41. The following factors affect the incubation on egg

1. Temperature

Incubator temperature should be maintained between 99 and 100 °F. The acceptable range is 97 to 102 °F. Overheating is more critical than under heating. An incubator should be operated in a location free from drafts and direct sunlight. Temperature is probably the most important single factor influencing the development of the embryo. A higher temperature will advance the hatch and a lower temperature will delay hatch. Younger embryos are especially susceptible to high temperatures because the upper lethal limit is very close to the optimum incubating temperature. High temperature will cause the embryonic membranes to dry out too soon. Chicks that hatch may have an unsteady gait.

2. Humidity

The relative humidity of the air within an incubator should be about 60 percent. During the last 3 days (the hatching period) the RH should be nearer 65-70 percent. Too much moisture in the incubator prevents normal evaporation and results in a decreased hatch. Too little moisture results in excessive evaporation, causing chicks to stick to the shell, remain in the pipped shells, and sometimes hatch crippled. Using a wet-bulb thermometer is a good way for determining relative humidity. If the wet and dry bulb read the same temperature, the RH would be 100 percent.

The RH plays an important role in egg incubation. It is through pores of the eggs that the embryos breathes and loose some of its humidity during formation. Inside an incubator, humidity is controlled by sensors or mercury thermometers (wet bulb thermometer), which constantly monitor the environment in the machine. If the RH inside the incubator is too low, there is a risk of high embryo mortality due to dehydration. However, if the RH is too high, the chicks may develop properly but when it is time to hatch, there is a high risk of "drowning". This means that the egg has not lost enough moisture, thus the internal air cell at the large end of the egg is either too small and when the chicks tries to take in its first breath, it will breath in liquid and drown. Large eggs suffer more from dehydration than the smaller eggs.

3. Ventilation

This is one of the most critical factors inside an incubator. The best hatching results are obtained with normal atmospheric air, which usually contains 21 percent oxygen. Oxygen concentration above or less than 21 per cent affects hatchability. Carbon dioxide concentration should not exceed more than 0.5 per cent inside incubator as higher concentration reduces hatchability and it becomes zero at 5 per cent. It is essential that the room in which incubator is installed should have adequate ventilation. The internal fan speeds or RPMs should be roughly 7200 rpm. It ensures that the air inside the machine is being circulated from the ceiling all the way to the floor in a circular motion eliminating any possible hot spots in the machine.

4. Turning of eggs

The turning of egg prevents adhesion of the embryonic membranes, thereby reducing abnormalities and malpositions. Proper turning of eggs ensures uniform heating of eggs. Eggs must be turned during most of the incubation period, except for last 3 or 4 days prior to hatching. Most of the modern incubators have a provision of turning the eggs, automatically, once in every 3 hour; however, it is observed that if the eggs are turned hourly, the hatchability improves.

Table 41. The incubation requirements for various poultry

Species	Incubationperiod (days)	Temperature (F)	Humidity (F)	Do not turn after	Humidity for last3 days
Chicken	21	100	85-87	18th day	90
Turkey	28	99	84-86	25th day	90
Duck	28	100	85-86	25th day	90
Muscovy duck	35-37	100	85-86	31st day	90
Goose	28-34	99	86-88	25th day	90
Guinea fowl	28	100	85-87	25th day	90
Pheasant	23-28	100	86-88	21st day	92
Peafowl	28-30	99	84-86	25th day	90
Bobwhite quail	23-24	100	84-87	20th day	90
Coturnix quail	17	100	85-86	15th day	90
Pigeon	17	100	85-87	15th day	90
Emu	52	97	30-40	49th day	No data
Ostrich	42	97	20-35	39th day	No data

5. Positioning of eggs in incubators

Eggs can be set either vertically, with the broad end up, or horizontally, on their sides. Follow the directions of the manufacturer for proper incubation.

6. The air cell in the egg

Soon after an egg is laid, a small air cell forms at the broad end between inner and outer shell membranes. A membrane separating the mass of the egg and the air bubble serves as a diaphragm to relieve stress and pressure resulting from thermal changes of temperature.

Table 42: Events in embryonic development of the chicken egg

Before egg laying	Fertilization, division and growth of living cells. Segregation of cells into groups of special function (tissues).
Between laying and incubation	No-growth stage of inactive embryonic life. (50,000 to 80,000 cells)
During incubation	
Day 1	
16 hours	First sign of resemblance to a chick embryo
18 hours	Appearance of alimentary tract
20 hours	Appearance of vertebral column
21 hours	Beginning of formation of nervous system
22 hours	Beginning of formation of head
24 hours	Beginning of formation of the eye
Day 2	
25 hours	Beginning of formation of heart
35 hours	Beginning of formation of ear
42 hours	Heart begins to beat
Day 3	
60 hours	Beginning of formation of nose
62 hours	Beginning of formation of legs
64 hours	Beginning of formation of wings
Day 4	Beginning of formation of tongue
Day 5	Beginning of formation of permanent organs and differentiation of sex; Aortic structure begins forming and thickening
Day 6	Beginning of formation of beak
Day 8	Beginning of formation of feathers
Day 10	Beginning of hardening of beak
Day 13	Appearance of scales and claws
Day 14	Embryo gets into position to break the shell
Day 16	Scales, claws, and beak become firm
Day 17	Beak turns toward air cell
Day 19	Yolk begins to enter body cavity
Day 20	Yolk sac completely drawn into body cavity.Embryo occupies all the space within the egg except the air cell
Day 21	Hatching of chick

Courtesy : A.L. Romanoff-Cornell Rural School Leaflet, Sept. 1939

Factors affecting fertility

Fertility may be defined as a percentage of eggs those have been fertilized. Factors affecting fertility are:

1. **Heredity**: Some strains of chicken produces better fertility than others. It is possible to increase or decrease fertility by continuous selection within a strain for longer period.

2. **Breed:** The fertility is lower in heavy breeds compared to lighter breeds. This may be due to poor mating ability, inbreeding and physical

incompatibility, etc. This problem can be partly solved by using artificial insemination, restricted feeding or continuous selection.

3. **Age of birds**: Fertility is usually higher in young birds than their older counterparts. Breeding males should be at least 6-7 months old for high fertility whereas the males of slow maturing heavy breeds may not reach maximum fertility until 8-10 months of age.
4. **Male: female ratio**: Both higher and lower male to female ratio will reduce fertility due to infighting between males and inability to cover more number of females, respectively. The recommended ratio is 1:15-16 in layers, 1:10-12 in broilers and 1:1-2 in quails.
5. **Semen quality**: The semen volume, sperm concentration and number of successful mating also alter fertility. It varies due to species, breed, strain or individual.
6. **Managemental factors**: Cocks those are kept in the darkness for longer periods give lower fertility.
7. **Laying pattern**: Fertility (and hatchability) is higher in the first year of laying than the subsequent years. This is again higher in first 12-15 weeks of laying then starts gradually declining.
8. **Climate**: Extreme high or low temperature in layer house reduces fertility due to poor mating frequency because of inactiveness of birds.
9. **Nutritional factors**: Deficiency of certain micro-nutrients such as vitamin A, Pantothenic acid, Vitamin E, Biotin and minerals like Ca, P, Na, Mn, Zn and iodine lower fertility.

Factors affecting hatchability

- Like fertility, hatchability varies with breed, strain and individuals.
- Usually hatchability reduces with increase in inbreeding coefficient, while out-breeding improves it.
- Management and nutritional status of breeding stock with special reference to minerals and vitamins considerably affects hatchability.
- Too high or low temperature in layer house reduces hatchability
- Hatchability is higher in eggs from younger flock and *vice versa.*
- Faulty pre-incubation storage conditions of eggs reduce hatchability.
- Eggs having abnormal shape, too small or extra large eggs, thin shelled and eggs with poor internal quality do not hatch well.

- Optimum temperature and humidity in the incubators are most important for desired hatchability.
- The desired levels of oxygen and carbon dioxide in incubator play major role in obtaining good hatchability.
- The reverse setting of eggs with narrow end up seriously lower down the hatchability.
- Inadequate and faulty turning during incubation lowers the hatchability.
- Use of separate hatcher with slight decrease in temperature and increase in humidity in the hatcher as compared to that of setter improves hatchability.

Selection of hatching eggs

i) Select eggs from breeders that are

  a) Well developed, mature and healthy.

  b) Compatible with their mates and produce a high percentage of fertile eggs.

  c) Reared under stress-free environment.

  d) Fed a balanced breeder diet.

ii) **Egg size:** Select eggs for hatching that are normal in size. Large eggs hatch poorly and small eggs produce small chicks.

iii) **Egg shape:** Oval shaped eggs hatch better than spindle and round shape eggs.

iv) **Egg shell colour:** Dark brown eggs tend to hatch better than light brown eggs. Avoid tinted eggs.

v) **Egg shell thickness:** For best hatching results egg shells should be between 0.33 to 0.35 mm in thickness.

vi) **Specific gravity:** A positive relationship exists between fertility of eggs and their specific gravity.

vii) **Defects in eggs:** Remove eggs with obvious defects, dirt, cracked or thin shells. Always set fresh eggs for incubation.

viii) **Shell texture:** Eggs set for incubation must have smooth, thick and uniform shell texture.

ix) **Cleaning of egg shells:** Slightly soiled eggs can be cleaned by lightly sanding the soiled area. However, washing also removes the protective cuticle, making the egg more susceptible to contamination.

Internal egg quality: Eggs should have good albumen and yolk quality and should be free from blood and meat spots or any other defects. *Tremulous air cells* reduce the hatchability drastically. The higher the Haugh unit reading (>80) better is the hatchability of the eggs.

Care and incubation of hatching eggs

The success of hatching depends on proper handling and care of the hatching eggs so that healthy and vigorous chicks are produced. Even before incubation starts the embryo is developing and needs proper care. Points to be considered to maintain better hatching egg quality are:

- Collect the eggs early in the morning and frequently during the day.
- Hatching eggs should not be washed unless necessary. If it is necessary to wash eggs always use cloth with water warmer than that of the eggs. Do not soak the eggs in water.
- Store the eggs in 55- 60 °F and 70-75% RH.
- Eggs should be placed in small end down position. When the eggs are stored for more than 10 days, hatchability will improve if eggs are held small end up. Eggs should not be stored for more than 10-14 days.
- Alter egg position periodically if not incubating within 4-6 days. Turn the eggs to a new position once daily until placing in the incubator.
- Allow cool eggs to warm slowly to room temperature before placing in the incubator.

Fumigation

Hatchery is one of the greatest areas of disease risk in the whole cycle of poultry production. For successful hatching operation, the overall design of hatchery assumes importance. The flow of air, movement of people and equipment should be such that it can never pass back from dirty areas such as the hatchers to clean areas and the setters and egg holding rooms. Two methods are used to disinfect hatching eggs under field conditions, namely fumigation or dipping in a solution of detergent or disinfectant.

Formaldehyde gas is generated by adding formalin to potassium permanganate by which we can disinfect the hatching eggs. The ratio of liquid formalin is approximately twice the dry measure of $KMnO_4$ (1g $KMnO_4$ /2ml of formalin). Sixty grams of $KMnO_4$ and 120 ml formalin for 100 ft^3 or 2.8 m^3 cabinet space. The temperature of 21.1°C (70°F) and 70% RH for the duration of 20 minutes time are the optimum conditions for fumigation.

Sanitize eggs and equipments before storage or use by fumigating. It must be relatively air tight and equipped with a small fan to circulate the gas. Stack the eggs inside the room so that air can circulate among the eggs. Remove eggs from the cases for good air circulation. Mix the ingredients (Table 43) in an earthenware or enamelware container. Circulate the gas within the structure for 20 minutes and then expel the gas. Allow eggs to air out for a few hours before placing them in cases.

Egg dipping in detergent- sanitizer or in disinfectants is highly effective in greatly reducing or eliminating the bacteria from the shell when performed correctly. However, there is little or no effect on those bacteria that have already penetrated the shell. Attention must be given to the temperature of the detergent which must be higher than the egg temperature.

Table 43: Concentration and time recommendation for formaldehyde gas fumigation

Sr No	Concentr -ation of fumigant	Quantity* of $KMNO_4$ (gram)	Quantity* of formalin (ml)	Hatchery component	Fumigation time in minutes
1	1x	20	40	Chicks in hatcher, Incubator room	03 30
2	2x	40	80	Eggs in incubator (1st day), Incubator room	20 30
3	3x	60	120	Hatching eggs (immediately after laying), Hatchery between hatches, Wash room, Chick boxes	20 30 30 30
4	5x	100	200	Trucks	20

*Required for each 100 ft^3 of space.

Sanitation of incubator and equipment

Thoroughly clean and disinfect the setter and hatcher after each hatch. Remove all egg shells, down, dust, and extra material with a broom or vacuum. Wash the unit with a warm detergent solution and rinse with a disinfectant solution. When becomes dry, turn the units on and bring to proper temperature and humidity conditions prior to filling with eggs. Quaternary ammonia is the most commonly used disinfectant for equipments like incubators and hatching trays. The incubator and its components should be cleaned and made free of organic matter before disinfection. Fumigation is another tool for disease control when the cleaning is poor, eggs are dirty, or machines are filled with eggs and it is difficult to empty and clean properly.

Hatchery hygiene

Transmission of diseases and infections from one generation to the next can occur through hatching eggs. Disease producing microorganisms can enter the egg by-

- Trans-ovarian transmission
- Egg shell transmission

Trans-ovarian transmission

Certain micro-organisms can enter the yolk before ovulation or the albumen as it is being secreted in the oviduct or they can be attached to the spermatozoa as appear on the surface of the phallus (male organ) which in turn can infect the female reproductive system. For example, M*ycoplasma, Salmonella* as well as microorganisms causing disease like Avian encephalomyelitis, Lymphoid leucosis, Chicken infectious anemia, EDS-76 etc.

Egg shell transmission

Certain bacterial and fungal contamination can also take place across the shell during the storage and hatching of eggs. The shell contaminating micro-organisms can be destroyed with various disinfectants as long as they do not penetrate. The egg shell transmitted disease causing agents are Salmonellas, Arizona, *E. coli*, Coliforms, Pseudomonas, Proteus, Aspergillus, Streptococci and Staphylococci.

Disposal of hatchery wastes

The main methods of disposing of the waste material are as follows:

1. **Incineration**: Incinerators at temperature above 1600 °F (870 °C) burns the waste materials to ash.
2. **Waste disposal pit**: The debris from hatcheries must be covered not less than 15 cm of soil.
3. **Dehydration**: The hatchery waste is hygienically dehydrated to make hatchery by-product meals which can support satisfactory performance when fed to chickens, particularly laying hens, because of its nutrients with high calcium content.

Sexing of chicks

There are two methods of chick sexing - Vent method and auto sexing

1. ***Vent method*** is very popular and originally developed in Japan. It depends upon the observation of rudimentary sex organ. In case of males, there are three bean shaped bumps, whereas, in females centre protuberance is missing. Chick sexing machine is also available which is a tube like structure having magnifying lens and eye lens to see through. One end of this machine is inserted in vent of chick and when lighted, it enlarges the view of sex organs by 3-5 times. However the disadvantage with this machine is that the sexing process is slower than the one with naked eye.
2. **In *auto-sexing***, plumage colour linked with sex chromosome are taken into account to determine the sex. For example, when a Rhode Island Red male is mated to Barred Plymouth Rock female, all the female progeny will be black and male progeny barred.

Grading day-old chicks

The chicks below the minimum standards should not be allowed to go to the customers. Some standards for chick quality are:

a) No chick deformities.

b) No unhealed navels.

c) Above a minimum weight.

d) Not dehydrated.

e) Down colour representative of the breed.

f) Stand up well.

Packaging and dispatch of day-old chicks

Chicks should be removed from the hatcher as soon as all are hatched and about 95% are dry. Further drying and hardening should be confined to chick boxes in a holding room with a temperature of 75 ^{o}F to reduce the danger of chilling and with a RH of 75 % to reduce dehydration.

Chick boxes vary in size and construction. The box size for holding 100 chicks in centimeters is 56 x 46 x 15 or 18 usually divided into four compartments. Most chick boxes are constructed of corrugated fiber or bamboo, some are made of plastic, which can be washed, disinfected and reused. The bottom of the chick box must be covered with some materials to which they may clamp their toes. The baby chicks should be dispatched in such a way that they should reach the customer's farm early in the morning.

Economics of hatchery business, Troubleshooting hatch failure

Chick production cost

The chick cost is highly variable due the differences in hatching egg cost, percent hatchability, hatchery operating cost and delivery cost. Many costs other than the eggs cost are involved in the actual hatchery operation. It includes labour, electricity, depreciation, chick boxes, repairs and maintenance, consumable supplies, services (beak trimming, sexing, comb trimming), general and administrative (office expenses, telephone, taxes, insurance, interests, etc.).

When egg type chicks are sold, only the pullet chicks are involved; the cockerels are usually destroyed. Thus, the cost of producing a pullet egg type chick is twice that of a straight-run (non-sexed) chick, since only half the chicks produced are pullets. Some hatcheries calculate their hatchery costs on the basis of a straight-run chick, and then multiply final figures by two to arrive at the pullet cost.

Factors affecting chick production cost

1. **Labour efficiency**- Automation and labour efficiency are instrumental in reducing labour costs.
2. **Wages**- The hourly cost of hatchery labour is an important criterion of hatchery cost.
3. **Managerial efficiency**- The manager should be able to direct the people and conduct good business procedure.
4. **Utilization of incubator capacity**- There should be cyclical demand for chicks.
5. **Size of hatchery operation**- Generally, the cost of hatching a chick is lower in larger hatcheries.
6. **Electricity**- As the amount of electricity used in the hatchery is large, the rate of power is important.

Economics of hatchery with 10000 egg hatching capacity at a time

A. Fixed capital assets

a.	Construction of Hatchery buildings with complete concrete wall and C.I. Sheet roofing	Rs. 4, 50, 000.00
b.	Electric power installation in hatchery	Rs. 20, 000.00
c.	Generator 10KVA with starter having main switch	Rs. 1, 75, 000.00
d.	1 No. Refrigerator	Rs. 19, 000.00
e.	Setter (12000 capacity) and hatcher (5000 capacity), one each	Rs. 6, 00, 000.00
f.	Construction of office cum store room	Rs. 1, 00, 000.00
g.	Miscellaneous	Rs. 52,000.00
	Total	**Rs. 14, 16, 000.00**

B. Working capital

a.	Payment to attendant monthly	Rs. 3000.00
b.	Procurement of graded eggs from recognized farm @ Rs. 10/- per eggs for 10,000 eggs	Rs. 1, 00, 000.00
c.	Transportation of eggs	Rs. 1, 000.00
d.	Carton for packaging chicks	Rs. 5,000.00
e.	Misc. (Vaccination of chicks)	Rs. 3,000.00
	Total	**Rs. 1, 12, 000.00**

(The cost of each item varies from time to time and place to place.)

Diagnosis of hatch failure

Eggs failed to hatch can be judged by breaking and examining them for certain diagnostic signs based on the appearance and comparative development of the egg and embryo. Break the egg into a flat container and evaluate the contents according to the following criteria:

Clears: Absence of a blood ring or embryo development indicates that either the embryos died early in incubation or the eggs were infertile.

Blood rings: Clear eggs with a blood ring or small embryo indicate that death occurred in the first three days of incubation possibly because of incubator malfunction.

Early-dead or mid-term embryos: Possible causes include excessively high or low incubation temperatures, improper turning, low viability of the egg caused by parental nutrition or inheritance, improper ventilation and suffocation, disease, poor egg shell quality, and contamination.

Fully formed and not pipped: The usual causes include low average incubation temperature, weak viability of setting eggs, improper humidity, genetic defects, contamination or temperature malfunction.

Malformed chicks: Genetic deformities may occur. High temperature during certain formation times may lead to deformities. Rough handling of incubating eggs may contribute to malformations.

Trouble shooting hatch failures: Eggs do not hatch for reasons which may or may not be the fault of the person caring for the eggs. Below are a few common reasons for incubation failures.

Infertile eggs: Procure the fertile hatching eggs from farms having at least one male with every ten females.

Parent stock: Weak and unhealthy or nutritionally deficient diet fed parent stock. The care for the breeder flock should be taken following sound poultry management practices.

Eggs are too old or improperly cared for before incubation: The hatching eggs should not be stored for longer than 7-10 days before incubation.

Shell contamination: Incubate only clean or slightly dirty eggs cleaned with sandpaper. Do not wash dirty hatching eggs or allow eggs to sweat before placing them in the incubator.

Temperatures too high, too low, or too variable: Check incubator temperature with an accurate thermometer, and adjust the thermostat accordingly.

Too little or too much humidity in the incubator: Obtain a hygrometer and measure the humidity before making further adjustments.

Eggs not turned often enough: Turn eggs at least two or three times daily. Commercial hatcheries turn eggs every two hours.

Improper ventilation resulting in low oxygen: Forced-air incubators should start with vent openings half-opened. Increase ventilation after ten days until openings are fully opened at hatching time.

Rough handling of eggs: Excessive handling and jarring of eggs while turning, especially during the first week, may be harmful.

Importance of hatchery records

To manage a hatchery efficiently and to keep costs to a minimum, the manager must have certain records after each hatch, each week and at the end of each month. Records should include the following variables: flock, strain, farm, date of set, machine(s) used, location of eggs in machine, number of eggs set, number of fertile eggs, number of early dead (0 to 7 days), number of middle dead (8 to 14 days), number of late dead (embryos 15 days or older), age of each embryo, malpositions (in embryos 19 days or older), number of pipping, malformations, number of eggs contaminated (rots), number of cracked eggs (transfer cracks and others), number of dead and culled chicks and number of live chicks. Clear, accurate records are essential for useful egg break even analysis.

Breakout analysis

A breakout analysis of hatching eggs must be done to evaluate the breeder flock's progress with respect to fertility and hatchability. It is an absolutely essential diagnostic tool for identifying the cause(s) of problems in hatchability.

These are three types: Breakout of fresh, non incubated eggs; (2) Breakout of incubated (5 to 12 d) eggs and (3) Breakout of eggs that did not hatch (hatch residue).

For breakout analysis eggs should be removed from the setter/hatcher tray, placed on egg flats, and identified as to flock, location, etc. The exterior of the egg is examined first for egg traits, pipping, and location of the air cell. The shell is cracked at the large end, over the air cell, and a hole opened in the shell and membranes to observe the interior of the egg. If the egg appears to be infertile or contains a very early dead embryo, the germinal disc must be located to make a definitive identification of fertility. If the embryo is relatively small, the egg can be broken into a dish for further examination. Eggs with late-stage embryos should be observed for pipping into the air cell, then opened with scissors from large end to small end without disturbing the position of the embryo. The embryo's position, the embryo's age, malformations, contamination, and other factors should be observed and recorded. Comparisons with live embryos of various ages can be done to train those developing experience in the breakout technique.

Breakout of fresh eggs is used to provide an immediate evaluation of flock fertility. The breakout following candling will include eggs determined to be

Table 44: A diagnosis chart to assist in solving incubation failures

Symptom	Probable Cause	Corrective Measures
Clear eggs with no embryonic development (infertile eggs)	Eggs damaged by environment	Gather eggs frequently (at least once daily).
	Eggs stored too long or incorrectly	Store eggs at 50-60 ^{0}F and 60% relative humidity. Incubate eggs within 7 days of lay.
Blood rings	Improper storage	Follow recommended egg storage and collection recommendations.
	Improper incubation temperature	Check thermometer accuracy and incubator functions. Follow recommended temperature settings.
	Improper fumigation	Follow fumigation recommendations.
Many dead embryos at early stages	Improper incubation temperatures (usually too high)	Follow recommended incubation temperatures.
	Improper egg turning	Turn at least 3 times daily.
	Improper ventilation	Increase ventilation rate in incubator and/or room, but avoid drafts.
	Pullorum disease	Use eggs from disease-free sources. Have blood-test of the breeder flock.
Early hatching (may have hemorrhagic navels)	High incubation temperatures	Follow recommended incubation temperatures. Check equipment for proper function. Guard against electrical surges or high incubator room temperatures.
	Improper egg storage	Store eggs at 50-60 ^{0}F. and 60% R.H. Turn at least 3 times daily.
Late hatching or not hatching uniformly	Low incubation temperatures	Follow recommended incubation temperatures.
	Warm and cool spots in incubator due to faulty design	Contact incubator company or obtain a different incubator design.
	Old or improperly stored eggs	Gather eggs frequently, cool immediately and store eggs properly. Do not store longer than 7 days.

(*Contd.*)

Symptom	Probable Cause	Corrective Measures
Sticky embryos (embryos may be smeared with egg contents)	High average incubation humidity	Follow recommended incubation humidity. Check size of air cell as an indicator for adjusting humidity condition.
	Low incubation temperature	Follow recommended temperature settings.
	Inadequate ventilation	Increase ventilation rate in incubator and/or room, but avoid drafts.
	Improper fumigation of eggs	Fumigate eggs by following the procedure carefully.
Embryos sticking or adhering to shell	Low incubation humidity (especially during hatching)	Increase incubation humidity by increasing water evaporation
	Excessive ventilation rate	Reduce ventilation rate but maintain minimum air exchange to prevent suffocation of embryos.
Crippled and malformed chicks	Improper incubation temperatures (usually too high)	Follow recommended incubation temperatures.
	Low incubation humidity	Increase incubation humidity by increasing water evaporation.
	Improper egg setting position or turning during incubation	Set eggs with small ends down. Turn eggs at least 3 times daily. Do not turn eggs within 3 days of hatching.
	Slick hatching trays	Use trays with wire floors or place crinoline on hatching surface.
Large, soft-bodied mushy chicks; dead on trays; bad odour	Low average incubation temperature	Follow recommended incubation temperatures.
	Poor ventilation	Increase ventilation rate in incubator and/or room, but avoid drafts.
	Navel infection (Omphalitis)	Clean and disinfect incubator and hatching units between settings of eggs. Maintain dry hatching trays. Properly store and fumigate eggs.
Rough or unhealed navels	Improper incubation temperatures	Follow recommended incubation temperatures.
	High hatching humidity	Maintain proper humidity.
	Navel infection (Omphalitis)	Clean and disinfect incubator and hatching units between settings of eggs. Maintain dry hatching trays. Properly store and fumigate eggs.

Courtesy: Publication 1182, Mississippi State University, U.S. Department of Agriculture

infertile, eggs containing early dead, and cracked eggs. The *hatch residue* breakout includes all eggs that did not hatch. Candle breakout and residue breakout should be done weekly or at least every 3 weeks. Regular, consistent analysis of these breakouts will result in flock histories that can be used to diagnose hatchability problems, minimize losses, and compare strains, flocks, farms, hatcheries, and many other variables.

Biosecurity in the hatchery

Biosecurity is defined as, '*the prevention (or control) of pathogenic microorganisms from contacting animal populations*'. Additionally, biosecurity is a tool to help minimize the effect of infections and decrease the impact of diseases. Biosecurity measures are taken in following respects.

i. **Location:** Ideally, hatchery should be located at least 1-2 miles away from other commercial poultry farms and away from public road facilities and other farm operations.

ii. **Movement:** Movement in the hatchery should be '*one way*' from clean areas to dirty areas to minimize movement of contaminants.

iii. **Construction:** It should be without access points for rodents or stray animals, crevices, free of leaks and damp floors, etc.

iv. **Ventilation:** Proper ventilation is necessary for control of various respiratory diseases.

v. **Temperature:** Appropriate control measures should be taken to avoid extreme temperatures.

vi. **Hatchery equipment:** Farm equipment can be a source of disease transmission and should be cleaned and disinfected regularly.

vii. **Vehicles, personnel and visitors:** Vehicles and visitors are major sources of contamination. Parking should be away from the hatchery buildings. Protective outer clothing, including boots and headgear should be worn at all times in the hatchery.

viii. **Protection from pests and predators:** Rats, mice, wild birds, fly and beetles can all cause contamination and spread diseases.

ix. **Control points at the hatchery:** Hygiene is a key management factor in the hatchery. Positive air flow minimizes the risk of transfer of contamination from the hatcher back to the setter.

x. **Egg transport:** Ensure clean trays and trolleys are returned from the hatchery. Egg transport vehicles should be cleaned between collection runs, if also used for chick delivery.

xi. **Disinfection:** Disinfectants are chemicals those can kill pathogens on contact. Detailed classes of disinfectants and their uses are described elsewhere in this book (Chapter: 28)

Computer applications for hatchery management

In large hatchery practices computers are used to manage the entire operation smoothly starting from receiving hatching eggs to delivery of chicks.

Over the past few years systems like, *Computer Based Monitoring/Alarm Systems* have become available and surely more will follow. This is a computerized system, provides continuous monitoring, alarm, control, automatic data gathering and analysis and chronology of hatchery events. In addition, the facility also explains to the operator what to do to correct the problem. Especially with complex and interconnected systems, this becomes important, to take the guess work and the hunt out of responding to an alarm. Also these systems have the ability to store data over time. Thus giving the hatchery managers the ability to analyze the cause-and-effect relationships between control or adjustment decisions and actual results, allowing fine tuning of future control decisions and increased hatchery efficiency.

Question Bank

I. Fill in the blanks with appropriate word (s)

1. .... and ....are basically two types of incubators available.
2. A newly hatched chick can survive without feed for ....days.
3. Blind cracks can be defined as...
4. Body checks can be defined as...
5. During candling on 7th day of incubation infertile eggs will appear ....
6. For good incubation, the CO_2 in incubator must not exceed...............
7. For incubation, chicken eggs should be placed in the setter and hatcher for ....and ....days respectively.
8. Generally, the air cell is present at ....end of the egg.

9. Higher the reading of Haugh unit value for albumen quality .... will be the hatchability of eggs.
10. Incubation period in J. quail is..........................
11. Incubation period in turkey is ....
12. Optimum incubation temperature for chicken eggs is................
13. The average weight of quail egg is......................
14. The ideal body weight of day old chick (egger) is ....
15. The RH of the egg storage room should be...................%.
16. The strength of formaldehyde gas required for fumigating hatching eggs immediately after laying is........................

Answers

1. Forced air and still air
2. 3
3. Hair line cracks
4. Fine cracks which have been sealed before oviposition
5. clear, or show a dark ring.
6. 0.5 %
7. 18, 3
8. Broader
9. Better
10. 18 days
11. 28 days
12. 99.5 °F
13. 10 g
14. 45 grams
15. 75 to 80%
16. 3x

II. State True or False

i) A fresh egg when laid by hen has no air cell.

ii) Blood spots inside an egg are caused due to rupture of small blood vessel of developing embryo.

iii) Eggs possessing strong shells hatch better than eggs with thin shells.

iv) Forced air and still air are basically two types of incubators available.

v) Hatchability based on fertile eggs is more precise.

vi) Is 'still air' incubators require higher incubation temperatures as compared to 'forced air' units.

vii) The spores on the egg shell get sealed by the cuticle and thus reduce the microbial penetration of the egg.

Answers

i) True	ii) False
iii) True	iv) True
v) True	vi) True
vii) True	

III. Encircle the correct answer

1. The position of egg during incubation should be............
   a) Broad end up b) narrow end up
   c) horizontal d) none
2. The percent weight loss of egg during incubation ....%.
   a) 10. b) 12
   c) 14 d) 16
3. For fumigation, the quantity of $KMNO_4$ and formalin required (per 100 cf) to get 3x concentration is.........
   a) 60 g and 120 ml b) 120 g and 60 ml
   c) 160 g and 80 ml d) 80 ml and 160 ml
4. Which of the following incubation problems might cause malposition?
   a) Improper egg storage b) Eggs stored too long
   c) Genetic defects d) Inadequate turning
5. A hatchery design would have the egg storage room adjacent to the:
   a) Chick grading and handling room b) Hatchers
   c) Setters d) Lunch room
6. An example of a sex-linked qualitative trait is
   a) Fast and slow feathering b) Egg production
   c) Egg color d) Breast fleshing
   e) Growth rate
7. In the production of quality chicks, hatching eggs must be collected at least how many times per day?
   a) 1 b) 2
   c) 3 d) 4

8. After an egg is laid, its hatching potential can at best be?

   a) Maintained
   b) Improved
   c) Maintained for short periods
   d) Improved for short periods

9. What do eggs lose during storage?

   a) CO_2 and ammonia
   b) CO_2 and water vapor
   c) Protein and shell quality
   d) Carbon dioxide and hydrogen

10. Chick size is normally what percentage of egg that was set?

   a) 55-60
   b) 61-64
   c) 59-72
   d) 66-68

Answers

1. a	2. b
3. a	4. d
5. c	6. a
7. d	8. a
9. b	10. d

IV. Write short notes on the following

a. Methods of sexing chicks.

b. Hatchery biosecurity

c. Control of egg borne diseases

V. Answer the following.

a. Describe in detail care and management of hatching eggs.

b. Discuss factors those influence the hatchability of eggs.

c. At what temperature must eggs be held during incubation?

d. How long does it take to hatch various species of birds?

e. Candling eggs - how is it done to determine whether an egg has a living embryo?

f. What do fertile and infertile eggs look like when candled?

g. When incubating eggs, what environment conditions must I carefully control?

h. What are the reasons for a poor hatch of eggs.

i. How to sanitize hatching eggs and incubator?

j. How does a chick embryo develop?

k. How long fertile hatching eggs can be stored before they must be incubated?

l. How soon after hatching should the chicks be removed from the incubator?

m. Should the dirty hatching eggs be washed before incubation?

n. What are the best methods to follow for sanitizing eggs and incubators to reduce bacterial infections?

o. Why the chicks may die in the egg after they pip or break the shell?

p. Describe a typical modern hatchery.

Index

D

E

F

O

P

Q

R

S

FSC
www.fsc.org
MIX
Papier | Fördert
gute Waldnutzung
FSC® C083411

Zeitfracht Medien GmbH
Ferdinand-Jühlke-Straße 7
99095 Erfurt, Deutschland
produktsicherheit@kolibri360.de